T0302335

The Pox Lover

The Pox Lover

An Activist's Decade in New York and Paris

Anne-christine d'Adesky

The University of Wisconsin Press

Publication of this volume has been made possible, in part,
through support from the **Brittingham Fund**.

The University of Wisconsin Press
1930 Monroe Street, 3rd Floor
Madison, Wisconsin 53711-2059
uwpress.wisc.edu

3 Henrietta Street, Covent Garden
London WC2E 8LU, United Kingdom
eurospanbookstore.com

Printed in the United States of America

This book may be available in a digital edition.

Library of Congress Cataloging-in-Publication Data

Names: D'Adesky, Anne-Christine, author.
Title: The pox lover: an activist's decade in New York and Paris /
Anne-christine d'Adesky.
Description: Madison, Wisconsin: The University of Wisconsin Press, [2017]
| Includes bibliographical references.
Identifiers: LCCN 2016049004 | ISBN 9780299311100 (cloth: alk. paper)
Subjects: LCSH: D'Adesky, Anne-Christine. | Women political
activists—Biography. | AIDS activists—Biography.
| Journalists—Biography.
Classification: LCC PS3554.A243 Z46 2017 | DDC 813/.54 [B]—dc23
LC record available at https://lccn.loc.gov/2016049004

This book is dedicated to:
Mary McLemore
&
Megan McLemore

In Memoriam

Let Me Remember & Honor
In my early ACT UP family:
Michael Callen
John Cook
Keith Cylar
Jon Greenberg
Robert Hilferty
Aldyn McKean
Kiki Mason
Sarah Pettit
Evan Ruderman
Vito Russo
Assotto Saint
Cleews Vellay

&
My parents:
Viviane Thérèse d'Adesky
Raymond Georges d'Adesky

&
My grandparents:
Serge and Nita Berthoin
Edith and Raymond d'Adesky

&
My French aunts and uncles:
Christian Berthoin
Colette Berthoin and Christine Serieyx
Gaston Wyss and Florence Meunier

Someday, the AIDS crisis will be over. Remember that. And when that day comes, when that day has come and gone, there'll be people alive on this Earth, gay people and straight people, men and women, black and white, who will hear the story that once there was a terrible disease in this country and all over the world, and that a brave group of people stood up and fought and, in some cases, gave their lives, so that other people might live and be free.

Vito Russo, May 1988

Contents

List of Illustrations ix

Preface xi

I ~ Paris 3

II ~ Roots, Baby 55

III ~ New York 71

IV ~ Paris, de nouveau 96

V ~ New York, de novo 143

VI ~ Paris, enfin 154

VII ~ New York 169

VIII ~ New York, Still 189

IX ~ London 199

X ~ Paris, avant tout 202

XI ~ New York 208

XII ~ New York 219

XIII ~ New York, Round 27 232

XIV ~ *New Orleans*   238

XV ~ *Amsterdam*   242

XVI ~ *Paris*   245

XVII ~ *New York*   252

XVIII ~ *Paris*   256

XIX ~ *New York*   263

XX ~ *Vietnam*   272

XXI ~ *New York*   279

L'Afterword ~ *The Circle Is Complete*   286

P.S.   297

Thank You   298
In Memory & Action   301
Suggested Readings   302

Illustrations

ACT UP, Stop the Church protest, December 1989   x
The river Seine   2
The man of Ades, Gentilhomme François d'Adesky   56
Family reunion in Chamonix, late 1950s   60
Author's parents, Raymond and Viviane d'Adesky   60
Author's family in France and Haiti   61
Lori E. Seid's Lesbian Love Lounge, Dyke March, 1993   79
Dyke March, NYC, July 1994   89
Author in Avenger drag at inaugural Dyke March, 1993   114
ACT UP, slide projection on Notre Dame Cathedral, 1994   125
ACT UP, slide projection on the streets of Paris, World Aids Day,
    1994   133
Statues in front of the Musée d'Orsay, Paris   134
Dyke March, NYC, 1994   150
Author posing for an intimate portrait series of NYC and
    AIDS activists   151
Author as a child in Fort Lauderdale, Florida   151
ACT UP's Women and AIDS poster by Gran Fury   158
ACT UP Die In protest, September 2013   179
Author and John Cook in Paris, 1993   184
ACT UP–Paris protests against National Front, January 2013   251
Marine Le Pen poster graffiti   255
Justice silenced   255
Author portrait, 1990s   266
Homage to the victims of terrorist bombings and Islamophobia,
    2016   296

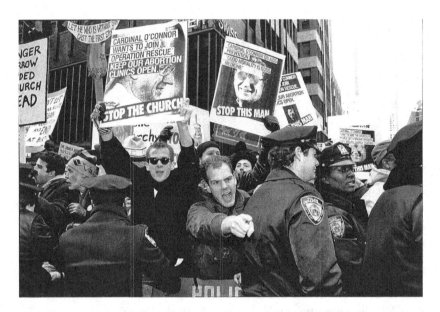

ACT UP, Stop the Church protest, Saint Patrick's Cathedral, December 10, 1989. (Ellen B. Neipris)

Preface

$\mathcal{D}$ear $\mathcal{R}$eader,

I've decided a brief preface is needed for this book, which might be best described as a highly personal history of the 1990s, a mash-up activist diary-cum-battlefield-notes-cum-travelogue of a particularly hot decade and two pocked cities, Paris and New York. It was an intense decade framed by my involvement in AIDS and ACT UP—a global epidemic and a protest movement that has strongly shaped my life and work, as it has for many friends and professional colleagues.

As you'll see, the AIDS epidemic serves as a contemporary backdrop and metaphor for what I call my poxed life. I fit somewhere in between the baby boomers and Gen X. We are members of an imploded generation, one that took in the energy of a massive death star and quickly transformed our terror and rage—*personally, publicly, crudely, boldly*—into a daily ritual of street protest and creativity and very gayish love. Some struggled with despair and depression and illness and addictions and found themselves in 12-step meetings a decade later, staying clean and sober and not having nearly as much fun, but definitely alive, and somewhat wiser.

A tsunami comes and threatens to sweep you away, drown you without hope of a breath. You make an instant decision to hold on, to try to hold fast to your loved ones. Or at some point you may let go out of sheer exhaustion, or you're forcibly taken by the current and seek another anchor point, a refuge. You worry about everyone else and vow to never stop searching or remembering the missing and the dead. Every day in the nineties such waves hit the shores of New York City and in Paris, where I spent much of the era working as a journalist chronicling the AIDS epidemic while getting sucked further into currents of activism. At some point I simply accepted that I had become an advocacy journalist. I was not neutral—not about AIDS. I still strived as a professional journalist to be fair and accurate and to recognize the many sides to an argument.

But the current of AIDS took me away in the nineties and deposited me onto other shores. There, I met my movement family.

Like other people, I was pulled to join ACT UP early on because so many people in my social circle were getting sick. I later spent time with the Paris chapter of the group. I also learned how to play hard while protesting, something that marked the inspired creative street activism of the Lesbian Avengers, a group that some close friends and I launched in 1992. It started with a rant and led to some wild actions. We got pulled into other issues and cross-movements over the years. But the scientific puzzle of AIDS and how to treat the disease remained my overriding professional focus over the decade. That's how I came to be awake and jetlagged and walking after midnight in Paris and the East Village of Manhattan for much of the nineties, en route to, or recovering from, a street action or a hangover or some combination of both.

So many amazing people showed up for what felt like a decade-long protest, a series of days and nights and zaps and moments and connections that unfurled as the most memorable parties do, replete with a colorful cast of characters who inspire, or entertain, or irritate, with dramas aplenty, with the ingestion of too many mood-altering substances, including coffee needed to brave another action. The slogans and fashion were inspiring, so was the art, and so were the myriad affinity groups of friends who dreamed up ever more outrageous outfits and actions. One joined a protest committee, learned some skills, made instant lifelong friends, had conference affairs, requisite boy and girl dramas, and messy breakups. There were nightly meetings, constant processing, and a million arguments about strategy. Humor helped us survive the nineties. So did dancing. Madonna provided a soundtrack for our generation; so did the Pet Shop Boys and Brit boy pop bands. Everyone loved Morrissey and always would. Amid our fun it was always about taking an action. Today, now—we have to respond!

It was also exhausting and heartbreaking. Every week, it seemed, someone's death was announced. Someone we knew or had just been sitting next to, a month or a protest earlier. Someone new had entered the hospital or hospice. Someone could no longer walk or was going blind. Someone was being evicted or couldn't get into the country to attend a critical meeting because of the US HIV travel ban. The AIDS drugs were no good. The clock was always ticking. ACT UP's protests grew more and more shrill.

Much of the drama of the nineties AIDS movement centered on the battle to access HIV treatment. This book provides a personal snapshot of a period activists define as just *Before* and immediately *After* the arrival of lifesaving combination antiviral drugs, particularly protease inhibitors that have had a Lazarus effect. It was an era in which close friends and loved ones landed on one or the other side of that beacon of hope, that redline of survival.

The Pox Lover is also a diary of overlapping investigations, including a bit of digging into my own family's roots and ties to unfolding and historical events in France. As the saying goes, the personal is political. But I appreciate the reverse too: the political is personal, so often, at least for me. Why or when do we care about political issues and causes? It's when we feel a personal connection to them. The more personal, the more one engages with the heart, the more one seeks deeper and more complex truths.

In this book, I've taken a highly personal approach to history, including events that took place before my lifetime, to better understand where I connect (and where I don't) to the larger picture and why this matters: How these connections have continued to shape my life and actions ever since. How the political battles that are paramount today—over terrorism and nationalism and the resurgence of fascism—can be traced to ideas and groups and people and political issues that emerged in the nineties. How we might learn from that decade of protest as we consider our actions now to stop the new wolves of the Far Right here and in Europe—the Donald Trumps and others.

This book is based on the intermittent journal I kept throughout the nineties (and after). Although it's tempting to revise one's views with the sage passage of time, I have avoided doing that. I've elected to use pseudonyms for individuals who are intimate relations but not necessarily public figures; most other friends, colleagues, and individuals are identified by name. After all, this is my version of our shared history, not theirs. We also know how unreliable memory can be, including nostalgia. I'm eager to hear from readers who can offer their view of events chronicled in this book.

That takes me to the subject of Monsieur Jean-Marie Le Pen, whom I began to track in the nineties. He's the repugnant, neonationalist founder of France's reigning populist right-wing party, the National Front. At the time, Le Pen was going after ACT UP in Paris as well as the Roma (gypsies), immigrants, and other undesirables. Le Pen remains an unrepentant xenophobe who lost the reins of his party's leadership to his eldest daughter, Marine, in 2000. She has recast the National Front as a softer traditional values political party, with herself as a modern Joan of Arc engaged in a holy war for the nation's cultural soul. A few years back Marine won a historic seat in the European Parliament. The November 2016 shock polls showed that if France held its presidential election that day, she would win, or might place second to an equally hardline rightist.

That makes 2017 a critical election for France, one that greatly worries progressives not only there but across Europe. What's happening there is happening here in the United States too. Marine Le Pen and her father are great admirers of our new president, Donald Trump; so are Europe's neo-Nazis.

I also had—have—a personal stake in such questions. I was born in Marquette, Michigan, in 1958, but my mother was French and my father was born in Haiti, from a Belgian family. Both were students in France during the Nazi Occupation, when the collaborating Vichy regime stripped 75,000 Jews of their rights and citizenship and shipped them off to death camps in Germany and Poland. Only 2,500 of them survived.

As a child, I encountered a certain parental silence whenever I sought to learn more about what my parents had seen or done as young people during the Occupation, what they were told in school, what they knew—as it was happening—of those packed trains headed north. I wanted to know my extended family history better, to better understand the postwar, postcolonial French culture and values that had shaped my parents and were passed on to me. I wanted to poke at the layer of silence. I only realized some years ago, for example, that the Nazi Occupation extended to the French overseas departments. It wasn't just in France; it was a colonial Occupation. Since I have relatives from those places too, I became more curious.

As luck would have it, France began to reexamine its postwar past in the nineties, including via the Papon trial—a critical event I attended. I was struck at the time by how much Maurice Papon, a former French official accused of sending Jews to the gas chambers, resembled my French grandfather. Papon seemed quite ordinary—a typical enough French bureaucrat. That's when I began to learn how many other ordinary civil servants helped him remain happily living in France, *complicit as fuck*, as we would say in ACT UP about Ronald Reagan in the early days of the AIDS epidemic.

Trolling around Paris, in between ACT UP protests and my reporting work, I began to dig. What connected a man like Papon to a woman like Marine Le Pen? How powerful was the National Front? Who was fighting back? Could fascism ever return to France? It seemed impossible, *and yet*.

What about in my New York, or in Florida, where I grew up? For years, ACT UP had been battling groups linked to the Moral Majority and the Christian Right that were well connected in Washington, that had big money and lobbyists. I was seeing old-new alliances between high-up officials of the Catholic Church like Cardinal John O'Connor in New York, born-again televangelists like Jerry Falwell, and antifeminist PTA-type church ladies being groomed for local office. Their political agenda was rabidly antigay, antiwomen, anti-AIDS, anti-immigrants: anti-everything-I-felt. It was very white but sought to recruit minorities in a ministry of hate. It would end with a prayer circle and a plea for more volunteers, money, and God's protection to carry on their holy work. The more I sought to connect the dots, the more dots emerged to connect.

⤙

Finally, my story here is an off-the-beaten-track travelogue, moving between my home in downtown New York City and regular visits to Paris, usually for work, but always for fun and romance too. My personal journey began spontaneously during an after-hours walk in Paris, a gorgeous city that I wanted to know better. It became a much longer nightly walk and journey—a decade in the making—often by that great river, the Seine. This body of water still serves as a personal balm, a calming mirror that looks unchanged beside the fast-transforming urban metropolis.

Today's Paris is not the city I trolled in the nineties. So many neighborhoods have had face-lifts, just as they have in New York. They're radically transformed, gentrified, cleaned up. Drugs are still all over Paris, still big business for urban gangs and new mafias, but a developer bought up much of the Marais where ACT UP gay boys would grab a cheap kebob and fries after a meeting before heading to a favorite hook-up spot—a French leather bar or a city cruising park. Many of those gay boys are also dead, as are many men and women from the former French colonies who died of AIDS in the period *Before*.

In the nineties, few in my circle were thinking about *le marriage gai*, or having *les enfants*, or the possibility of *le divorce* that is predictable following the gay honeymoon of same-sex marriage, as it has for heterosexuals. They were staying up— like me, like all of ACT UP, like AIDS activists from Kigali to Bangkok—from dusk to dawn, helping another night unfurl. *Why sleep?* That seems to me one of my mantras of the decade.

Why, indeed, when one needed to stay awake, to remain vigilant, to say no (or *non*) to some greedy drug company action, or ready a press release, or plan a zap? Sleep was for another person, another time, an older generation. It wasn't only cocaine that kept the East Village and the Marais awake in the later nineties; it was the need to grab at life, to create, to connect with others, to remain fully alive, and to keep the heartbreak at bay.

Before I say too much more—spoil your fun—let me simply invite you now to take a walk with me. A stroll. Where we'll end up depends on you as much as me, you'll see. If you're like me then perhaps you'll find that as you read this diary, my working journal, you'll begin making your own connections, taking your own notes. Maybe you'll discover our stories are linked in ways you would never imagine—as I found mine linked to distant events and even odious people in history. I, for one, won't be at all surprised. *Au contraire.*

Luckily, I've had a most delicious and odd travel companion during my long walk. A historical tart. Not a proper guide at all, in fact, but a rather suspect narrator; extremely biased. Definitely not your *New York Times* type, and not a sleeper either. No; the type that inevitably steers you toward what's likely to be risky, forbidden, and, therefore, probably fun.

All I ask here, at the start, is what was asked of me: that you keep an open mind. That's the best compass of all, I've found. I ask that and your willingness to take a trip, to dig in, and risk getting your hands a little dirty. To have some fun. *C'est tout.*

The Pox Lover

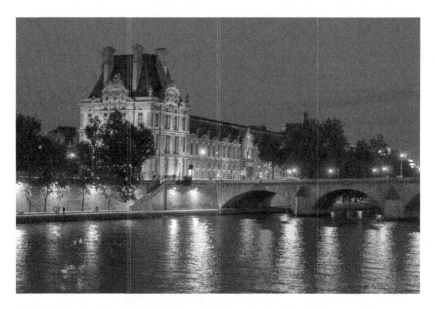

The river Seine: watery spine of Paris. (tomcraig@directphoto.org)

1

Paris

Those who are most dangerous are the ordinary men.

Primo Levi

~ 1

AUGUST 1993

It's summertime in the City of Lights. Evening is edging toward me with the soft breeze that blows in from the faraway Atlantic, bringing the smell of the sea. It lifts and dries the hair on my legs. My eyes take in a familiar sight: the prow-shaped tip of the Île de la Cité, the vaulting spires of Notre-Dame, the graceful linden trees in full bloom below a sky so pale and white it masks a quarter moon rising above a horizon of bridges. My feet leave damp prints on the steps where I linger, staring at the magnificence of the view. Before me, the Seine is a broad, brown strip of celluloid exposed to the sun, flashing Mylar silver with undertones of purple, brown, mustard, and blue that fade and become translucent near the surface of the water. Close to the bank, the river is a slab of slate, impenetrable as the gray day.

Beyond these steps are others leading up or down the bridges in the distance. A set of cracked and refurbished ribs extending from the spine of Paris, of the Seine. I study the whorls on the river's surface, how the current forks around an oncoming tug then grows quiet as it gently rocks the moored houseboats. I long to live on a houseboat, to wake up every morning and gaze up at the blackened faces of a siren. There's something about this water, this whole scene, that moves me, that inexplicably soothes me.

⟋⟍

I arrived here earlier today and came immediately to this spot, to the worn footsteps used for centuries by invaders hoping to wrest control of Europe. I'm

3

here on a mission of sorts myself. Not an invasion; more of a rendezvous. But, like a spy waiting for further instructions, I don't have a clue about who or what to expect, not even what I might look for. I'm simply possessed with a vague sense of destiny, of needing to be here, in this exact spot. Things have conspired to get me here, back to this familiar city, to this known set of landmarks. Things, and events, and time. Time is before me, in the unmoving sky.

Time has left a blueprint on my face; I'm so much older. Not the person I was before, or even the person I thought I would become. In the mirror of the river I recognize my own face but not the stranger's. That other face has lost its easy ability to laugh. It has seen too much. Its cheeks are etched like an old man's after too much war. I'm going to look like William Burroughs when I'm older, I think: angular, serious face; deep creases that began when I was twenty. A face blotted with purpose, with veiny eyes that look red and tired and sad.

It's not just jet lag. I haven't been sleeping, a perennial problem. It's been a crazy-busy spring and summer. I've been moving too fast; so many protests, so much organizing. And there's always so much I want to research and write. I feel drained by my life in New York. Always fun, always exhausting New York. I seriously needed a break.

I look away and look back at my reflection. Now I can see the child, too, inside my own eyes. A child harmed by loss and invisible wounds. A child tired of work who seeks to nap. A laughing child who wants to jump into the river and take a swim, ignore the dangers of the adult world. A child seeking adventure. A child enchanted and soothed by the memory of this bridge, this water, this city, this sky. A wandering child seeking home.

For weeks, for months, for years, it seems, I just haven't stopped. I've kept myself in motion: working, acting, reacting, organizing, protesting. Taking care of my friends who are sick. Researching the science, endlessly reading drug trial results, talking to doctors. Trying to figure out who's brilliant and who's just a good lab technician, whose approach to the viral mystery of AIDS is going to deliver a drug that really makes a difference. There's so much happening and yet there's not a breakthrough. And now it's over. I've spontaneously walked away from the mountain of my magazine editorial work at *Out* and my life and girl troubles and responsibilities in New York to let myself breathe for a spell.

I watch the water, swirling and slapping the concrete bank. It enters my eyes, washes over my hot brain. My head is so full of faces, voices, months of conversations, too much stress; all of it has exhausted me to the point of immobility. I've lost the desire to speak; my tongue lies heavy as a dog in the shade of my mouth. All I want to do is sit here and let the days and months slide into the river. For the moment, all that matters is before me: *nothingness*.

Hours pass. I've dozed heavily, drooled on my shoulder. The feather-pillow sky has fled, leaving dusk in its wake. But the air is warm, welcoming. I look around. There are people walking in the distance and on the opposite bank of the river. They don't notice me.

I feel lazy, malarial. I watch the streetlights flick on across the way, illuminating the grand state buildings, the sculpted balconies. History is a friend, beckoning from every corner. But I'm rooted to my spot, heavy with something more than fatigue. During my sleep, something has happened. Something that was lurking under the patina of my days has been stirred. I can't touch it, can't locate it, but I know it's there. A feeling: old, deep, vague.

When I close my eyes I feel it rise up. When I open them it disappears. I play a game, opening and closing them. And then, without warning, I begin to cry.

The feeling is so sharp yet muted that I find it hard to breathe. A hot tide rises, tightening the muscles in my chest and face, arms, and legs. Soon, I'm overcome with grief. With a feeling of loss so profound it makes me tremble and cough, causes me to look around to see if anyone has noticed. But no one's paying attention to me. *I'm alone with my sorrow*, I think. *With all this death.* The blood-sorrow is pumping inside my ears, raging, pounding in my temples like a distant surf. My arms and face are coated in a fine sweat. The tears spill down my cheeks, gather on the end of my chin, slowly drip onto my shoes and the sidewalk. I make no effort to wash them off. Instead, I stand, stricken, and hear myself make a small noise like a young cat clearing its throat, a high-pitched, private, racking sound.

After a while, the feeling has ebbed. Through my tears I see the river. It looks unchanged after so many years. I've aged; it hasn't. I walk close to the edge and, crouching, wash away the crusted salt tracks.

Gone are the sounds of the night: the honking cars, the staccato laughter of tourists. I stare at the water, at the bridges, at the lights bouncing along the quai. A tranquil scene. I hear my mother's voice calling to me from far away. I hear the dim echo sound of a cowbell—a signal to come and eat dinner. I'm that child again. I'm running ahead of her, baguette in hand, eating it greedily. A moment later, I see my father. He's but a boy, laughing, shouting, and running along a narrow street in a pale T-shirt, a wooden slingshot stuck in the back of his Tyrolean suede shorts, his pale legs freezing in winter. He's been shooting at boats in the Seine. Now I hear him too, looking for me, calling my name. Now come the others: Grand-père Papou and his second wife; Grand-mère la Comtesse; my French aunts and uncles; little-known and long-dead great cousins, all mingling around an outdoor table in the countryside. I'm seeing Chamonix, an Alpine pastoral, where I spent many childhood August vacations.

Another wave of emotion, more faces, snapshot childhood moments. The Seine is drawing something out of me: a fragile, invisible thread of memories and people. A stream of faces flows before me, coming forth with such clarity that I feel pain at seeing them again.

I see the boys. My friend Jon Greenberg, such a gentle man, who taught everyone about holistic medicine and the beauty of herbs. He just died. He went to Haiti with me for Mardi Gras; so did Anna Blume and Laurie Weeks, a wild time. We didn't sleep for five days, just danced and drank Barbancourt rum and went to visit people dying of AIDS in their homes, bringing them some solidarity. Jon drank *clairin*: rotgut, killer local moonshine. He danced with old ladies and old men, twirling them around. He was fascinated with vodou, with the *loas*—the Haitian saints—his own spirituality deep. He was so happy in Haiti, so interested, so friendly with everyone, so open and soul caring. And later so sad to be dying.

ACT UP held a public funeral for him. We carried his casket through the streets of lower Manhattan. That was so recent: July 16, only two weeks after Tim Bailey's public funeral in DC. Who can forget Jon's parting words to the world? *I don't want an angry political funeral, I just want you to burn me in the street and eat my flesh.* We cried, we chanted, we danced, we celebrated Jon. But we remain angry.

I'd been at Tim's protest funeral too, watched his brothers and other pall-bearers from his affinity group buddies, the Proud Marys, tussle with the White House security cops, trying to grant Tim his dying wish: to be heaved over the gates, to ACT UP in death too. It almost felt appalling to watch that casket being fought over: a desecration. The cops were upset; they didn't like their role. We all felt the power of death, the sacredness of that body. Tim hadn't been a close friend like Jon, but I'd admired him. Both were pioneers.

The scene shifts. I'm with Jimbo, a buddy from my high school era and good tennis player. He was a close friend to my oldest, bestie friend M, the woman who became my first girlfriend in college and remains family now. Jim got sick after M and I left Florida, for Barnard and the Big Apple. He did make it out of our hometown, Daytona Beach, but how far north I don't know. He was so southern, with such a twang. *Heeey y'aaall* . . . And so gay, in retrospect. Prancing around in his little red diving Speedo, a super buff boy all the girls wanted bad. Probably a lot of boys too, now that I think of it. He dated girls then, publicly. Senior captain of more than one sport. Prom king, I think. This was the mid-1970s. KC and the Sunshine Band played at my high school senior dance, at Disney World. No one ever talked about fags, unless it was a slur; I don't remember the word *dyke* ever coming up. It wasn't in my vocabulary. I later learned about other tennis pals from those days who died of the fairy disease, as the rednecks in Daytona still call AIDS.

Here's Jimbo now, handsome, killer bod, a superstar on the swim team, standing quietly in his Speedo high above us on the diving board, all concentration. He executes a perfect dive, perfectly aligned hands and feet, no splash. He's beaming with happiness. Now here are the other tennis boys, Robert and one whose name I can't remember. He liked to store a joint in his teased-out Afro, an early bad boy. His daddy was rich; he drove us to the beach in a sky-blue Benz. Their friends: long-haired, shirtless, sun-burned stoner boys, jumping into the ocean in tennis whites that became see-through, making us laugh, making us want to look. I'm watching them swim far out now, laughing at me who's newly afraid of sharks, urging me to come in. *Don't be afraid, Anne. We'll protect you!*

They probably never got out of Florida either, never got to know the big open gay life of a big city like New York, the community of tolerance and love I found as an adult. The Florida boys of summer whose parents couldn't confront what happened to their beautiful sons. They died of a sudden illness, said the obits. But the neighbors knew, I bet. Or some knew. I'd hear the hometown gossip from M, who stays in touch with our old friends in Florida. At least some of them led gay lives and had boyfriends, however closeted, however limited to the dive gay bars with the Doobie Brothers burning up the juke. Unmarked bars where the entrance was in the back and where the rough biker crowd that rolled into Daytona every spring would cruise by, revving their engines hard, roaring their displeasure at the fairy bar. I didn't know about this back then, learned it only much later, when I finally realized, a bit foolishly, that there had always been gay bars in my hometown. I'd just been ignorant, raised to be homophobic like everybody else.

⌐

The sun is so hot, almost as hot as in Haiti. I'm in Paris but I'm seeing the harbor of Port-au-Prince. The national penitentiary, where I visited not long ago. The sun is broiling. There's no shade, no cool cells for the inmates to take cover. The prisoners are all just left lying out in the open, wearing shorts and no shirts, wearing flip-flops, sitting in the dust or along the broken walls, eyeing me,

wondering: *Who is this blan who has turned up? Why does she speak our Kreyol?* Watching
me walk to the farthest corner of the yard, where I can't tell at first if the cluster
of men are sleeping or dead or so sick they're unable to shift positions, to sit up
properly, in order to broil in the sun.

They're so thin and covered with sores. They're lying on their own shirts,
their own rags. The flies are in their eyes and noses and they're too tired to
bat them away. They have that wasting disease and no one in the prison says
this but even their families stay away. These men are so sick, their bodies are
just playing a trick on them to keep their hearts beating. I see their faces anew,
the same hollowed-out faces as the AIDS ward at Saint Vincent's hospital in
Manhattan I know so well by now. Haitian faces that gladly accept a little water
from my plastic bottle, but have trouble drinking much of it. It spills out of
cracked lips, their tongues whitish, covered with candida. Thrush, a tell-tale
sign of advanced AIDS. Bodies that smell like death already. Eyes that meet
mine and say simply, *I know. And there is nothing anyone can do for me.* Split lips that
murmur *fè lapriyè pou nou* as I leave. *Pray for us.*

The sorrow floods me like love. I'm choked up with the fullness of my life;
for all that's been lived and is gone forever now. All these people I've loved and
known. I want to see them all again. I want them all back, every single one.
Even those I haven't lost but no longer love with the same intensity. All of it, all
of them, overwhelm my heart. At dawn, I walk back to my room, dazed, still full
of my life and its small history, seeing all and no one. For once, I fall instantly
asleep without dreaming.

I awake with a start. It's past midnight. I dress in darkness and walk quickly to
the water's edge. It gleams with garlands of loam in the neon wake of passing
tourist boats. I feel very tired but am already acutely awake, like an insomniac.
There are scattered people here and there. I reach the Pont de l'Alma and
slowly head north, along the Right Bank, up to the Musée Arabe, then across
the bridge to the Left Bank. I leave the riverbank, leave people and activity
behind, venture down unlit pathways that dwindle to dead ends, walled-up
doorways, new construction.

I walk the city like a somnambulist—with a calm, steady energy, lidded
eyes, and no desire to speak or interact with anyone. Devoid of hunger or thirst
and not afraid. Drawn along by an internal hand, by the sight or the sense of
the river never very far away. I use the river as a compass, imagining the water
as it once flowed beneath the quiet streets, here, under my feet. The city is dark
but alive, full of shadows and furtive movements. Through it I pass like a
shadow.

By dawn I've completed the entire perimeter of the city. I've spoken to no one. But my mind has been a silent reel of vision, projecting a million thoughts and voices and images, all of them evaporated by daylight.

It's quite humid, a heat wave that forces almost everyone indoors. My clothes stick to me but I'm not bothered. The sun is a shiny disc through the gauze of a cloud. I stare at the pattern of the clouds on the surface of the water. Today the Seine is greener but doesn't move unless forced to. A small tug nudges a flat black barge twice its size and overloaded with cement, but the motion of water is illusory. Everything appears two-dimensional, without depth or contrast. I use my fingers to create a frame: I see a Cubist still life, a cut-out, a pastiche of shapes and color—white triangle overlapping black rectangle with gray cone over forest green. Newsprint squares for the administrative buildings across the water. Where's the requisite pipe for my Picasso landscape? It doesn't exist.

My eyes are bad but I don't like wearing my glasses and I forgot to bring a camera. Not that I need to record any of this; it's enough to capture the image for myself, mentally. I've adapted to my nomadic, ascetic routine. For days I wear the same thing: a pair of now-dusty pants and a tight dark-blue T-shirt, thin socks, heavy black boots, no bra or underpants. I lie on my back on the banks of the Tuileries on a stretch of concrete my Paris friends call the gay beach and roll my pants down below my navel, roll up the legs, roll up my shirt and sleeves, take off my boots. Expose my belly, my legs and hairy armpits. I dip my feet into the river.

I can't get enough of this heat. Everyone else seeks the shade, but not me. I do the opposite. During the hottest part of the day I place two coins on the side-walk, and when they're burning I put them carefully on top of my closed eyelids. I want to feel the sun, as hot on my flesh as I feel inside.

Another sweltering day. My skin wears a fine mantle of salt; I'm sweating from every orifice—nose, ears, navel, butt crack. I wander through the streets, then rest, wishing for nothing. But listening—listening very carefully.

A voice has entered my head and, with it, a presence, an essence. A low, raspy voice, like a muffled growl, whispering to me from the shadows of my nightly walks. A voice that never grows louder or more distinct. A face that's so elusive I have to close my eyes to glimpse it. A muse, I think.

What I glimpse is an old woman with a wild, unkempt face, with eyes like slits. A savage and wily creature. A crone. *Me*, I think, laughing to myself. *My future self.*

Who is she? A messenger of some kind? A fellow wanderer? She's old and weathered, but strong. A survivor. Someone who lives close to here, to this littered spot, this shadowy netherworld. For decades—or centuries perhaps? It's not all that clear at the moment. I can barely grasp her face.

I open my eyes a crack and trace the ripples of the Seine striking the wide pillars that hold up the bridge. Right there, over there, just beyond that barge, behind the tarpaulin left behind by some construction crew, there she is. Right now I can just discern the outline of her dirty smock.

She's laughing. I can hear the laughter in my head: a satisfied chuckle. Her teeth are stained betel-juice brown and broken in front. She's wearing a dark necklace of some kind and what looks like a seaman's bag, a frock made from canvas sacks that she's tied together with a thick, black belt. She looks a bit insane. *Who are you?*

A face stares back at me, hard to capture. Two liquid drops, gray black and piercing. A level gaze. Not friendly, not hostile. She's spitting on the ground, grinning. A mixed-blood creature with wide, high cheekbones and thick brows knitting together over small eyes. I hear her voice, hear the sandpaper rasp inside my ear.

Sel.

She has a low voice; it's hard for me to hear it.

Sel? As in sel de mer?

Sel. French sea salt. Coarse, briny, discolored. Her face is shiny with sweat, the skin of her cheeks and arms almost transparent, like a dried sardine's.

Stranger—I hear the rasp again more clearly now—*friend. Come here. Listen to me. I have something to tell you.*

But before I can respond, she's turned and is moving farther away, toward the low horizon. *Wait!* I think. *Where are you going?*

⌐

I have to concentrate to not lose her—it; not to lose sight of her slightly bent figure in my mind's eye, moving away quickly. If I get up from my spot, will she disappear?

She's grumbling now, cursing, talking to herself. What's she saying? Something I can't understand, in a language I don't recognize. Greek, or Latin maybe.

I decide to get up. I take the stairs two at a time, leading up to the massive Hôtel de Ville. There she is now, all the way across the square. I walk carefully, watching for the rats in the bushes, for men leaning into the shadows. I've been to this square many times, but I've never looked at it carefully, as I do now. *For her, for that face.* My heart is beating. I'm short of breath but feel exhilarated. Around the corner, down an alley. The image is gone. She's gone. *Dammit.*

I walk around a long side of the Hôtel, spy another bench. I'm already tired.

A few minutes later I hear: *Sit down, my friend. Let me take a closer look at you.*

⌒

How long did I doze? The woman, the apparition, the trick in my mind as I think of her voice, is gone. She smelled vaguely of musk, of old potpourri flowers. Closer up, her hands and arms and lower legs were covered with tiny scars, scabs, and what looked like old vaccination marks. *A salt licker. A sailor's bastard child. A woman with a sailor's uncouth mouth.* I try to recapture her image. No luck.

I get up stiffly. My left leg has cramped from dozing on my side. My shoulder feels numb. I can't believe I fell so hard asleep. I'm covered in a coat of tourist-bus grime. Someone—maybe more than one person—has passed close by me. I see the trace of dirty footsteps around the base of the bench. I quickly pat my pocket for my money and keys. All safe.

⌒

During the day this square, the Hôtel de Ville, is packed, but at night the hustlers take over, young women and men standing alone or in small groups, smoking and talking, meeting each other's eyes. I've seen them night after night. A pair looking me over as they do now, lazily curious, wanting to know my business. *Am I buying? Selling? Do I want drugs? What's my pleasure?*

From my new bench, with my back to the river, I look up, trying to make out the identity of the statues of France's famous men: philosophers, scientists, artists. I don't see any women. The Hôtel is huge and ornate, the size of a city block, but so poorly lit I can't make out the faces above the second level. I mentally review what I can remember about this landmark, now a museum to French history. Not much. For days, I've been carrying around a pocket guide-book; an out-of-date edition with yellowed pages. It makes a cracking noise when I open it.

I read about the Hôtel for a while, daydreaming about the royal court, the parties. Visioning the protests, the laboring classes clamoring for the king's head.

For centuries the Hôtel de Ville was central to trade and commerce, the receiving point for goods coming from abroad—from the East, the Orient, and Africa—for boats loaded with spices and newfound treasures designed to please the noble classes. The Bourgs, first sons of the French bourgeoisie, held their meetings inside the Hôtel. And here, from that bridge down there almost all the way to the cathedral, the kings of France held their giant feasts in gilded marble ballrooms where prostitution thrived.

All around me, generations of dissidents were shot or executed. Over there, under those trees, visiting Cossack princes once paraded in tall fur hats during turn-of-the-century fairs. They wore leather codpieces under their frilly pants. Across the square, a decisive battle was fought between the French Resistance and the occupying Nazis. High up, out of that second-story window, the great but shy aviator Charles Lindberg greeted fawning crowds after his celebrated transatlantic flight.

The internal newsreel sputters out; the screen goes blank. Later, when I open my eyes again, resolved to move, I hear a rumble of thunder in the distance. The air is very humid. It feels like it could rain, but the sky is clear. I search for heat lightning in the distance. The pair of hustlers who were eyeing me earlier has left. So has almost everyone else. The heat has probably driven them inside.

Hello, friend.

Her voice bothers my ear, like before. In a second I'm wider awake. I sit up, look all around. There are two older women sitting a few benches away and, past them, a group of men standing.

Friend, over this way.

There's a narrow street behind the Hôtel that leads to another building. I walk gingerly, avoiding garbage, smelling old urine, stepping on crumpled glassine bags and syringes. I see that the Hôtel remains a place of real commerce, of vice and fleshy trade. At the corner, I stoop down, smelling the flow of decay. It's the river, far below, a distinct smell of sulfur and mud.

The newsreel is playing again. All along these streets, before they were paved, the Seine moved, slow and thick, a great latrine into which everything was dumped, including the bodies of those who fell into disfavor with the king. The Hôtel was the main site of execution. A huge guillotine once stood there, in that far corner, visible from across the river even to the maids of the rich who lived in the mouselike rooms now favored by students. From their garret windows, they could view the spectacle of the crowds, shouting for the accused, demanding action or mercy, spitting at the royal executioner, getting trampled in the frenzy of the moment.

I've hardly slept, but no matter; I'm flush with a sense of history, envisioning it all, ignoring the wet sucking noises of a passing stranger, the flat, polite stare of a Hôtel security guard. For a second, I spy Joan of Arc, high on her horse in her shiny armor. I hear the snap and hiss of twigs set afire, smell the thick smoke, the unmistakable nauseous smell of burning flesh. I recall a scene from a play I saw in New York about Saint Joan played by the actress Linda Hunt. A mixed face, not unlike Sel's, some Indo-Euro-Slavic mix.

Where'd she go now?

I've lost Sel in my reveries about Joan of Arc and Linda Hunt. The voice, that weathered face, is gone again. *Zut.*

After a while I give up. I walk the long block around the Hôtel and find a café selling coffee to go, a newish, welcome feature in France—then take a fresh seat on a high ledge facing one side of the square. Close by is an enclosed inner courtyard, padlocked behind large, steel doors to discourage visitors. Through a crack, I can see dozens of dirty and broken statues: a beheaded Adonis, a young Venus streaked with pigeon shit, fat cherubs with various lost or damaged limbs. The statues probably belong to the Hôtel de Ville, either copies or originals in need of repair. I'm glimpsing Paradise, a surreal Eden, a crowded garden party of mythical creatures, each one sensuous, muscular, or impossibly plump, curved, the Lover or Beloved.

A low chuckle. *Sel.* She's been here all this time, spying on me, looking at what I'm looking at, through my eyes. *What are you seeing, stranger?* she asks. *What are you reading in your little book? Lies*, she says gently. *Whatever it is—all lies.* I feel her eyes looking back up at the Hôtel, at the famous men in their gilded robes.

Her voice is a too-hot breath in my ear, a gust of humidity. *Our greatest men are pederasts*, I hear her whisper. *Those that aren't chasing after too-young girls. All my good brothers.* Her laughter is the cackle of geese. Of shattering glass. *Even the corrupted men of the cloth who sent them to an early heaven. Their bodies stank like mine does. They bathed in perfume to mask the odor of their diseases. Their wigs and bodies were full of lice. What's really behind these immortalized faces are scandals, peccadilloes, dark crimes, perversion. That's what's made this country great. Don't let anyone tell you otherwise.* She's licking her lips, satisfied. Her own hair, I see, is speckled with pigeon mites.

The *café à porter* is too hot to be drinking on this sweltering day, but it's delicious. I can barely hold the cup. The steam settles on my face. I look back up at the massive Hôtel. I wonder who stands ignoble above me.

Behind me materializes a group of German tourists, led by a pert young guide whose high voice irritates me, reminds me of what I dislike about bourgeois French women, which is their mannered affect: a singsong way of speaking, a pretention of false cheer masking coldness and a critical spirit. The woman eyes me with a quick smile and suspicion, then leads the group quickly past. What am I doing here—trying to break in? She looks back once, disapproving.

Screw you, lady.

I look back into the locked courtyard. The stone flesh of Hermes; the perfect breasts and huge, muscular calves of a Madonna, one missing part of her right arm, making it harder to cradle the Baby Jesus. Another saint is missing both lower legs. The loss makes him vulnerable, more appealing, more human. I like these broken saints and virgins.

I imagine myself painting a giant encaustic portrait of the scene inside. Fallen icons for the ill and disabled. A tableau for the dying poxed boys. One of Saint Anthony of Padua, the patron saint of the sick and the lost, revered by sailors. A wealthy young nobleman from Lisbon who opted for the simple life and later died of ergot poisoning, aka ergotism, now named Saint Anthony's fire. A poisoning caused by the ingestion of alkaloids from a fungus found in grains like rye and some cereals, *Claviceps Purpurea*, as well as some known drugs. A slow, painful death that used to be associated with witchcraft.

Saint Anthony's feet and hands likely grew twisted, purple and dark green as the poison spread, constricting the flow of blood, causing pains, seizures, and convulsions, causing mania. He probably walked like the lifelong alcoholics with advanced cirrhosis and diabetic neuropathy who lumber through our cities with numbed feet swaddled in dirty rags. Peripheral neuropathy has become a side effect of some of the new HIV drugs. I have friends with AIDS who can't feel the ends of their fingertips or toes. They lose their balance; walking is a gentle act. I hope Saint Anthony hears their prayers.

I learned about the saints and popes in my Catholic elementary school, about the politics of canonization. One of my favorite myths about Saint Anthony concerns his tongue. He died at thirty-five and when his body was exhumed thirty years later, it was reportedly dust but for his tongue, which glistened as if still alive and moist. It was a sign of his gift for oratory, for preaching. The tongue is now on display for veneration in a big reliquary, along with his jaw and vocal chords. It's a popular relic. The true believers are so obsessed they have been lobbying papal officials to test his gifted tongue, to see if it's truly living, like their belief in Jesus's resurrected body. I'd love to be the scientist testing that theory. I also like the idea of dying boys praying for their diseased gay tongues to survive, to perversely lick at life again.

I modify my fantasy church portrait, paint a series of gold circles in the corners of the canvas, each a mini looking-glass reliquary with a glistening *lingua viva*, a waxy tongue, inside. Add lost objects and Mexican *milagros* scattered around his blackening body: keys and jewels; fingers, toes, and teeth. *Sancti ad corpus gangraena*. Saint Anthony, Portuguese saint of loss, of *saudade*. Add a recording to the portrait that one listens to with a press of a finger, as in a museum. *A morna for the lost tongue*, sung by the great barefoot goddess of Cape Verde, Cesària Évora.

I saw you before, her voice interrupts my vision. *Earlier. Walking near the Pont Saint-Michel. I thought you were a man at first. In fact, you reminded me of an old trick.*

⸻

My wild guide is a walking archive of hidden histories, of sedition. For years she's camped out on these park benches, her scarf tied with a knot and placed on the ground beside her like the elderly homeless women around here. But Sel is only pretending to beg, though she'll take the money. Begging is a ruse. It keeps the police from growing too suspicious, and others from paying too much attention to her—a surefire way to be ignored by the passing public. She has other things on her mind. Important things. She's like me, stalking someone elusive, something lurking behind the curtain of the ordinary day. An enemy, possibly. Her friends are social outcasts who survive along the edges of the Seine, inside abandoned buildings, or far below ground within the labyrinthine Catacombs. An underground force that emerges like Sel at night and disappears into its hidden entrails by dawn.

I'm on my feet now, as certain as Saint Joan of this voice, this inner muse, my sense of a mission. Sel's some kind of a messenger and I'm to be a vehicle for her words. That's how it feels, that real. But what's the mission? What's the enemy?

I have a voice inside my head, talking to me, I think. *That much is true.*

⸻

Is this going to become a novel, a monologue, a play? I can only guess. Try as I do, Sel won't fix herself more clearly in my mind, her story, her history. But she's led me again to the river, which today stinks of faintly rotting eggs. Eggs pickled in brine, uncapped after decades.

Later, wandering home again, I begin to notice them more, pay closer attention. Some alone, some in louder groups. Some with children lying on dirty blankets, bored and restless. Smoking cigarettes, drinking. Some trying to remain invisible in daylight, looking beyond or past me as if I'm the one who's a ghost. I hear words I don't recognize, a cadence of languages from the East, possibly Slavic. Worn out refugees from an ethnic Balkan conflict that's heating up again, forcing a new generation to flee war. A battle playing itself out here inside their tired minds and bodies.

Her tribe, I think. *My tribe, too.*

~ 2

For over ten years, I've spent my working days studying an enemy I can hardly locate. A modern pox; one that touches all things, all things in me. I can look back at my life and see the swath it has cut, wide and far, across the lives of my loved ones and friends and legions of strangers. A disease and an epidemic that has irrevocably changed my life and my focus. Walking without direction, as usual, I keep my eyes pinned on the Seine. I trail my fingers along the uneven concrete surfaces of the wall that runs parallel to the river. In this humidity, my fingertips feel plump, hot, overly sensitive.

Only a few weeks ago, these same fingers were stroking an ill man's face. Johnny, my good friend. Stroking his thinning hair, quietly reassuring him that I'd be back, that he wouldn't die suddenly and unexpectedly while I was away. Across the sea, he's another insomniac, afraid of sleeping, afraid of never waking up again. He left a message yesterday, eager to know if I've come across something to help him — a potential cure. He wants to know what I've learned at the recent AIDS conference. A man who's bored and tired of being so sick, who can't bear the heat of another New York summer without being able to go out in shorts because of his purple Kaposi's lesions — the gay AIDS cancer, KS — and who's jealous that I've gotten to escape to Europe and especially to Paris — gay Paree, as he puts it — a city he considers the most romantic in the world. And that I have a lover to walk with me at night along the Seine. I should be shot, he tells me, or at least forced to drag him along, IV in tow. Neither has happened. Instead, he's a shadow; another voice besides Sel's that I hear constantly, that I talk to.

Even here, so far away, I feel his suppressed terror, his longing, his over-whelming panic and grief. Emotions like food that stick in my chest, painfully, when I think of him, as I do now. I've said my prayers that he won't choose this moment to die. The thought flits across my mind again: *no, not while I'm here. Please.*

———

Before me, the surface of the Seine reflects the sun, sliding down the huge glass windows of a department store. The river runs red like the biblical Red Sea behind Moses. In my mind, I watch the fleeing Israelites and the walls of water closing down upon the Pharaoh's men, drowning them in a red bath. Here too, the long artery of Paris is shot through with infection, with taint. It seeds this city with death, with a loss of life unseen by the average citizen or tourist. It pulses, hard and visible, in the thick vein of Johnny's neck like a small frog swallowed by a snake. As a tourist boat passes, I search its wake for the flailing arms of Egyptian soldiers; a trail of locusts; pale, bloated frogs floating belly-up. Death is pumping inside my chest, stealing away my earlier happy mood. I want to physically push it away with two hands, part the Red Sea with mine, push Death back through it to the other side. *Stay away*, I say. *Give it a rest.*

Sel is with me now, merging her thoughts with mine, listening to me talk to myself. She's pointing to different parts of the city. *This is the battlefield, right here. A battle others ignore.* Over there, on the isthmus of the Île Saint-Louis, I read earlier, is the Hôtel-Dieu, the famous public hospital where past victims of plague sought shelter, only to be tossed into the river by the king's frightened soldiers. How many, like Johnny, are dying of AIDS there now? How many stand at the windows looking out, dreaming of suicide, of running naked, screaming, down the broad pavement? We are having an inner conversation, Sel and I, but there's no separating our thoughts. When I listen, I hear her voice; when she speaks, I hear myself.

The hot feeling is inside me again. *Johnny*, I plead, casting a pebble at the nearest tourist boat, *don't die. I'm not ready for you to go.*

There's a taste of metal in my mouth—salt . . . blood, I realize with alarm. I touch my nose; it's bleeding. I try wiping it away, plugging it up with a finger. It forms a thin, viscous coat of red mucous around my fingertips, like an embryonic sac. I think of Johnny's blood—infected, lethal, getting harder to tap inside his weakened veins. He's diabetic, on top of the HIV. A lifetime of injections. I think, *He'll never see Paris again.*

At the river's edge, I dip my hands in, rinse my face. I watch as the nose blood mixes with the water and dissipates like a dye. I take a tentative sip, studying the water carefully. *How polluted is it, really?* It tastes slightly sweet. *From the Seine and Sel into me*, I think, burping. *Let it flow.*

Now that it's late summer, the gay beach is filling up. The beautiful men of Paris who've come here from the provinces to escape marriage and their families are undressed along a stretch of the quai, exposing compact French bodies, stout legs, designer *culottes-maillots* bikini briefs. A group of svelte Asian boys play mahjong. Two blacks—that's what the fashionable French call their dark citizens: *les blacks*—eye the men who pass with feigned disinterest.

No one knows how many men here are infected, and since so many are in the closet, or bisexual, or married, no one will. The ancient stigma of the pox is attached to this disease and only a brave few have rushed to warn the others. Most are still hiding, if they can. This is especially true among les blacks—who aren't just the Africans and Haitians but the Chinese and Vietnamese. To a racist here, les blacks are anyone who isn't native, who doesn't deserve citizenship, who should be kicked out.

AIDS has invaded the houses of the poorest and most invisible in Paris, those who've bargained their frugal life's earnings—and sometimes their lives—to secure a semblance of a visa and working papers for France. Who work under the table for slave wages and with the constant fear of deportation by well-bred Parisians who consider themselves enlightened, not racist. Who are lured by con men and policemen and narcs on the take to invest their life's savings in a bogus passport and an underground journey along a circuitous route, entering from northern Africa to Greece or Sicily or Croatia or from Russia or the far coasts of the Black Sea, down to Finland, then over to Belgium. There, after months of anxious waiting, if the broken saints of their journey are listening, they may make it to France, where a fresh trap is sprung.

The border of France is a noose, a tripwire ready to spring, to capture them, to expose them, to snuff out the new lives they have dreamed about. And by then they're penniless, dreams and fortunes lost, or actual slaves, especially the girls. Thousands slip past the noose anyway, stolen and sold by the clever mafias of the East and West into lives of indentured service or brothel hell. Somehow, the French authorities do not see them, do not track these young girls and boys, are not acting to liberate these modern slaves any more than did French colonialists of the past.

France is not mother, father, protector. Not anymore. Not ever. That great colonial lie has been laid to rest at last. No one who comes here from distant lands believed it, anyway; only those who once peddled the dream. Those who still harbor delusions of grandeur, who delight their children with stories of pampered idyll in the former colonies like Algeria—the dreaming, repatriated *pied-noir* generation. A rather racist term itself. The white civil servants sent to the French colonies to run things, to seek their fortune, to become the newest generation of masters. Then forced by history, by their leaders, to abandon ship, to be kicked out by the Algerians demanding independence, violently routing them, chasing their masters all the way to the heart of Paris until freedom is won. Forced to return home to the cold winters of France, to smaller horizons, to defeat. Some hold the tripwire tightly in their hands; they'll always vote to keep the blacks out of France. They'll go to their graves still clutching that nationalist, racist mantra: *La France pour les Français! France for the French!*

And right now, some of them are quietly cheering the return of Jean-Marie Le Pen, the old wolf who was their soldier in Algeria and is now their man in Marseille. He remains so tireless in his efforts to keep out the Maghreb, the Arabs. He and his blonde, blue-eyed, dutiful Catholic daughters. Patriots, indeed.

I hear myself lecturing but don't care. Sel's listening to me. Sel and Johnny, who must be up right now across the Atlantic, readying for another drip bag of toxic chemo medicine, as well as Sebastien, a distant relative. He called earlier today, asking about the trip. The men and women who rule France don't want to pay to care for, or educate, les blacks, even native-born blacks with polished

French manners, I tell them. Never mind those with this pox. All they want is for the carriers of the disease to go home—to go die at home. Black, white, yellow; second-, third-, tenth-generation French—it doesn't matter. *Send them away, and quickly!*

Sel has seen all of this, I think; watched it blow upriver like a storm leveling everything, leaving a shell of a city. A hulk, a house of cards, not this glistening, regilded Paris; not the sparkling pyramid of I. M. Pei and the billions spent to renovate the Louvre. *Va voir*, I hear her suggest. Go see for yourself.

I could do that. Go talk to those people I passed last night, near that make-shift squatter camp. Or go out to the suburbs, the banlieues, to Saint-Denis, where the Roma families are newly getting evicted. It's been in the past week's papers. A fresh police crackdown on the newest illegals. The new *sans papiers*. Or maybe later I could head south. To Bordeaux or to Marseille, where a generation of high school dropouts share good wine and trash can fires in the winter. Who, like the junkies all over Europe, use the fire to heat their spoons and cookers and shoot heroin from Hong Kong and Afghanistan into the backs of their knees. Into all the cracks of the body; the places that bend: crook of elbow, twist of neck, splay of fingers, toes, underarm.

I should go. I could go. But I'm tired, aren't I? That's why I'm here. I'll go next trip. Or not. I could easily spend a few days at this gay beach right here.

There's a worsening heroin problem in Paris, one the authorities are determined to wipe out. I've been following the story in the papers. The antigang unit here is tracking its distribution by Chinese and Russian and Afghan gangs using the oldest methods: violence, blackmail, informants. They're determined to break the schoolboy-junkie and secretary-addict of their wasteful habits, the kind they support by joining the parade of women and men in short dresses along the Boulevard de Clichy. A section of the city I've taken to visiting in the early evening.

It's here that the junkies come in search of a new, more powerful mix of Afghan brown heroin cut with resinous Mexican black tar, then further cut with cheaper powdered heroin that mixes well in tap water and is proving deadly. It can attack soft tissue, seed it with infection by spore-forming bacteria like tetanus and a new class of bacteria, clostridium. The injection wound becomes black and crusty in the center, tender red underneath, but without much pus, like a mini-volcanic explosion cooled to hard ash as the skin turns necrotic. It's killer junk. I first came across it in a health report. Geeking out as usual with fascination about the science, the incredible reservoir of possibly nasty bugs that have been found in people shooting speedballs of coke and this new dirty heroin.

Most are strains of staph—*Staphylococcus aureus*—a common enough bacteria, but one that goes rogue inside the fucked-up noses of cokeheads. Obviously we should be really worried about the possible crossover with HIV, the extra vulnerability of the already immune compromised. I wonder if ACT UP–Paris is aware. If not, they probably will be soon.

Many of my friends here are gay and longtime members of ACT UP–Paris. Several of them, like Johnny, have today's scariest sexual pox. They're willing to show up at the AIDS pickets, but they haven't really dealt with the drug aspect of France's AIDS crisis. I do see it as a class thing; the world of drugs and poverty and immigration is still largely foreign to the middle-class, white gay men who make up the activist core in Paris. That's certainly true in San Francisco and New York. Most of my gay boy friends are aware of the junkies and the married women at risk, but when pressed for details, they don't know where the crack houses are, or the safe houses, never mind the whorehouses. They've never visited the childcare centers here established for immigrant women from Algeria or Senegal whose husbands abandoned them or died after passing the pox on to their unsuspecting wives. The many pretty, young and older Muslim women, married off as children to polygamous older men, now sick behind their veils. The first, second, third, fourth child brides. Successive crimes that lie behind the cloak of AIDS, but are not yet the subject of ACT UP protests, at least not that I've seen.

We need to talk about this though, who's still being left outside the movement. It's women, yes, and we've been organizing around that so much in New York. But it's also the women who remain socially outcast in our communities. Here it's the African women, the diaspora immigrants from the French colonies. And as in the United States, the transwomen and the druggies, both of whom turn tricks and get high as acts of survival. Who knows what they're escaping. A lack of love somewhere. A world that hates them. It's usually nothing pretty. I haven't seen them much at ACT UP yet either.

The men of ACT UP–Paris, I say to Johnny, as if he's here listening, *are not the children of '68, of Sartre and Socialism. They're the children of your generation. The 1970s and '80s. These French gay boys are former wanna-be-again yuppies.* It's just that the pox has stripped them of their privilege, their sense of a sure future. But the sense of entitlement is there; it's intact. Not all of them. I know a few who are great guys, really good politics, who get it. But a lot don't. *They are fighting for their own lives, not more.*

Now we have another pox ready to scar and harden the flesh. Clostridium. I wonder how the sore compares to KS, which also gets black and hard and ashy too, with advanced AIDS. Look at our friend Vito. He became so ragged, his face so ruined by KS. He had KS for, what, five or six years before he died?

Brutal. I love how Vito used to say to me, *Well I look like shit, sweetie, but I'm feeling okay today.* He was the real sweetie: a great activist, great film historian, good strategist, a feminist, and so proudly gay. We lost such a great guy.

How bad will this dirty heroin outbreak be? They need to track the source fast and get rid of it. Instead they'll probably just start locking up the junkies, throw away the key, make 'em go cold turkey in a cell instead of a hospital. Or maybe they're more humane here in France. There's free public health care, after all. *Fucking clostridium.* It never stops. There's just too many poxes for us to track.

The sun is lower, the air a bit cooler. The color of the river is closer to rust. The color of dying blood, I think, of dried blood. How long does it take for the blood to become dust in the body? Days? Weeks? Months? With a start, I realize I've gotten so involved in these morbid thoughts that I've lost complete track of time. It's almost seven; I'll be late for my dinner date. I leave Sel to jump on a bus. She walks away in the far corner of my mind, like in the final scene of a classic movie: an old woman leaning on a closed black umbrella, hunched over, wearing what looks like a faded-gray, cotton coat, her feet in worn sandals, like the old Turkish woman I saw earlier begging for money near the metro.

See you later, old lady.

~ 3

I'm on my way to meet Belle. The love of my life. Potentially anyway. We got involved in a sudden romance that began as a hot weeklong affair at last year's AIDS conference in Amsterdam and quickly evolved into something much deeper. When I met her, I was still grieving a stormy long-term relationship with a woman I'll call the Aerialist, another deep love. She's my official ex, but my heart has taken a long time to mend. I've had other lovers in there too— affectionate affairs—but up to now, I really haven't let myself open up, not like this. With Belle it was an immediate, mad girl crush. *Hot hot hot!* And the best: it felt so reciprocal. None of the bad drama I'd been having for so long. Just a sense of total pleasure at meeting someone fantastic, and loving everything that's happening. The honeymoon phase.

To complicate matters (or make them more interesting, depending on your perspective), I also had a short affair with another woman in Amsterdam, also in ACT UP, and from New York. We've kept seeing each other a bit. I like her a lot but it's more FWB, friends with benefits. A philosopher. A lover of Hegel and thick, dark, expensive red wines. She became a new friend of Belle's too, and, for a second, they too felt the haze of hash-induced desire while we all trolled around together in Amsterdam. We're so postmodern, aren't we?

A quick caveat: I don't consider myself promiscuous; if anything, I delude myself that I'm loyal, even old-fashioned in my sense of fidelity to lovers. And, of course, love often comes when one doesn't expect it; when one doesn't even want it, like heartbreak. Typically, in my case, love rides in on heartbreak's back. Throughout much of my turbulent relationship with the Aerialist—through our periods of struggle and separation, during stints of nonmonogamy where we had other lovers and tried to give each other space—I was already mourning her, mourning us, the loss of another love. And I'm still mourning that relationship somewhere, it seems. Maybe grief is the only way I can feel the love, a tortured form of nostalgia.

But with Belle it's different, and easy. We're natural companions. We just pick up where we leave off—in conversations, in letters, in bed. She's a big reason I'm back here in Paris: to see her and my relatives, and to try to convince her to come to New York this fall for a visit. I want us to be together for longer than a few weeks, to know what we might have beyond *une grande affaire*.

Belle was—she is—gorgeous, with penetrating sea-glass eyes, a megawatt smile, and dynamic energy. She's smart, with good politics. She caught my attention immediately at one of the first Amsterdam action organizing meetings. She's just one of those great personality people; very positive, very caring. She's been a leader at ACT UP–Paris, a *pasionaria*. I liked the way she listened at meetings, deeply, putting her hand on her chin and concentrating. She likes digging into the issues like I do and debating. Really she's just a doll.

I think we just smiled at each other with our eyes at a certain point in Amsterdam and that was it. We knew we were going to have an affair. Isn't it incredible when such moments happen? *Boom*, that's it. Or that's how I remember it. She just stood out, wearing the classic ACT UP–Paris white T-shirt with bold, black letters, wearing jeans and some Docs. There are so many great people in ACT UP—cute girls, definitely—and at these conferences they are from all over the world along with all the brainy, creative scientists and everybody else who shows up for the mega-meeting-party-research confab.

That's something people who aren't in groups like ACT UP may not appreciate about activism: despite the serious subject and critical life stakes, it can be so fun, and the people who are drawn to protest and social change, so interesting. I'm finding the same thing here in Paris, although there are fewer women in ACT UP so far. That's changing though. Anyway, it's one of the perks of joining ACT UP that I would never have anticipated. I've made so many friends and had my share of sexy fun. It keeps us going. There's just a lot of love in this movement.

—⌐

As I expected, Belle's holding court, leading a discussion about the latest ACT UP–Paris battle, one centered around the group's nascent needle-exchange program, which the government has bitterly opposed. It's a bit like New York. The AIDS activists here are following ACT UP–Amsterdam's lead, handing out bleach kits and disposable needles at several sites, albeit only a fraction of what's needed. Since many of the Paris activists are older gay men, they know the street scene well enough to figure out where to leave condoms and safe-sex kits: along the water's edge, at the entrance to the city's big parks, where most of the gay cruising takes place, favorite tricking spots like the streets around the Russian embassy and the Bois de Boulogne. The locations are being discussed as I arrive. I take mental notes.

Several people wave and blow me kisses. Belle takes my hand for a second but doesn't stop talking. About a dozen people are here tonight. They've unpacked a small picnic: cheeses, ham, grapes, six or seven different kinds of wine. Belle hands me a glass, smiles again, doesn't break her stride.

We need to recruit, Belle says to a thirtyish man with a shaved head and two silver rings in his left ear, who seems to agree. A handsome boy. He's wearing jeans and a white T-shirt and very nice black shoes. American-style, but designer wear. Gauthier, I note for Johnny, who appreciates such details. He nods as if he were being rebuked. A mama's boy, I decide. I hear someone say his name. Luc. He gives me a quick, shy smile. *We need to work in coalition with the groups who run the methadone clinics*, Belle adds. *The people we want to reach don't know us — they're not going to trust us.*

I take a seat. It's a familiar discussion. *We're too insulated*, designer boy Luc agrees. *We really don't know enough about what's happening. I know they arrested some people last week behind the Gare du Nord. So where did all those people go? We have to connect AIDS to homelessness, to the housing problem. That should be a top priority, shouldn't it?* Not everyone agrees. *Let's stick to AIDS*, a voice behind me says. *We can't solve all those social problems. We're not a welfare agency.*

I turn around and take note of the voice. An older, round-faced man with thin lips and a mustache. *Oh, now that's ridiculous!* Belle says sharply, but her voice is light and high. *I completely disagree*, she adds, giggling a little, not wanting to sound so shrill. *That kind of attitude really turns me off.*

The round-faced man shrugs. He looks around. She's too powerful for him. *I know what you're saying*, says another, *but we have to focus on how the epidemic is spreading. I think she's right. We can ally ourselves and stick to the communities we know best. But we should definitely create some kind of partnership.*

The others get into the debate. I catch Belle's eye. *Go on, tell him.* It's what I like about her. That passion.

I look past the group at the river. It's beautiful. This is an ideal spot for a nighttime picnic. Romantic. Magical. Something Paris has that New York sorely lacks. *You should go to these places,* Sel whispers, interrupting. *Don't wait for these people to take you. Va voir.* Go see.

Be careful, Johnny chimes in. *Those places are dangerous. You'll get yourself killed.*

It's a good idea. But I'll need a male escort. I shouldn't go to some of these places alone—not to the parks. I'm butch enough that I can pass, but some parts of Paris aren't safe at night for anyone. I've heard stories of muggings, of tricks who turn out to be undercover cops, who aren't afraid of beating up a gay man or a hustler because they know they'll get away with it.

Just a little longer—Belle signals to me—*then we'll eat. Okay?* I wink back at her. *Go on, then.*

⁓

Our group is camped out directly across the river from a spot where, in past centuries, Belle tells me, they held a royal ball and where, every summer now, the fags and dykes and especially the drag queens have revived the event. I share my wine with Aldyn, an activist friend from New York. He holds the dubious honor of being the most famous long-term survivor of AIDS, an ACT UP poster boy. We hung out together in Berlin, where he was a media star. It was the first time I really got to party with him. I like him a lot.

Aldyn is handsome and charming and looks the picture of health. He immediately informs me that he's slept with some of the boys here tonight, including Luc, and enjoyed every minute of it. *Am I becoming a slut?* he whispers to me. Aldyn makes me laugh. *You're a man of taste,* I whisper back. *They're all cute. Right,* he agrees. *That's what I've been telling myself. I'm a discriminating slut.* He's one of the rare white gay men from New York whom I consider pretty evolved and a feminist. He's forty-plus and looks thirty and hasn't stopped educating himself. When it comes to AIDS, he readily admits his fear of death but hasn't stopped living or having lots of sex.

I'll go to the park with you, Aldyn offers later, when I mention that I want to explore the city's seedy corners a bit. *But if anyone tries to pick you up*—he smiles—*I might get jealous.* I like how open Aldyn is about his desires. I wonder if he's slept with Belle. I think they slept in the same bed before I got here, but she does that with most of her friends, male and female. Their connection comes across as more sensual than sexual. I wonder if Aldyn sleeps with women. I've never asked him. He seems like he could, or would, if he liked someone. A free-spirited gay man.

He begins to give me the lowdown about the parks, about the different cruising scenes. He rarely goes out alone to the bigger parks. He says the gay

men of Paris are everywhere, especially in the shopping centers, and, by his
own estimate, they're all bigger sluts than he. I like listening to his stories. By
nightfall, I'm a little drunk and I've had too much to eat. So have Aldyn and
Belle. She waves good-bye to the group and leads me over to a shady corner to
neck. Then, after eleven, she leaves me. Even though it's late, she has to attend
to some errands and meet another friend for a quick nightcap. We make plans
to meet later at the apartment, or much later, at a bar. I'm in Paris. The night
out begins at dusk and ends at breakfast. Even though Belle and her friends all
work day jobs, they simply don't sleep and, every so often, they catch up on
weekends. *Very Brazilian*, I think.

I walk with Aldyn. We follow the Quai de la Mégisserie past the Île de la Cité,
the first city of Paris, then cross onto the Île Saint-Louis to mingle with the
tourists, then across the Pont de Sully, where, rather suddenly, there are more
men again and less of anyone else. From there along the Quai Henri IV, then a
left, up the Boulevard de la Bastille, which could be called the gay Boulevard de
Clichy except that there is little to distinguish who is selling and who is buying.
This is what Aldyn tells me, playing the gayboy guide.

Everyone's on display, including me. Tonight I'm wearing a long, loose
shirt. My breasts aren't large and I'm very androgynous. The men eye me with
curiosity. What are you? A man or a woman? Some species of *travelo*? The
evening air is refreshing. I enjoy the walk. Aldyn tells me he once tried to hustle.
It was more for the experience than the money, he says. Because he was such a
good boy, one who liked the idea of the forbidden, of gay sex being something
risky, potentially dangerous. Aldyn's not foolish enough not to have regrets, but
his regrets are for the future, not the past. *I'd do it again*, he says. *Except I'd have
more sex and I'd start a lot earlier. And I'd charge a little more money. I was a cheap trick.*
He laughs.

I'm thinking about whom Sel spends her days with. With gay boys like
Aldyn, recovering drug addicts, and older French women who once looked like
Belle and now resemble Jeanne Moreau in her fifties, with twice-divorced unfaithful husbands and less faith in the church, or with working-class kids who
are underemployed and ready to resort to a little underground black market
activity; to a trading mentality instead of a credit card one, if the opportunity
presents itself.

We head up toward the Bastille and, as we do, ducking down the dim
streets, Aldyn asks about my time, what I've been doing. I tell him about my
loose idea for a novel set in Paris, one that's both contemporary and historical,
one that begins right here and takes place mostly at night, featuring a cast of

marginals and narrated by an older woman—a voice, I explain, that's come into my head and is ever present. Aldyn was an actor and singer before he became an activist. He's a Broadway junkie, knows all the musicals. Went to Harvard and did Gilbert and Sullivan, has been in a movie. He knows all about giving oneself over to a character, to a voice, to an experience. *It sounds great,* he says enthusiastically. *Will you write a part for me? I'd like to play a lesbian. Or at least a cross-dressing fag.*

Like so many of my friends, Aldyn loves being a gay man and enjoys having a dick, but he's always felt close to women. They're nicer, he claims, more interesting. Maybe because they don't have a dick swinging between their legs, I think. That could be irritating.

I'm coming back as a lesbian, Aldyn informs me now. *As a femme. I've got the legs, you know.*

He does have shapely legs.

I like how frank Aldyn is about death, how matter-of-fact. How much he isn't dwelling on the possibility of sickness, but is wresting as much pleasure from his life as he can. I like his pseudo-Zen Buddhism, his patchwork spirituality, taking for himself all the best parts of every religion. He's not focusing on death but accepts the possibility, the likelihood that it may happen early, even for him, the poster boy for survival. He looks healthy but maybe he's a bit thinner than he used to be, now that I look more closely. In Berlin he rode around on a bicycle, shirtless. He's got a nice summer tan.

In Berlin, Aldyn was a keynote speaker. He skewered President Clinton for having kept Haitians with HIV in quarantine at the refugee camp in Guantánamo, Cuba, where we have a naval base. Housing Works has been involved too, helping to resettle those who make it to the United States. In April, ACT UP got twenty-two Haitians out of there. The protests are working. A judge ordered the camp closed back in June and seventy-eight more PWAs were brought over and resettled with help from ACT UP. The remaining should be out soon. I wonder if they'll stay in Cuba or come to the States too? Cuba has great and free public health care, but they quarantine people with HIV and TB. And they don't love the gays either. They'll come to the United States, I bet.

Come back as Shiva, I suggest to Aldyn, *or some goddess of love.*

A pagan diva; he nods, envisaging it. *Garlands of flowers, lots of worshipers, candles. I could live with that. What should my name be?*

The name springs forth.

Lolita, I say out loud. *The Goddess of Broken-Hearted Youth.*

Aldyn smiles, his eyes half-closed. *Lolita,* he repeats, pursing his lips. *Protector of the dreams of young boys. I'd never let anyone do anything to them they didn't want. All their secrets would be safe with me.*

Pedophile, I tease him.

Never, he retorts. *I like my men hearty, like soup.*

And hairy, I add.

Hairy like soup. He laughs. *Hair of the soup.*

He bats his eyes at me, moving his arms like seven snakes around his torso and head. Vogueing. Doing what I can best describe as a very energetic, awkward Dance of the Seven Veils.

Go boy, I think, *nothing can stop you now.*

As he spins, I suddenly see Johnny's face, veiled, attending his own funeral. *Stop it,* I hear my mind say.

To Aldyn I say, *I got a call from John. You know, my friend Johnny? He's not feeling that great. The KS, you know. It's getting really bad. He wanted to come with me, but he can't handle the heat. Wearing shorts. It embarrasses him.*

Aldyn doesn't say anything, but he's nodding to himself. *John has nice legs,* he says after a while. *I remember that.*

I'm reminded that Johnny likes Aldyn, confessed a quick-burning crush on the poster boy last year. We joked about it for a few weeks. Aldyn takes my hand for a second. *Hey, did I just lose you?*

~ 4

The night air is a balm. My mind opens up like a lotus blossom. Who is Sel? A healer, someone who's picked up her knowledge from the street and from books? A radical homeopath; a woman who digs up the clay from the Seine and uses it as a poultice for the skin rashes that come with the pox? I've been studying AIDS vaccines and immunity, the concept of *self* and *nonself,* what proteins might be turned on or off with gene therapy to kill HIV with neutralizing antibodies or to boost protection via cellular immunity. *Active versus passive immunization.* Reinfusion of one's HIV-infected blood, designed to stimulate a greater protective response to the virus. What we're studying in long-term survivors like Aldyn who may have some natural immunity to HIV or may have been exposed to a weakened virus that doesn't replicate as well, that's somehow kept him healthy for longer than others.

Maybe Sel can represent someone completely tainted, who willingly exposes herself to infection rather than eradicate it. That's what Jon Greenberg used to talk about. A fantasy. He tried to do what he could, experiment with his own body, eschew Western drugs in favor of nature's medicines. A *body-mind-soul* approach to healing himself, or at least dying naturally. Jon was madly popping B-12 when he came with me to Haiti, sharing it with a Haitian man we visited in his home. The man was standing on his bed, raving, when we arrived. He clearly had dementia, a sign that HIV had crossed the blood-brain barrier. That's what vitamin B-12 can do too, so Jon believed. I wasn't as sure, still am not totally convinced. But it couldn't hurt, I felt.

The Haitian man died two days later. Our visit and Jon's vitamins had given him and his family a dose of hope, just before the end. Who can argue that wasn't an act of healing?

Maybe Sel could be the extreme embodiment of the ACT UP philosophy of living with your disease. She won't try to rid the body of her pox, but absorb it, acclimate to it, become attenuated. Another idea Jon liked to fantasize about. How to embody a living vaccine. Or is she the opposite? A lethal Typhoid Mary, the social threat so feared by public health officials? Could she be both? A metaphor for the beast and the antidote in one body? It's an intriguing idea.

⸺

I tell Aldyn how, earlier, the river ran red, how this biblical metaphor came true in my mind. *Can you see it? Can you imagine how incredible Paris would look?* I ask him. *Truly medieval,* he agrees, laughing. *Are you always so visual? Or did you do a lot of LSD when you were young?*

Visual, yes; crazily so. A big daydreamer. Big, big fantasy life. It got me in trouble at school. I was always spacing out and talking out loud to myself. I still do that. *My friends call me the absentminded professor because I'm always off in some reverie,* I tell him. *But no LSD.*

What I don't tell Aldyn is that I've always been afraid of hallucinogens. My older sister had an overnight mental breakdown in college after somebody spiked the party punch with mescaline at an after-school social. This was Harvard, the early seventies, close to when Aldyn was there. She was at Radcliffe. A Virginia Woolf scholar. A near-genius, Mensa-smart sister who loved books and documentary film and had perfect grades and was in love, maybe for the first time. She is five years older than I am. She was extremely depressed at the time over a serious boyfriend who'd decided he couldn't marry her because she wasn't Jewish; he'd cut it off. Plus he was bisexual, we later learned. Maybe he knew something she didn't? When we finally came to rescue her, three months after the acid party, she'd covered the windows of her basement dorm with black curtains shutting out the light, the world, and was sleeping through her summer classes. Her roommates hadn't wanted to call us, to alarm the family back home. When they finally did, it was too late.

At that party my sister went right down the long black hole, à la Alice. It was a bad, bad trip. A no-return trip. She never recovered. She became another sister, one I love dearly while mourning the sister I lost overnight. It took years for the doctors to give her a diagnosis of schizophrenia. It also instilled a fear I carry of hard drugs, of loosening my mind too much.

Look at me, I say to Aldyn. *Can you imagine what LSD would do to someone like me? I don't need LSD. I need something to keep my mind and feet fully rooted in the here and now. I don't need anything to take me down more rabbit holes.*

He laughs. *I hear ya. You only want the* good *drugs.*

That's not a bad slogan. I make a mental note to share it with Belle. ACT UP could use it in their new outreach campaign to addicts. *Enough junk. We only want good drugs!*

⁓

I want to hear more about Sel, Aldyn says later as we approach the area where he says the cruising is hot. *She sounds kinda wild as a character. Keep me posted.* He's still moving his hands like a courtesan, still dancing a little. *Feel free to write me into your book too. I don't mind being immortalized.*

Ahead of us, I see Sel, waving through the streets. She looks more like a bag lady than some literary muse.

Let's have a quick drink, Aldyn suggests before we part. He points to a bar. *Quick and dirty.*

A drink before the cruise, I joke.

Before the Titanic sinks, he adds.

⁓

It's late and I've missed the last metro train. I walk slowly home. When I get to Belle's building, she doesn't answer the buzzer. I pray I'll remember the outdoor combination code, the location of the inner lights in the hall with timers that click off too fast, leaving one cursing in a dark stairwell. Inside, there's a message on her answering machine for me from Johnny. His voice sounds sweet—a bit anxious, but in better spirits. *I hope you're having a fabulous time without me. I heard the heat is a bitch. Did you find me a boyfriend yet?*

⁓ 5

I've received a call from Philippe Madelin, a French journalist friend from my earlier Haiti reporting days. He's expecting me for lunch on Saturday. He wants to catch up on Haiti, wants to know when my Haiti novel, *Under the Bone*, is due out. He's been working on his own book about dictators. That's how we met, sharing info about the deposed Haitian ruler Jean-Claude "Baby Doc"

Duvalier and his regime, a rapacious clan that was ousted in a coup in 1986. The Duvaliers and their in-laws, the Bennetts, have settled in southern France, protected from extradition back to Haiti—so far.

I'll get to meet Philippe's wife, Marina. I have to come to their house because he's recovering from an operation and can't walk far yet. Philippe is a classic muckraker, an unrepentant leftist who freelances and also works for French television. His specialty is documentaries, investigative reports, and true crime. I met him via a mutual friend, Bruce Dollar, an American investigator living in New York who was hired by Kroll Associates to help the incoming Haitian government recover millions of dollars stolen by Baby Doc and his minions.

Postcoup, I'd spent some time digging into the stolen Duvalier fortune. I'd had a lucky break. In the days after Baby Doc fled (with the help of the Americans, let's not forget), I went to a palatial house Duvalier shared with his pampered wife, Michèle Bennett. It had been ransacked by the jubilant masses. One had to tread carefully between piles of human shit that the people had dropped, purposely, on the floor and remaining furniture and smeared on the walls and mirrors to make it amply clear how they felt about their deposed leader. *Duvalier Kaka!*

In the stripped bedroom, behind a dresser missing its drawers, I'd discovered Michèle's personal address book, chock-full of names and telephone numbers as well as a bank ledger missing some pages, and other personal papers. It was a reporter's gold mine. It led me to other people who'd fled Haiti overnight, high-level officials later accused of grand theft, as well as names I recognized as friends of my relatives in Port-au-Prince. The names were linked to bank accounts in the United States and Switzerland, to paintings hidden in U.S. warehouses, and to boats docked along the Miami river—all potentially assets that could be frozen. For a while I worked with a fellow journalist and Haitiphile, Amy Wilentz, on what became file folders of an enormous pattern of theft. We shared our leads with the incoming Kroll team, trying to confirm what we could. Bruce and I became friends and later, Philippe.

Philippe has had his own field day digging into the story, following Duvalier's posh postcoup life of exile. He now wants to know more about his dragon-lady wife, Michèle. She used to live next to my grandmother in the Bois Verna neighborhood of Port-au-Prince and visit her as a young girl. Haiti is a small island; after a while, everyone knows everyone or it feels that way. That's also why it's hard to keep secrets. It's the land of *teledjol*, the gossip mill. Right now the word on the street is that Baby Doc is bored and broke now that Michèle has finalized a long-sought divorce.

⌒

On the telephone, Philippe gleefully tells me his book is done. In it, he's linked the younger Duvalier to certain mafia figures active in the south. *Ils sont tous des crétins*, he says: they're all morons.

⌒

Philippe appears messy but has an eye for detail. The directions he gives me to his house are precise. He lives on Boulevard Gouvion-Saint-Cyr, not far from the Arc de Triomphe and the Étoile, a rather posh district for a man of modest means. He opens the door looking, as always, like a wild man: slightly unkempt, his mane of white hair combed back to cover the balding spots. He's still in his fifties, I think, and has youthful energy, despite his recent hip replacement that's left him limping. He veers a bit to one side, I notice, like my old Volvo used to.

Allez! he says, grinning, ushering me into a large, sunlit apartment. His work studio is cramped, full of books, stacks of newspapers and documents everywhere, journalistic paperbacks stacked loosely on a shelf beside his computer. *It's in here.* He strikes the machine with enthusiasm. *I'm going to give Duvalier a good kick in the ass!*

Philippe introduces me to Marina, who's Jewish and a militant and appears to be older than he. I like her immediately. She's prepared a delicious lunch for us: couscous, hummus, pita bread. They have a modern marriage, but I notice immediately that Philippe sits while she cooks and serves the meal. I tease him about it right away. *It's true, it's true,* Marina says, laughing. *He's a chauvinist. Tell him, tell him.*

The conversation is all about politics. First Haiti, then Israel and the Middle East, then the French crackdown on Arabs. Marina works in an organization that sounds to me like the French equivalent of B'nai Brith, helping to raise funds for Jewish causes.

She's tough and biased and passionate about the Middle East. Israel, she agrees with me, has become a nation of fascists. She bemoans it. What happened to the left, to the peace movement? She feels for the Palestinians. *They have rights too, don't they? Of course. Absolutely. Israel must make peace!* But Israel is close to her heart. *Will Palestinians share the land, make peace?* she asks us rhetorically. *No, no. I don't believe it.* She's pessimistic. *You are naïve in America,* she says, smiling tolerantly. *Arafat doesn't control those men, those young men who murder and don't care about the Jews.*

We argue back and forth. Philippe pours the wine; Marina declines after a second glass. The two of them make a good pair, I can tell, passionate about ideas and books, highly opinionated, buoyed by a good argument. After an hour, we all agree to disagree.

———⊃

After lunch, Philippe asks, *Now, what's this business about the Seine? What kind of book will it be?*

First I tell him about New York, then about Berlin. The week I was there, a demonstration was taking place because, earlier, neo-Nazi youths had thrown Molotov cocktails into an apartment building filled with new immigrants, gravely injuring a young girl. Cities like Rostock and Chemnitz had become magnets for racist attacks. At night, the violence exploded outside the rave dance clubs that had sprung up on the eastern side of the city, in the dark basements of abandoned buildings and warehouses. Gangs of jobless, bored, angry kids from the East prowling around at night, looking for trouble, or kicks. I saw it everywhere: shaved punks with pale arms tattooed with the Iron Cross and the graffiti everywhere: *Bin Deutsch und Stolz. Arische Nation. Weisse macht. Ausländer Raus! I'm proud to be German. Aryan nation. White Is Might.* Like I've seen here in Paris, inside the metro: *Foreigners Out!*

Attends, Philippe says, trying out his rough English, *I must write*. He comes back, taking notes of what I'm telling him. *Okay, j'écoute. I'm listening.*

———⊃

Philippe takes notes like the stenographer I dream of being, jotting down my trip report in some shorthand I can't make out. I tell him about New York, the protests, what I've been up to since my arrival. About the gay community I've encountered here, the AIDS activist scene, Belle's social circles. How I've met a few lesbians and been turned off by their separatism, their detachment from AIDS as an issue that affects women. How I'm a bit tired of activist meetings in general, tired of narrow identity politics, of the way everyone gets so invested in their own little shadings of gender, how it's all a form of nationalism cloaked in a different wrapper. How it reminds me of the activist schisms I encountered in Haiti. How Paris is the same as New York in that way, people making religion out of their political causes, their gender identity. Using it to exclude as much as to include.

I show him pictures of where I stayed in West Berlin, where the gay neighborhoods struck me as disappointingly bourgeois: a lot of nice little cafés and bookstores, but none of the edginess and creative energy that I found in parts of East Berlin, where, skinheads aside, the social scene was more alternative and mixed and less consumer-oriented. How the gay men I met in Berlin were all into the stupid bodybuilding, designer drug scene that's taken over

New York. How I'm not interested in the gay ghetto mentality, the separation of the sexes, the tendency to fetishize and transform sexual behaviors or body modification into rigid lifestyle and fashion statements. How it becomes so dull so quickly.

Et les filles? Philippe asks, ever the sleuth, reviewing my snapshots. *Les femmes allemandes?* The German women?

I didn't meet that many women in Berlin, I explain. Women my age— midthirties or older—were hard to find, though we tried. They disappeared into couples that don't go out at night; nested. So said one young woman I literally bumped into, dancing till dawn in the huge, pitch-black bowels of a former bank-vault-cum-disco. It was my favorite night of the trip. *The discotheque was surreal,* I tell Philippe. *Straight out of a Kafka novel. You'd have loved it. Everyone is into trance music. Although Michael Jackson is big there.*

Throughout all of this Philippe nods approvingly. He's delighted by my report. He loves to slum, especially mentally. With his bad leg, he can't dance right now. *More pictures,* he demands.

I hand him more. New York, the East Village, the protests with the Irish gay activists from ILGO at the Saint Patrick's Day parade; ACT UP civil disobedience actions in Washington, in front of various drug company headquarters. Pictures from the New York gay pride parade and the big Dyke March in Washington, a historic event. Some twenty thousand women invaded DC, organized by the Lesbian Avengers and women in ACT UP chapters of the West Coast, Philly, and other cities.

He studies the picture: a snapshot of New York Avengers with yellow-lined red capes like superheroines at the DC Dyke March protest. Wielding trash can metal shields painted with suns and the letter *A* like Amazon warriors, using the lids to drum and set a rhythm for the march. The phallic Washington Monument rising behind our group, framing the issue of sexism that is a key reason the group was created. The Avengers, a fun new street action group that some close friends and I in ACT UP and ILGO launched last spring, tired of the gayboy-heavy focus of ACT UP, the lack of lesbian visibility. We love ACT UP. We are ACT UP. But the singular movement focus on AIDS has ignored the health and other needs of the *L* in the LGBT movement. We wanted to change that.

I don't say any of this to Philippe, just add, *It's a new fun group. Like protest street theater but serious. There have been some murders and hate crimes and the media hasn't said much.*

He nods, digesting this. I'm not sure what he's thinking. Again, I feel my inner closet rise up and have to check myself.

He smiles. *You've been busy. Allez, more.*

Together we look at recent snapshots: pictures of Belle, Paris, the river. Then more pictures from the Berlin conference. Punkers with hot-pink Mohawks and metal in their lips and faces. Older skinheads. *Super hardcore*, I say.

⁓

I tell Philippe about my time in East Berlin, about an old friend of mine, Paul Outlaw, who's African American and gay and moved to Berlin from New York in the eighties to escape the racism of the United States. He had warned me. Ever since the wall came down, the energy has changed. He has personally been threatened several times. He can't even walk down the streets of East Berlin at night; he has to take cabs to go out when he's there. The neo-Nazi kids are openly violent: they've caught blacks and cut swastikas into their arms. And the police don't go after them; the police are afraid of them. Paul feels the East Germans are more nationalist and xenophobic than the West.

Philippe has gotten up to get a loupe—a magnifying glass of some kind. He looks like a detective, scanning the Berlin pictures, deciphering the graffiti I've snapped on city walls. I can feel him tucking these details away, ever the crime reporter, the writer, for possible future use.

There are other pictures of Paris on my camera—the neighborhoods around the Gare du Nord, where I walked earlier. I show them to Philippe. We drink some more. I describe my nocturnal wanderings, the new markets I've discovered, and my newfound pleasures, which include dining along the river-bank after midnight. I avoid getting too personal, though, not discussing my romance with Belle or details of the breakup with the Aerialist. But I give Philippe a little update.

I met someone new. Recently.

And the other one? Philippe responds. He's stopped taking notes, pours us a refill instead. *It's all over now?*

Philippe is a supersleuth with a memory for the smallest details. I don't recall ever telling him about the Aerialist, or our troubles, for that matter. But it seems I have. Or that he's managed to fill in the gaps.

Fini. Finished. *I'm still sad.*

Ah, oui, Philippe agrees. *That's divorce.* He pauses. *But you never lived together, did you? I don't remember that. That can make it worse.*

No, I say. *We never lived together.* To myself I think: *Live together? She had trouble agreeing to sleep over the next night, even after months, even after two years.*

And this new one? Is she also beautiful? Philippe adds for Marina, who's joined us. *All of her girlfriends are beautiful. Don't you think?*

Marina smiles. If she's embarrassed, she doesn't show it. She studies the pictures. I hand her a picture of Jersey.

Very pretty, she says. *Is she Jewish?*

Philippe smiles to himself, shaking his head a little.

Defensively Marina adds, *She looks Jewish, or Italian. Italian?*

As a matter of fact, she is Jewish. I laugh. *But she's not a practicing Jew. Secular, cultural. Not religious.*

Marina digests this information silently, still studying the picture. I have no idea what she thinks of me, her husband's younger lesbian friend from America. I wonder if he even has other gay friends; somehow I think not. But I could be wrong.

Very pretty, she says again, smiling, handing back the picture.

⌒

I've never talked with Philippe about being a lesbian or what I sometimes consider myself—bisexual (because the occasional handsome boy or man can turn my head and turn me on a little bit, and when this happens, I always ask myself: *Do or Be? Do I want to* sleep *with him or* look *like him?*). And with Marina hovering close by, I'm a bit uncomfortable. My friendship with Philippe began on a professional basis and has steadily evolved along an axis of shared interests, of lefty politics, of investigative journalism, of Haiti and historical crimes, and an appreciation for government scandal. But it's never gotten to the point of deep confessional. I find it hard to talk about my sexuality simply, without qualifying it. The categories seem too restrictive. I want to change the subject when Philippe prods: *And the other one, who lives here? Are you still friends? What's her name? Still happening?*

I smile. Belle.

She's fine, I say. *But you know—it's complicated; the distance. I do love her a lot, though.*

Philippe turns to Marina. *She's in love with someone here. Do you see how complicated her romantic life is? Very complicated. C'est la jeunesse. That's youth.*

Marina smiles at me.

Catholic, I inform her, anticipating the question about Belle. *But not practicing either.*

Unless AIDS activism can be considered a religion, I think to myself. *It does demand a steady practice of faith.*

Ah, she nods, then shrugs, as if to say, *Well, she's not Jewish but we won't hold that against her, will we?*

You're happy. Philippe laughs, summing up my predicament. *That's good. Let's have a toast.* He raises his glass. *Welcome. We're glad to see you.* We clink glasses. *À l'amour.* He adds, switching to English, *To love.*

To your book, I add. *All success.*

⌒

Philippe drinks more than I do, and faster, which is impressive because I can put wine away when I'm in the mood. We're on a second bottle. *I've had insomnia, I tell him a while later when he and I are alone again. So I started walking. That's how it started.*

I explain to him how I've been taking long walks along the river, all night, from dusk to dawn. *You know how it is—when you're not ready to write yet but your mind is talking to you, and you can hardly keep up.*

Of course, he says. *The beginning is always the hard part. We enter into the forest and then we get lost, right? We writers. We have to find our path to get out. That's why I tend to stick to journalism. So much easier.*

I tell him about the research I've started doing about the Seine and its history. How I want to know strange things like how many people have killed themselves jumping in, odd facts like that. How I need to get into the historical archives. Some of them are restricted. You have to be an academic or somehow secure permission. I'm not even sure what I'm looking for yet, I tell him. And I don't have that much time. *Can you help me?*

Philippe looks up from his notepad, eager as a child, challenged by the prospect of digging up hard-to-find information. Not to worry. He refills his own glass. *I have a contact at the historical library. I'll call her for you. She'll know where the books are likely to be. How far back do you want to go? The eighteenth century? The twelfth? Any particular period? It doesn't matter: my friend will know.*

Philippe loves to tell stories. He doesn't like simple ones, prefers elaborate tales. He launches into a long one about how he met the historical archives librarian, who once lived in Haiti. He wonders if we might have crossed paths, been there at the same time. She'll want to meet you, he concludes. *So you see how it can't be just a coincidence.* His eyes twinkle as he says this. *You were meant to do this book.*

Marina steps in a bit later with coffee and dessert. We take it into the living room. I listen to them talk about their vacation plans, about Philippe's recent operation, which has left him walking with a cane (an improvement over his crutches). In another six months he'll be walking without it.

Marina is gracious, a smart, serious woman. *I have an early meeting tomorrow,* she says, taking her leave of us before we've finished the coffee, *but don't be a stranger. Come back. Whenever you want. But wait—take some pastry with you.*

She disappears into the kitchen again. Philippe slips away too, back into his office-den to look for something. I watch through a doorway as he rummages through his papers. I get up to check out the view from the window. In the kitchen, Marina is wrapping the pastry. I look in. She smiles at me, the tolerant smile of a wife who knows her husband is a little too much sometimes. Through a wall now, Philippe is telling me about Chirac, who, he says, is billed as a conservative but whom he personally considers a fascist. Marina is nodding at this.

A kind of fascist, Philippe clarifies, his voice rising, *not like Le Pen. But the same instincts, you understand. Un salaud. A bastard.*

We've been communicating a little about Le Pen and the shifting politics in France. I'm aware of right-wing leaders' recent attacks on gays, an assault on some black students in the south. How some ACT UP boys scuffled with a group of skinheads putting up Le Pen posters in the Marais. About Ras l'Front, an antiracist group that's organizing against Le Pen's party. I hope to visit their offices if time permits.

Philippe returns at last, holding some scattered clippings about the National Front and its recent legislative victories in the south. *Look at how much press he's getting now from the big papers,* Philippe says, *even if it's mostly negative. He's very dangerous.*

I hear Marina echo from the kitchen, *C'est vrai—dangereux et fou!*

Le Pen's main strength is still in the south, Philippe adds, *but it's expanding in the north, in Alsace-Lorraine, near Germany. It's due to the lousy economy, but he's taking advantage of it. And the Socialists, what are they doing? Those in charge are idiots.* Philippe is in his glory, scanning each clipping with a nod before giving it to me. *They've decided to launch an austerity program.* His voice is sarcastic, disgusted. *Once it fails, Le Pen will be even stronger.*

Philippe has been a student of French politics for over thirty years. He still considers himself a Communist, and he's angry about the failure of the Left, of Socialists, of Socialism, of the once-strong French Communist party, but he won't give up.

If we resign ourselves, we're screwed, he says, adding, *foutu. Foutu, foutu. How do you say it in English?*

Ruined.

Ruiné. Philippe nods, grimacing. *C'est justement ça. That's it. We're giving Le Pen every advantage with such stupid policies.*

⌒

We're finishing our coffee. Philippe is distracted. He couldn't find a news clipping he also wanted to show me. *Do you know about Chirac and his big plan to clean up the Seine? He's crazy, you know. Chirac held a ceremony where he threw some fish into the river and promised it would be as clean as Perrier by the year 2000. It was a great publicity stunt. Idiotic, but original. I'll find it for you. Give me your fax number here. You don't have one? Well, I'll bring it by. We'll have a drink together, next week. D'accord?*

The wrapped pastries are still warm. Marina embraces me with four kisses, not three, when I finally leave. I've promised Philippe I'll ask my exiled Haitian friends living here for fresh details about the whereabouts and latest activities of the Duvalierists. Tell them about his book. He wants to meet them.

⌣

On the way back, riding the metro, I think about Mayor Chirac. He sounds like a Reagan technocrat with his PR campaign to purify the Seine. I look around the subway car, wondering who supports it. Probably everybody. Who doesn't want to swim in the river?

What about Le Pen? I'm worried about what Philippe's told me. I think about what I've recently witnessed in Berlin—the rise of xenophobia there and all over Eastern Europe, of protofascism, of former Yugoslavia, again coming apart at the seams. What I also found in the hippie capital, Prague. The new mecca of European youth. Another place luring disaffected teenagers drawn to the growing death-metal music scene. *All the angry young men*, I think.

I'm so distracted I miss my subway stop and am forced to walk an extra ten blocks to Belle's apartment. On a corner, I stop to buy a small notepad and scribble as I walk, pausing often, taking notes. My brain is hot, my thoughts flying. My hands are damp with sweat, smearing my words. I have to stop, focus.

I read my own words back: *Sel hears about Chirac's campaign to clean the Seine. She decides it's a metaphor for fascism. She'll embody impurity. She'll celebrate all that is impure about France, all that's rotten. She and her clan will be the scum of Paris. They'll wage war on the mayor and his minions. Their weapon is their filth.* But how to avoid the wrong analogy with AIDS? How to avoid falling into the right-wing stereotype of AIDS carriers, of sex, as criminal? Must figure out.

I'm concentrating so intently that I arrive back at the apartment with a migraine. I immediately ask Belle, *Did you know Chirac wants to clean the Seine? To make it as pure as Perrier water? That's what Philippe told me.*

No, she didn't know, but it doesn't surprise her. *C'est un cochon*, she says of Chirac. She murmurs this as she embraces me, slipping her hands under my shirt. Her palms are cold against my skin; I walked so fast that I'm sweating and I've got a headache. *I think I drank too much*, I continue as she hands me a glass of water and pushes me onto the sofa. Her breath is hot in my ear; she's licking it and talking to me. *Le Pen's got it in for everyone*, she says. *The homeless, the drug addicts, the prostitutes, the elderly on social security, the workers. He's an asshole. Vraiment.*

I can't swallow the aspirin; I don't like bubbly water. I'm the only American I know who prefers E. coli in tap water to Perrier. Instead, Belle gives me a drag of her cigarette and a shoulder rub, lifting my shirt off completely. *Tell me about your visit. But kiss me first.*

~ 6

Belle and I love each other like an old couple: two people soothed merely by the presence of each other. We lie together quietly. I'm wine sleepy. She's pulled closed the curtains, put on a blues record—Nina Simone—and lights her umpteenth cigarette. The room is dim. I can feel her smiling. *I love you*, she's telling me silently.

Sel and the Seine and Chirac are banished from my mind. Belle and I lie together, immobile. She eventually falls asleep. I look at her face. She's like a Modigliani: heart-shaped face; long, pale, voluptuous torso; hands folded over full breasts; full hips; strong legs. I study her, wishing my silent thoughts could penetrate her dreams.

Je t'aime aussi. Bien que tu ne veux pas venir vivre avec moi à New York. I love you, too. Even if you won't come and stay with me in New York.

Why won't you come? I move closer to her face, trying not to wake her. *Share my life, even for a little while? Why, really? What is it? You don't want this, right? I'm tired of only seeing you for two weeks at a time. I want more. Maybe I only want it because it's not possible. But that's how I feel about you, deep down, cross my heart. That's how I could love you, if you wanted it, if you let me in. That's how easy it can be with you, sometimes. So simple. So close to my soul.*

I can't sleep. There's a tape in my head. I'll wake her if I keep moving around. I get up. In my suitcase is a journal I've been keeping since we met in Amsterdam. I pick it up and open to a random entry, then another, searching them for a message. *Was I feeling this way a while back, months ago? I was, wasn't I?*

I read it. *Meeting Belle is a gift. Accompanied at once by some knowledge that she can't give to me in certain ways, can't care for me in certain ways that I might have wanted, that I still want if I'm true to myself. Does this knowledge of what can't be create the feeling of a loss? Or does the fulfillment of a part of my romantic ideal invite the need for more?*

I hate journals, I think. *Dreck.*

⁓

I flip off the lights and sit in darkness. Belle is lightly snoring. *Will she visit me in New York? Only if she gets some money*, I think. But I know money isn't the reason. *Maybe she isn't really gay.* I feel ashamed by the thought. But it persists. *What if it's true? Or if she's bi? So what? She's crazy about you, but she doesn't want to come to New York. I don't see you moving here either. Of course, she hasn't asked you to. But would you?*

Would I? I don't know. *I think I'd try.*

I look outside. This is the twelfth arrondissement, a residential district of large, undistinguished apartment buildings, broad avenues. Past midnight, the boulevard is fairly deserted, and it feels less like Paris than some American city, where neighbors don't know each other. The apartment belongs to Belle's parents, who are away in Australia for a few months. The apartment is modern, with Scandinavian-style furniture and bright colors. We're imposters, living in someone else's house. Children playing adults. This is a boring neighborhood, I think now. Too quiet at night. Nowhere to go if I wanted to, right now, for a consolation cocktail. For a chat with a stranger at the bar, to swap life stories. That's what I like about New York. Twenty-four-hour New York.

How long can it go on this way? A few days here and there? I'm asking the bartender in the window, my dim reflection. *It's been so good, without any great complications, any demands. Is it good because we live on separate continents? Probably. Right?*

Go to bed, I tell myself. *Stop this silliness.*

⁓

Back in bed, I can't help it, I replay the tape: her life is in Paris, mine is in New York. We aren't moving to live with each other. She knows that I've met some-one new—Jersey—and that I want a serious relationship. With her, but if not her, with someone else. She knows that things with Jersey are heating up.

She also knows I'm still grieving the Aerialist. She's told me, frankly and from the start, that she's no good in relationships; that she's inconsistent, gets smothered easily. That she has a habit of disappearing—that's how her past lovers viewed it, anyway. She doesn't like to disappoint people and she needs her freedom. And we live an ocean apart. Of course we can have other lovers. *Just keep a little left over for me.* That's been her response whenever I've broached the subject of our future.

So where does that leave me? She loves me, but. *But, but, but . . . I want more. I want to be with her for more than two weeks.*

I look over at her figure, shrouded in sleep. I want her to wake up, to console me, to talk. I'm hungry. I want something from that great little food stand in the Marais. A croque monsieur. Or some *frites*. Nothing's open now in this neighborhood. *Merde.*

The sun will rise soon. Sleep, I think. Try. Just try.

⁓

What time is it? Early still? Outside the window is a familiar panorama of gray-beige rooftops. The sky is the color of a pigeon's feather, a dirty-gray water-color wash. It looks like it will rain. Thinking of everything I have to do makes me tired. But sleep is elusive. I slip quietly out of bed, sit on the floor while Belle sleeps, turn on the computer. After a while Belle stirs, then gets up to smoke a cigarette. She gives me that look. The invitation is in her eyes. *Come back to bed!*

When I wake again it's noon and a fresh cup of coffee is being handed to me. Aldyn is couch surfing, playing houseboy to his favorite lesbians. He prances about in his briefs, then jumps in between us in the bed. *Let me tell you about a dream I had,* he says. *I was having sex with this incredible-looking boy.*

Are you sure it was a dream? Belle teases him.

Uhh, wait, let me close my eyes. You're right, he adds, eyes shut tight. *It was all too real.*

Was the boy's name . . . by any chance . . . Luc? I ask.

Luc . . . who? Aldyn looks around innocently. *Oh, that Luc. Well, maybe. I couldn't tell.*

Raconte, Belle orders. *Tell. Spare us no details.*

~ 7

I've only planned a short visit and can't extend my ticket. There's not much time to do my research. I review my short list: the historical library, the National Archives, a guided tour of the Hôtel de Ville, the Catacombs, the sewers, the police museum, perhaps one of the big cruising parks at night if we can borrow someone's car. I want to go to the Mosque to drink mint tea, a must when I'm in Paris. Belle tells me there is an AIDS demonstration this week, and an ACT UP meeting. Friends have invited us for dinner, for drinks. She wants to introduce me around. And before I get back to New York, I hope to complete a draft of my article on Berlin for *Out.* A look at gay life in the postreunification nation.

The museums of Paris are still on summertime hours, as are many of the public institutions. The tour of the Hôtel de Ville takes place on Friday; so does the tour of the sewers. I've seen the Catacombs before, but I want to revisit them, through Sel's eyes. To see if I run into the drug gangs that have set up shop in their unused arteries. That's where the new shooting galleries are, according to one of Belle's friends. But first I have to see the river. Get my daily fix.

Belle accompanies me. We ride the subway to the stop at the square of the Hôtel de Ville and walk down to where the houseboats are docked. She tells me it's the most expensive real estate in Paris; there's a huge waiting list to rent a slip. You have to have connections.

It's not going to rain. It's the Paris of my childhood memory, damp, with brazen pigeons searching for crumbs at your feet. The air is salty. I can't understand how this can be, since the sea is so far away.

Would you live with me on a houseboat? I ask her. *It's my dream.*

Okay, she grins, without missing a beat. *But only if we get married.*

Oh, break my heart, will you? I chase her down the street. *If I catch you,* I scream after her, *I'll throw you in the river.*

Catch me, she yells.

Finally! I've caught her. I'm kissing her, openly, hungrily. I'm dancing a little, I'm stroking her face, and she's laughing at this sudden demonstration of passion, at the covert, curious glances of passersby. She loves being out in Paris, she loves this about being with me; she likes holding hands and making out for everyone to see. That's what she says to the men who linger for too long. *Oui, c'est jolie les lesbiennes, n'est-ce pas?* Yes, lesbians are pretty. *Maintenant, va-t'en! Foutez-nous la paix!* Go on! Leave us alone!

The Bibliothèque Historique de la Ville de Paris is a dream library, located back from the street, behind an inner courtyard. I present my passport to a gentleman sitting at a small desk by the entrance and receive a slip of paper to fill out: a daily pass. The library is very quiet—all seriousness—but it is busy. Through a large set of doors, I see a study room lined with desks and chairs, a reading lamp before each seat, and, to one side, large windows looking onto gardens. It's a civilized library, one that might have belonged to a king, or, more likely, to the royal historian, the king's personal scribe. Many of the seats are filled. I'm in the main room, accessible to the public; here are the file drawers with the call numbers and subjects. On a floor above them are the stacks, where the precious material is carefully guarded. I ask for Philippe's friend, who, luckily, is in. She's the *jefe*—the senior librarian.

She's also expecting me. Philippe, supersleuth, has tipped her off. She isn't sure exactly what I'm looking for—nor am I, of course—but she's at my disposal. She's a young woman, pretty and energetic; late thirties or early forties, and she's curious about me. Philippe has told her I'm a journalist, that I have Haitian roots. She too lived in Haiti for a few years. When she smiles, she screws up her face as if she's about to cry. I like her.

We talk about Port-au-Prince, about the political situation there now. It turns out she lived one street away from my grandmother's house on Rue Duncombe. The street bears my grandmother's family name: Duncombe, after Lord Duncombe in England. More dubious royalist roots. She wants to know more about my Haitian family background, but my time is short. Another day, we agree.

Life is funny, isn't it? she muses, pulling me into a quieter corner, away from the ears of the rest of the staff, her juniors, who are, I see, discreetly eyeing us. *We have a limit on the books you can take out*, she whispers. *But bring the cards to me. I'll give you whatever you want.*

Scratch a French bureaucrat and you'll find a latent revolutionary, one with a secret maternal fondness for the wild-at-heart, the anarchist. After a bit more small talk, she checks her watch. *You have a lot to do and there isn't that much time. Why don't you get started?* She points out the photography books about the city, and the books about the Hôtel de Ville, walking briskly past rows of lateral file drawers. They can't be taken into the reading room; they must remain over here. Here are all the call numbers, arranged by author, subject, title.

I don't know where to begin. *Anywhere*, I think. There's enough material here to write a hundred books on the Seine, and at least that many touch on the famous Hôtel de Ville, which is cross-referenced with Place de Grève—the square where workmen used to hold their strikes. Some of the entries are written in pencil, in a handwriting that resembles my father's, long flourishes on the *f*'s and *g*'s and *k*'s, and crossed European *7*'s. These are followed by the date of the document or period in question.

Despite what she's quickly explained to me about the system, I have trouble figuring it out. What's *réserver*, what's on *microfiche*, what's a rare document locked behind the grill of the stacks and, I assume, encased in some airtight box to prevent its deterioration. I'm also confused about how to fill in my request. This isn't the alphabetized Dewey decimal system but some vestige of Napoleonism; treasures pillaged from foreign lands that have found their way here into the hands of some discerning archivist with no intention of revealing his precious secrets to a bumbling layperson like me. I glance at my watch: only three hours till closing time. I'll never be able to read half these books. I glance at the Xerox machine; it's being used. *Merde!*

⌐

I politely ask for Philippe's friend again. She comes down the staircase from the stacks and takes my cards, then disappears. I'm all innocence. I have asked for twelve books and two rare manuscripts, a highly illegal request. I'm elated. I should have been a librarian, I think. I love the smell of old books.

While I wait, I peruse old pictures and artists' prints. This is the Paris where Sel would have fit in: a putrid place, overcrowded with peasants from the provinces hawking cheese, fish, vegetables, pigs. I look at the early drawings of the Île de la Cité: the fourteenth-century bridges, the Place de Grève—long the civic center of the city, the place where the poor and unemployed came looking for jobs and to protest the lack thereof. There are finely detailed sketches of parties, famous balls, foreign kings arriving by boat to be greeted by crowds bearing fruits. Here, the bridges of Paris are streets unto themselves, built several stories high. Every bridge houses a different market: wheat, livestock, timber, grapes from Champagne.

The Seine is a giant slug, a stagnant lake, a breeding ground of filth and disease. Mayor Chirac is right. There are fires and revolutions, plagues, skirmishes. Syphilis flourishes, *le mal francoso*.

I feel so happy. Libraries restore my soul.

⁓

I jump forward in history to the fin de siècle. Paris is the center of progress, of invention, of sophistication and fashion. Artists, scientists, diplomats, courtesans. I study the wide-angle photographs of the 1867 International Exposition. There are elephants, exotic animals brought by ship from India, Brazil, the Arctic. The pasha and the harem titillate French sensibilities.

Paris, the Glamour Years. A heavy coffee-table book. I look at pictures of the city during wartime, up to the German Occupation. An idyllic place. The café society, graced by the towering elegance of the Eiffel Tower, lit in 1925 with neon letters advertising Citroën, a precursor of modern advertising. The streets are all narrow and cobbled; the nightlife is fantastic: cabarets; circuses; dancing; men with long, waxed moustaches and capes. I admire the bustles and corsets, the Russian soldiers wearing high ostrich-plumed hats, the skinny artists painting the portraits of the rich at the Place du Tertre in Montmartre in exchange for bread.

I recognize the most famous names—writers and artists, a few photographers and entertainers: Jean-Paul Sartre, Simone de Beauvoir, Dolly Wilde, Gertrude Stein, Sylvia Beach, Romaine Brooks, Isadora Duncan, the photographer Nadar, André Gide, Albert Camus, Josephine Baker.

I pick up another picture book. Here is the classic photograph by Robert Doisneau, *The Kiss of the Hôtel de Ville*, capturing two lovers in a spontaneous embrace. It's become an emblem of romance in a liberated France. Only later would we learn it was staged; actors were employed by the photographer. Like battles and victories often are, history can be staged. Hitler, a showman politician, certainly knew that.

⁓

I look at the Seine, the backdrop of so many scenes, painted and photographed from so many angles, through so many delighted eyes. I've barely scratched the surface of my subject and already I'm overwhelmed. Maybe I'm just hearing voices, like any other crazy person who's recovering from a hard relationship. *Do all writers feel a bit mad at a certain point? Probably. Or it's just as Philippe said, I'm entering the dark forest.*

As I watch his friend arrive with a stack of long, skinny volumes, I begin mentally scaling back my ambition. I have to be a more selective reader. I'll focus on the river and the Hôtel de Ville; anything else I get to will be a bonus.

As it turns out, the petty criminals of Paris have helped me. Several books I requested are missing. *An increasing problem*, says Philippe's friend, who keeps my cards to note the theft or loss.

I tend to admire the criminal spirit, maybe because I'm afraid of the law and I am, for all my protests, the product of a Catholic upbringing, however remiss. But I draw the line at stealing books. Especially rare ones. For a minute, mentally, I become a despot. Cut off their hands, I think. The first phalanx of the little finger. *We must protect the libraries!*

I skim through books. Esoteric titles such as *Sewers: Notes on the Cleaning of the Sewer Waters by Aluminum Sulfate, Application by the City of Paris, June 1870*. And Maxime du Camp's six-volume *Paris, Her Organs and Functions, XIX Century*. I'm disappointed about the dense du Camp book. I recognize his name as a premier gossip who penned dishy diaries about the goings on of the royal court. Nor will I be able to get a look at the missing first-person recollections of the Great Sanson, the famous Butcher of Paris, a fourth-generation member of a seven-generation house of royal executioners. He was also known as Monsieur de Paris—Gentleman of Paris.

⁓

I'm speed-reading at a feverish pace, the way I learned to in fifth grade, reading down the middle of a page of text, hoping my mind will catch the details on the side. In an hour, my notepad is a wonder of shorthand notes but nothing as neat as Philippe's. Since I have an atrocious short-term memory, I wonder if any of it will mean anything to me later.

Lutetia. Conquered by the Romans. Nickname: City of Mud. Governing philosophy: *Tout à la rue*. Everything in the street.

I lift my head to glance around me. What are these other Parisians reading, writing, debating? In France, in Europe, there is still a tradition of studying, a respect for and enjoyment of books. Less so in America. The book is becoming a dinosaur, and I, a writer, am one of a dying breed. I have to push such thoughts out of my head. I am at the beginning of a great journey, an intellectual, creative adventure.

Right.

And I have a wild guide: Sel. One who knows that the municipal authorities in Paris used to gather animal and human feces and store them for making saltpeter, a grisly fact that fascinates me. Human guano—*poudrette* in French—produced by the open fermentation of fecal matter. The name of the city dump, a slaughterhouse with high gibbets, was Montfaucon. With what strikes me as endless creativity (however morbid), one Jean-Pierre-Joseph d'Arcet discovered that its cesspool contents could be carbonized and used as a deodorant. I pick up a new term: *méphilisme*—death from gases of decay. This condition affected sewer workers, who developed pulmonary problems from *le gaz méphitique.*

⌒

Montfaucon. It hasn't appeared in any of the guidebooks or city tours I've come across. I'm fascinated, determined to learn more about this gallows-cum-deodorant factory. Something, some writer's instinct, tells me Montfaucon could play a role in Sel's story. I've put my trust in a sly creature who, I now see, is going to make me work. Did Sel once live at Montfaucon? Were her relatives hung there, their bones drying on a wooden gibbet to mix with the soil that was then cut into squares to dry the armpits and perfume the thighs of royal ladies? I jot down the ideas. *A family tree of the hanged, drawn, and quartered.* I like that last image.

⌒

Closing time. Paris is so civilized. I can leave my unread books on a special reserve shelf and read them tomorrow.

Paris is an ammoniapolis, an armpit of humanity. The Seine is an evolutionary cordon of sweat, urine, feces, bone. A chamber pot of once-royal piss. A *pisiculture*; a great fermenting soup of ideas and crossed purposes and dark deeds. A beautiful city built of shit.

~ 8

Four o'clock in the afternoon. I take the subway and rise up above the street, enjoying the moment when the slate-gray rooftops appear, and the tall, narrow apartment doorways; the signs for the local boulangerie. Paris aboveground offers new views; an interesting tangle of streets that suddenly reveal a familiar corner. I'm running late again, and I've lost the piece of paper upon which I marked the address of the demonstration. I only know the station. I'm walking close to where I lived at the age of thirteen, during the loneliest period of my life.

This is the administrative part of the city, a district I associate with sharp-beaked shopkeepers who eyed me suspiciously back then—my boyish clothes, my foreignness, my teenage American habit of jogging along the great manicured lawn of the Esplanade des Invalides, from one end to another, starting from the Gare des Invalides, the train station where I plotted for months about how to reboard the Air France shuttle bus bound for Orly airport and back to the United States.

Back then, I felt alienated and alone within the rigid French family in which I'd been placed for the school year. In their eyes, I was infecting Paris, a heathen diplomat from the United States, a rotten wasteful culture. A badly dressed *garçonette* with poor eating habits and a hideous written French grammar who was sure to corrupt their children with the Rolling Stones and a taste for sweets. *Chocolate truffles? Oui, s'il vous plaît. Yum.* The mother of the house disliked me as much as I grew to dislike her. She was plain ole mean, or, as my mother later admitted, in her inimitable French accent, *a real beeetch.*

I move at a clip, past the neat row of plane trees, leafless and forlorn in winter, and past Napoleon's tomb.

Who was Napoleon? A short man, rude, a Corsican bully who probably had a small dick, the source of his macho inferiority complex. That's what I used to think, jogging so long ago on my lonely Sundays, wondering about the state of the skeleton inside—if it really existed or if the tomb was empty.

Looking around, I note the changes. The area looks more modern, less, well, French. Paris in the nineties is a slick piece of technology. Glass everywhere. But stylish, I have to admit. Ultramodernity.

I study the giant wall advertisements like those that arch above the subway tracks. Huge, bronzed young women with glistening thighs and arms still boast the benefits of using any number of beauty products to smooth, moisturize, or massage the skin. The French are aesthetes and hypochondriacs; having failed to wash for centuries, now they minister to their bodies with slavish attention. In the historical library I learned about the French penchant for Victorian glass ampoules, for dissolving aspirin, for any product that reflects a scientific, clinical approach to healing. Above my head looms a giant natural sponge; the copy reads like a botanical text.

Rien n'a changé là, I hear her say. Nothing's changed there.

Sel! She's back, reading over my shoulder.

Purification: it's a national, cultural pastime, she adds. *Look how many times it appears in that advertisement. Six. They can never get enough of it.*

⌒

Outside the metro, I'm lost in the streets, never an unpleasant activity. Finally, I'm the one who's spotted. Belle shouts to me from a café doorway. Before any ACT UP action, the group meets at a café to plan strategy and finesse details; afterward, they retire to another café to discuss how it went. I like the French method of protest. *Caffeinated direct action.* But nothing too rushed.

There are familiar faces from a previous AIDS conference, and they're grinning at me. I realize Belle and I have become a gossip item. They know things about me and I wonder what they are, what they know about our affair, the state of our romance. The world is small; the world of AIDS activism even smaller. *All roads once led to Rome*—I smile back at my new friends—*now they lead to ACT UP.*

I'm not planning on getting arrested today. It's a picket action; I don't think CD—civil disobedience—is on the menu. But things can happen at these protests. I'm not ready for that now. I've had my fill of sit-ins in recent months and I'm on a work vacation this trip. Of course it could happen; it's happened before when I only planned to cover an action as a reporter. I'm not sure how the French judges treat a CD action. So far, with the help of ACT UP's lawyers, I've been able to clear the myriad protest misdemeanors off my record. I've never spent long in jail. I continue to pass as a model citizen, at least on paper.

Waiting for the picket to start, I recall the Stop the Church demonstration. December 1989. It took place at Saint Patrick's Cathedral in New York, organized by ACT UP and WHAM, Women's Health Action Mobilization, a feminist group. A good example of when I couldn't sit quietly, literally; it was too damn cold. *How could that be almost three years ago? Feels like yesterday.* Five thousand of us showed up to protest the Catholic Church's opposition to AIDS education in New York public schools. We were targeting Cardinal John O'Connor, a true homophobe who'd repeatedly blocked LGBT groups from participating in the annual Saint Patrick's Day parade. He's been a nightmare in this epidemic.

That day I hadn't fully committed to civil disobedience, which had been planned for months. There were dozens of affinity groups who planned to block Fifth Avenue—the nightmare scenario of urban cabbies. It was after Thanksgiving and before Christmas and I remember I had a lot of work. Maybe writing for *OutWeek*? Can't recall. Life's a blur. I know I hadn't committed myself to any affinity group but was keeping track of my friends in the Marys. My plan was to watch them do their bit, maybe slip into the church, see how O'Connor responded. He'd declared ACT UP a moral enemy. Worse, the antiabortion group Operation Rescue was coming to support the cardinal.

When I got there, I learned that O'Connor had secured a restraining order barring the action. *Great.* He'd raised the stakes. The first of the affinity groups was already blocking the avenue, and more were waiting, planning to block it in waves. ACT UP's Ray Navarro, who was getting sicker already then, was dressed up as Jesus. He was acting as a host and commentator for DIVA TV, doing interviews with activists and the crowd. Ray really looked a lot like Christ. I say *looked* because he died a year later, just after our Day of Desperation action if memory serves me.

At Stop the Church I ran into Robert Hilferty, a filmmaker friend, theater buff, and arts journalist. He was really excited by Ray's outfit. *The drama, the drama,* he'd say about our actions, loving it all. He was filming for a documentary he's made about the protest. *Are you getting arrested, Anne?* he teased me. *You know you will. Watch out. Those Catholics girls bite.*

It was so bitterly cold; the church was a little warmer inside. I slipped into a pew midway down the aisle before the sermon and communion. Word was some ACT UPers had planned a holy wafer action of some kind. So I waited as O'Connor began to preach. Then realized, with disbelief, that he just planned to ignore the whole thing. *Ignore ACT UP? Ignore the thousands massed outside and the TV cameras, as if one could? The gall,* I thought. *This man really couldn't give a shit! He's fine to see gay men die.* I looked around for ACT UP, straining to see who was going to speak out, stand up to him, to the leader of New York's Catholics who refused to give clean needles to drug addicts with AIDS. I wondered if those who'd planned to do CD inside the church were already arrested, maybe in an earlier service. *Where was everyone? Where was ACT UP?* I saw a few familiar faces. Everyone was quiet.

My heart was pounding. That much I remember. There was that moment of truth when I realized I might have to drop my reporter's role. As much as I disliked getting arrested and never looked forward to getting locked up, staying silent was no longer an option. At the same time I felt bad for my neighbors in the pew. After all, they'd probably just come into the church to pray, though some were tourists. I felt them freeze when I finally stood up. They all looked straight ahead, refusing to meet my eye, following the cardinal's example. I hadn't rehearsed what I'd say, but there I was, without a bullhorn but projecting. Loudly enough, I hoped, to make O'Connor hear me.

ACT UP is here. We're here. You can't ignore AIDS. The whole world is watching!

Behind me, to the left, near the back, I heard other protesters chanting too. *The church needs to support sound prevention programs including condoms and needle exchange. You need to stop demonizing people with AIDS. Educate, don't discriminate!*

ACT UP was there, after all. I was ACT UP too, wasn't I? I'd stopped being a reporter, once again. There were only a few of us but we were loud. The people in the church were shocked, captured by the drama. *Sit down!* O'Connor thundered. *ACT UP!* We thundered back. *Fight AIDS!*

It took the security guards quite a few minutes to reach us. Some dodged the security guards rushing in, the police. I opted for a dignified exit, sort of. I didn't sit down and get dragged down the aisle as some did. I was forcefully escorted out of the cathedral. In no time, my hands were cuffed, the plastic cutting off circulation. But I felt exuberant, justified. O'Connor's policies *were* wrong; the church *was* on the wrong side of this battle. I still felt bad for the churchgoers, but, I rationalized, at least they'd gotten to witness an important event, a historic event, and to hear our demands.

And some had listened. Exiting the church, I heard the swell of people shouting, wolf-whistling, clapping. Not only the ACT UP crowd, but ordinary passersby, cheering.

In the end, it had all been worth it.

⌐

Today ACT UP–Paris is protesting a blood scandal and demanding the resignation of top officials at the Centre National de Transfusion Sanguine. They're accused of knowingly distributing blood products contaminated with HIV to thousands of hemophiliacs in 1984 and 1985. French officials wanted to develop their own blood screening test back then and avoided buying one manufactured in the United States—a deadly delay.

It's still not clear how many people are affected; between 4,000 and 4,400 hemophiliacs were given the transfusions and a growing number have died of AIDS or are ill now. Their families seek justice, as well as compensation for their losses. And a public apology. They want the public officials put in jail.

AIDS is a drama of egos and greed and, in this case it seems pretty clear, criminal negligence. Socialist Prime Minister Laurent Fabius is complicit in this affair; so is Health Minister Edmond Hervé and Social Affairs Minister Georgina Dufoix. A number of lower-ranking officials at the national center and the health ministry are too. It's been all about money, bottom line, not public health.

I assume some of them are inside the ministry building where we're protesting, possibly cowering in their offices. Or looking down at us, wondering how they'll make their getaway.

⌐

Before the action starts, I listen to the proposed chants. Street protests are hardly new in France, but rhymed slogans are never easy and, here, they sound off. The language doesn't work, somehow. It's a similar problem with French rock and roll and, now, rap. ACT UP. FIGHT BACK. FIGHT AIDS! That's easy enough. *The government has blood on its hands?* I offer suggestions for rhymes, but I'm not a poet. *L'état fait couler notre sang?* The state spills our blood? The chants are awkward.

___

I take my place in the picket line, holding up a familiar sign: a visual haiku— bloody hands on one side of the poster, a coffin on the other. How many times have I held signs identical to this one? I've totally lost count. *Berlin . . . Amsterdam . . . City Hall and Grand Central Station in New York . . . the White House in Washington . . . Kennebunkport, Maine, where we protested against George Bush at his summer home last year . . . that was a fun action . . . Wall Street . . . the CDC . . . the NIH in Bethesda . . . the INS in lower Manhattan. And all the Avenger actions. Saint Pat's parade every year. . . .*

Et voilà, here we go again.

___

It's a short demonstration after all. The sky is blue, the day warm. Some of the staff from the health ministry step outside to watch. They're amiable and supportive, it turns out. There are no cordons of policemen and the car drivers that pass are a bit stupefied but not hostile. Instead of honking horns as they do in New York, people get out of their cars, then get back in. AIDS activism is still new enough in France at this point to warrant polite curiosity and even some nationalistic pride—*Shades of '68! To the barracks, to the picket lines. Vive la France!*

The patrons of a nearby bar are gathered in the doorway. Several, I find out later, are stone drunk. When we join them in the bar, the regulars nod to us somberly. *Une sale affaire,* one mutters. A dirty affair. The government is wrong on this one; someone will have to pay. The minister will be forced to resign; you'll see. They say it to themselves. They're all men, a half dozen nursing beers, green Pernod, and other vile-looking drinks in tall glasses. They stare at us, women and men with shaved heads and leather pants, drag queens in tight frilly dresses who daintily remove latex gloves dipped in red paint up to the knuckles. The younger generation, unashamed and happy to shock. Like AIDS activism, a novelty; a bit of afternoon entertainment. The barflies say nothing, a bit estranged but bemused. *À la votre,* one of them lifts his glass. *Allez, allez.*

___

I'm thinking about blood again, tainted blood. Johnny's blood, poxed with HIV, diabetic and full of cancer drugs now too. My mother's blood, shot through with infection, her marrow radiated before she died of breast-turned-liver cancer, her bilious liver swollen to twice its normal size and hard as a lemon under her skin. My older sister's blood, pumping through brain cells, running along scrambled neural circuits, leading to dead ends—repeats of memory and speech. My own blood, newly fish-poxed.

I think about the victims whose names are on some of the posters here. What a crime the agents of the state carried out, knowing their decision spelled a game of Russian roulette, knowing the chances were good that someone would be given some contaminated blood. Is it power that let them detach from their decisions, feel they didn't hold the gun, put it to the head of a vulnerable patient, spin the gun's chamber, even pull back the trigger? Is it any less a murder in their eyes if it happens a decade later, when they've moved on to other jobs, up the echelons of power? I'd like to ask Messieurs Hervé and Fabius to comment, *s'il vous plaît.*

Sel has something to say about this. I imagine her for an instant, leading a battalion of hemophiliacs, a regiment of schoolchildren, to battle with the state. Not with a genteel picket like this one in front of the ministry, but like Joan of Arc, the hero of every French child. As an obsessed general waging unholy war. Sel gathers up the French hemophiliacs who haven't died yet but sense death is near. She urges them to mobilize, to recognize their newfound power to infect the rosy-cheeked children of the powers-that-be, to demand that France spare nothing to save them. Sel's battle cry: *Tout à la rue!*

⁓

Across the street, I see a small boy holding his mother's hand. They were watching the protest from the sidelines earlier. The child looks sickly, like he could have thin blood. He stares in our direction until his mother pulls him away.

His name and possible story flash before me. Charles. Nickname? *Piglet.* A young street sidekick who turns up from time to time, who hangs with Sel, the old lady who's nice to him. A slowly dying boy she's grown fond of. A child who's reached a level of sagacity before the age of reason—twelve—and is still alive, to his own and everyone else's surprise, particularly Charles's mother's. A wise child, ready to revolt, to escape his mother's fears and doomsday prophesies.

I feel a small hand grab mine, cold and velvet soft. Pudgy. Fleshy mounds and fingertips. So pale. Light-blue veins like worms in the wrists. Fingernails bitten to the quick. But strong fingers—surprisingly strong for such a delicate flower of a boy. A child with hidden, stubborn strengths. One who may even betray Sel, his protector. This last thought comes to me as a surprise. *A Judas child.*

The boy is now at the end of the street, still struggling with his mother, looking back at the protesters. In my mind, Charles-Piglet smiles, a shy soul, timid bold eyes under long lashes.

Salut, petit Jude.

⟆

Later, a panaché or two later (beer and lemonade mix, *delish!*)—I'm relaxing. I'm glad it was just a picket. The ACT UP crew is happy too, chatty. The action was a success. They've gotten some media and some of the ministry people engaged them. I listen to their conversation about next steps, about outreach to more hemophilia groups, what else can be done.

I borrow a marker from the barman, grab a napkin, make a reminder note to myself: *Factor VII.* Then grab a few more napkins. I draw a body, extending itself over Paris, lying along the length of the snaking Seine with the Eiffel Tower in the background. I sketch arteries and veins of the river extending from the body's ribs into streets and neighborhoods. I'm seeing a possible Frida Kahlo–like painting, the Seine coursing through a pale hemophiliac body. One losing blood from many orifices.

I start again. The body, horizontally lain, becomes a human boat, with a giant mast and white sail of IV blood marked with a red cross on it and stamped F-VII. A wooden pirate's vessel with Joan of Arc as the maidenhead, protector of the holy voyage. Ideas, ideas, always too many when I get excited or too tired. I probably shouldn't drink too much; this panaché goes down so easily.

Damn. I've spilled my beer drink. I've ruined my drawing. I crumple the napkins up and throw them away. I write the reminder on my hand instead: F7.

⟆

One thing I learned today, that got my attention, is that intolerance of certain drugs including penicillin and cephalosporins is a sign of a possible deficiency of Factor VII. Those happen to be the two drugs I'm highly allergic to. What does that mean?

A little backstory: I only learned about my allergy to cephalosporins a while back. I'm forever warned. I can't take Comtrex, which is an over-the-counter bacterial drug that comes from a mold, *Cephalosporium.* I took it for a bad cold when I was working at the NYC AIDS hotline on First Avenue, as a telephone counselor. I'd felt a flu coming on and popped two tablets of Comtrex. I'd never taken them before. The next thing I knew, my friend Anthony Viti, who was sitting across from me, began to yell at me. He'd been watching me start to droop in my chair. *What's going on?* He didn't even call 911 because we were directly across from Bellevue hospital. He just grabbed the office chair I was sitting in that had wheels and raced me across the street to the emergency room.

By then my right eyelid was drooping, a reaction I learned was called *ptosis*. Then the muscles of my right cheek fell a little too, like a stroke patient. I began to feel numb and slow, like I was encased in lead, and my toes and hands and knees didn't react when a resident ran a prickly tool over them like a mini spur testing my reflexes.

The attending residents were medical students, skeptical of Comtrex. *Is she an addict? Was it an overdose?* But Anthony was adamant, hysterical: *No, she just took a flu medicine! I swear!* Soon a senior doctor got pulled in, took a quick look at me, and yelled at a nurse to give me a shot of cortisone. Boom, I began to come right back. It was really scary, especially for Anthony. *I thought you were dying!*

Maybe I was or would have. That's how I learned I'm very allergic to cephalosporins, which are cross-reactive with penicillin, a mold that put me into a coma when I was an infant. I used to wear a penicillin allergy bracelet and still should. And now I wonder, could I have some minor deficiency of Factor VII? Am I a borderline hemophiliac? I do seem to bruise more easily now, but I thought it was just getting older.

I told you: the political is always so personal to me.

There's one more thing: I was struck today by the concept of the body that simply can't contain its life force, can't control itself. The body that can bleed out. I don't know why it seems like the ultimate metaphor for our contemporary political body, now being poxed by AIDS, but it does to me. We're bleeding out from all corners of the globe. This epidemic is still out of control.

11

Roots, Baby

~ 9

It's time I shared a bit of family history—mine, not Sel's—so you can better appreciate why I'm tempted to pitch a tent in the garden outside the historical archives for a few months. I've started dipping into the Vichy period, including Vichy Marseille. Looking for my French relatives. I'm especially curious about the deeper roots on my father's side, which began in Alsace, near Germany, and eventually spread across the world, not only to Haiti but the Belgian Congo too, divided now into the Democratic Republic of Congo and Rwanda. I've got relatives across Europe and South America and Africa that stem from this complex family peregrination, this postcolonial migration.

I also have relatives who love genealogy. They've done the heavy-lifting research for me—for us, the still-living family members. They've traced my father's family roots and family name to a nobleman once named Ades, who lived in a place by the same name, in the north of France. This ancestor was either an aristocrat or part of the landed gentry who served in the French army. This was at a time when the Polish king, Stanislav, an ally of the French kings, had established a seasonal court in Alsace-Lorraine, near the German border.

In my personal files at home, I keep a document, creased and copied over so many times that the words are hard to read. It's just a Xerox copy, but the dark stamp of a royal seal is still visible, like a thumbprint. It's signed in 1798 and represents the thing that people fought over for centuries: a title. It confirms that one Monsieur François d'Adesky, *gentilhomme* from Alsace, ably served in the military campaigns of one Louis-Stanislav-Xavier, *fils de France* and uncle of the king, and Charles-Philippe of France, another son of France. He fought for the royals throughout 1792 and was rewarded with membership into the French nobility.

The backstory on this fancy fellow is what amused us—my siblings and I. *The romance of it all.* According to the family lore, this long-ago ancestor fell in love with the handmaiden of Stanislav's wife, the Polish queen. But he still

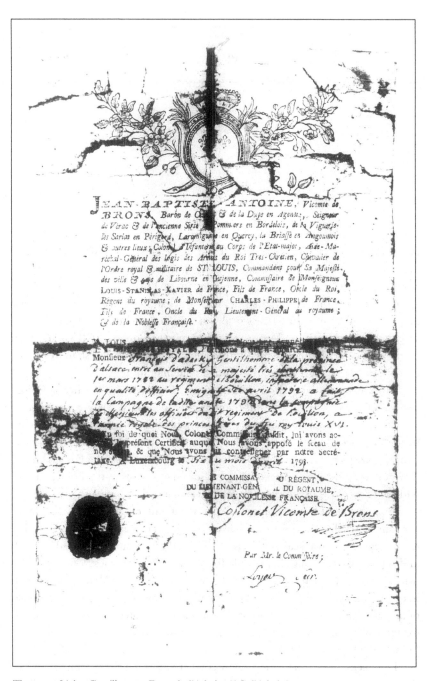

The man of Ades, Gentilhomme François d'Adesky. (AC d'Adesky)

lacked the requisite title or enough land, and other je ne sais quoi that made up a proper royal dowry in those days, that would allow him to marry up and become part of the Polish court. So Stanislav gave him a break, gave him the royal nod—and, most important, that little piece of paper: his title. The family Ades acquired a *d'*, as in *de—of*—as in of Ades, the man from Ades. With a Polish twist to make it d'Adesky. The family gained a royal coat of arms: three roosters. *A trinity of royal cocks.* I know—awesome family roots, haha.

Somewhere, we'd also been told, some branches of our family were Jewish, and later became Catholic during one of the many periods where being a Jew was no longer safe. During the French Revolution, our ancestors were divided in their loyalty: some remained royalist, fighting for the monarchy; others supported the republic. A house divided. A personal family history I find repeated over the generations in my own family. By and large, the male ancestors served in the military or were doctors. But which of them broke class ranks, rebelled against the nation? Not easy to know. There's no information about any dissidents, or any of the women.

Eventually, one branch of the d'Adeskys ended up in Belgium, which is where my Haitian grandfather was born. He had two brothers. One went to Africa (then the Belgian Congo); one stayed in Europe; and the third—my grand-père d'A, as we called him—was sent to Haiti. This was just after World War I. He served as the Belgian consul during the U.S. occupation at the tender age of eighteen.

According to family lore, my Haitian grand-père d'A was shipped abroad because he was a hothead soldier who disagreed with the war and had tried to blow up one of the kaiser's tanks in protest. That sounded romantically brave. In order to avoid his arrest, the family secured a spot for him on a ship headed for Haiti and worked their Belgian family connections to have him named a consul to Haiti. I later imagined him as a character in a Graham Greene novel.

But that may be what my father used to call *une petite exaggeration*. Recently one of my relatives in Europe—one whose memory is much better than mine—explained that our grandfather had killed a young man like himself. He liked to box and he liked his drink. One night he engaged another soldier in a boxing match and the other fellow died. It might have been a tragic accident, but it spelled disgrace and possibly prison for my grandfather. Swiftly, he was put on board a freighter for Haiti and a new life. He did indeed become a youthful *consul d'affaires* for the Belgian nation. He also met my Haitian grandmother, who was seventeen when they married. The rest is a story for another book. I bring it up because it represents a common thread I've uncovered: the holes in the family biography, the bits that don't always line up to present a pretty picture for posterity. I may even find this version of events has flaws if we keep digging.

⌁

On my mother's side, I know even less of the backstory. She was born in Grenoble, into the Berthoin family. I learned not long ago that the family estate there is still quite something. Skiing was a family tradition and my mother, a complete couch potato as the adult who raised us, had been a young champion skier. The family was well off but not super wealthy, falling somewhere in the upper-middle class of the French bourgeoisie.

Only recently have I discovered contemporary relatives who, I'm still learning, were heavily involved in politics before and after the collaborationist Vichy period. One, a cabinet minister, Georges Berthoin, played some significant role. He seems to have crossed paths long ago with the infamous Monsieur Le Pen in the European Parliament. But that's getting ahead of today's story.

I want to tell you first about my French grand-père—my mother's father, Serge Berthoin. We called him Papou. He's the relative I'm looking for, a bit randomly, in these history archives. I'm certain I'll find him, for some reason. He wasn't famous. He was a businessman, an entrepreneur. But I have an instinctive feeling I'll find him here anyway. You'll see why. Like my Haitian grand-papa, he seems to have had a brush with the law, one that forever altered the course of his life. Here, too, the details of truth have been hard to nail, but the hints are enough to push me to dig.

My French grand-père was a true gentleman, well educated, culturally worldly, with excellent social skills. A man at home in the world, modest yet proud. He had impeccable style. The grandfather I knew was a tall, elegantly dressed boulevardier type who liked to flirt and drink his espresso at an outdoor Paris café with a folded newspaper in hand. Think Jean-Paul Belmondo in *Breathless*. A rake with an appreciation for women; a playboy of sorts. Eternally young in spirit, rich enough, and so stylish. That was my Papou—tall and lanky, with folded white, silk neck scarves, looking unruffled, a ready twinkle in his eye, always open to a new adventure. He cultivated his persona, and, in time, he became that debonair gentleman, that dandy with his cravats, that man about town. He was style consummate.

He, like my mother, smoked Gauloises, unfiltered, his manner unhurried. Like her, he continued doing so until the very end of his life, unfazed even later by my mother's death from cancer, enjoying one of his last remaining vices. Papou embodied the art of living very well; a true bon vivant. Many of his habits were acquired early in life, when he was wealthy and could afford to go gambling at the crap tables in Monte Carlo or rent a vacation apartment in Nice. He savored the moment, lingering over his espresso like there was absolutely nowhere better to be, and never would be.

I was born during the second storied half of his life—the period he referred to as his *troubles*. I only learned about his sojourn in jail when I was a teenager and, by then, his troubles were long past. He could smile about the whole thing, even make jokes. He had been arrested by proxy, I understood, tarred, unfairly jailed for something another person had done.

⌐

I actually know little about my grandfather's childhood, but it appears typical enough of his social class—the aspiring, urban, upper French bourgeoisie. He received a good education in private schools, did well, attended university, studied business. He spent the long August holidays in Cannes or Nice, by the sea, and later in Chamonix, at the foot of Mont Blanc, an alpine ski resort. Much later, he purchased a small leafy lot there with a brook running alongside it and built three rustic chalets that reminded me of the story of Goldilocks. The smallest chalet barely contained two people; the other, four; the main chalet was big enough to accommodate the family and inevitable friends who would be discovered in the morning, sleeping off a hangover on the porch, camping style. As children, we'd be sent to chill bottles of wine for the adults in the icy little brook. The wine sometimes floated away and we'd have to go far to retrieve it. These were magical moments of childhood summer; idyllic.

Papou loved a sense of magic in his own life and was ever open to the possibilities of a moment. He was very spontaneous when it came to possible fun, an adventure. Even at seventy, he loved nothing better than to drive his convertible at very high speeds, something he used to do from Monte Carlo back to Paris at dawn.

He never stopped living large either. In the eighties, I lived in a big loft on Avenue A on the Lower East Side, right above the Pyramid Club. It was a hot gay club at the time, where a lot of drag performers like RuPaul started out. Papou came to visit me for a week. He was pretty old then but still full of life. I decided to throw a big party and invite all my friends to meet him. Of course most were gay. I wondered what he'd think; I was not officially out to him, though of course he knew.

Well, he was delighted. *So excited.* He sat in a big chair in the middle of the loft with dancing and gossip going on all around him and held court. He kissed so many people. And the next morning, walking around the loft in his silk robe

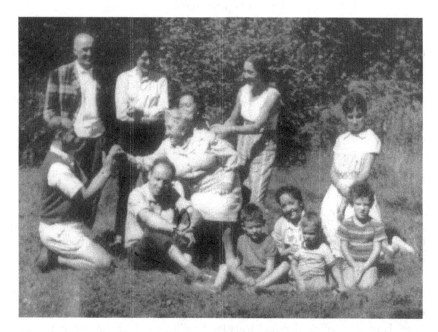

August family reunion in Chamonix, late 1950s. *Top, from left*: My grandfather Serge Berthoin (Papou); my mother, Viviane d'Adesky; two unknown relatives; *middle, seated*: my great-grandmother; *front*: (*kneeling*) my father, Raymond d'Adesky; (*seated*) my uncle Christian Berthoin; my cousin Claude Berthoin; unknown relative; my brother Serge; my sister, Kathy; (*standing*) my aunt Florence Meunier. (AC d'Adesky)

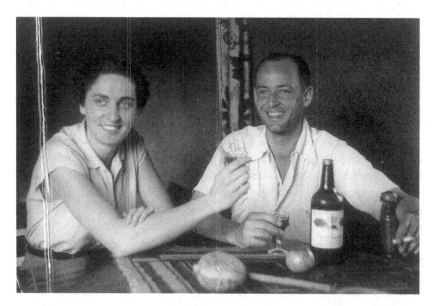

Life essentials: Haitian rum and espresso for my parents, Raymond and Viviane d'Adesky. (AC d'Adesky)

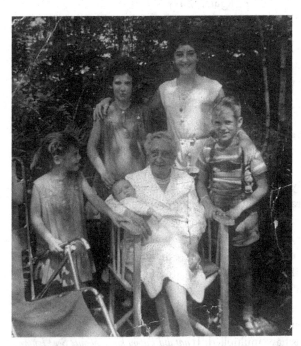

My great-grandmother, aunt, and relatives in France. (AC d'Adesky)

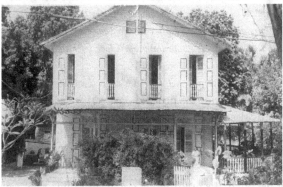

My grandparents' gingerbread home on Rue Duncombe in the Bois Verna neighborhood, damaged and later demolished following the 2010 earthquake. (AC d'Adesky)

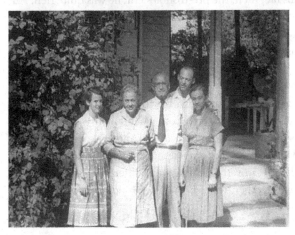

My Haitian relatives (*from left*): my aunt Chantal; Grand-mère d'A; Grand-père d'A; my father, Raymond; my aunt Evelyn. (AC d'Adesky)

with his slippers and Gauloises and black coffee, he innocently asked me: *What about tonight? More parties? I'm ready.*

Truly, he was a role model.

⌒

Papou was also a natural entrepreneur, with a knack for lucrative prospects and for business. During, or just after, the war, he actually managed to become the main representative for Lloyd's insurance in France, an opportunity that made him quite wealthy. I have my own questions about what he knew and did back then, since France's Jews were being evicted and their houses and properties usurped by Vichy officials during the war. But no one in my immediate family knows more at this point. We have some distant cousins in France—the Grenoble set—who might be able to tell me more about the Berthoin side.

After a little initial sleuthing of my own, I found Lloyd's turns up among many, many European companies whose records continue to be examined today as part of the attempt to provide reparations to surviving Jewish families of that period—to find and return the stolen loot.

So now the questions have multiplied: *What did Papou know about? See? Ignore? Feel afraid to confront? Anything? Was he in any way complicit in the ongoing plunder of Jewish properties, or the failure to return confiscated estates that continued after Vichy? How do we measure what people don't do, or say? It's something we'll look back and ask about AIDS too, won't we? I hope so.*

I should note here that I don't have any evidence or reason to think my grand-père did anything bad, but I know he profited during the war, as many people do. War, after all, provides ample opportunities for enterprising souls. He was always quick to spot opportunities to make money and would often tell me about good business ideas he had had but couldn't pursue for one reason or another.

For the first part of his life, then, the pre-troubles era, he was quite rich. An apartment in Marseille, rooms in Paris, and vacation homes in the south. He wasn't especially political, but, if I believe my mother's stories, he did help the French Resistance during the war. Here, again, the details are *très* fuzzy.

⌒

Voilà what took place, as far as I know now, based on my initial childhood shaking of the family tree: Before the Occupation, when Hitler was making his ascent, my grandparents divorced. They had married and had two children—my mother and her older brother—but they apparently bickered. A lot. I'm not surprised. They strike me, in retrospect, as very different people, and my grandmother, Mamie we called her, well, she had her good points, but she was also a diva. Demanding; a bit imperious. Already rich due to her marriage with my Papou. I have no idea why they divorced. Maybe Papou was away too often, gambling in Cannes. She did comment later on his natural penchant to flirt. *Je ne sais pas.* I only know it had to be something major for them to divorce, because she was a high Catholic, and this was simply not done. An annulment was better and she probably tried that first. But eventually they divorced.

She soon remarried a very wealthy Frenchman who loved Italy. A man who had wanted to be a monk but chose another life. A man of faith, someone she could trust, she felt. Dedy, a nickname. She met him in Marseille, where she and Papou now lived apart. Dedy's family had land, vineyards. He was a count of sorts, with actual papers to back his own nod to royalty—an important point my grandmother often mentioned in passing, as if this was a casual thing to her. It wasn't. She loved being the Countess of Sessevalle and later settled into a castle in Chiusa, in the Dolomites of Italy. The castle of Branzoll. A gorgeous, fairyland place. They had two girls who became sisters to my mother.

When I was very young, we stayed in the Branzoll castle. We have a grainy black-and-white picture of it in our family scrapbook. I mostly remember it was very cold and had mice that I worried were rats. I slept poorly, under heavy blankets. But I was impressed. I don't know when it was sold, or if the Germans occupied it. I think I remember hearing something about that.

Papou also later remarried a very kind woman, my step-grand-mère, Nita. When the war came, and Occupation, the south remained a Free Zone and they took refuge there. They had another daughter and Papou became step-father to a son from his new wife's earlier marriage, my uncle Gaston Wyss. The family divided their time between Marseille and Paris.

This is where the stories my siblings and I were told as children begin to diverge. I've done my best to synthesize what we collectively agree on, what's still up for grabs, and what's pure speculation on my part.

Perhaps not surprisingly my grandmother thought nuns would do a better job educating her children because only nuns and priests could be trusted to prevent Catholic children from having premarital sex. I know my mother and her brother were put in full-time Catholic boarding schools early on, something that made my mother feel very lonely. She tended to see her parents, now living in separate cities, during the long holidays.

When the war broke out, the children were sent south, to stay with a friend of Mamie's. Papou stayed around Marseille and, as I mentioned, his Lloyd's insurance-cum-realty business did quite well. Mamie stayed in a family chalet in Megève, close to Switzerland. She ran a boardinghouse there.

⎯⌐

This is where the family war story gets more interesting. Mamie had a best girl-friend who was Jewish and lived in Geneva. That's how Mamie came to play her part in the war—her claim to some historical fame—a role that may or may not have led to my mother and other relatives being lined up to be executed by German soldiers. That's the jewel in the crown of this small saga I'm recounting.

I'm told that my grandmother and her friend managed to ferret out some thirty Jewish children to safety in Switzerland, using her boardinghouse as a way station. It's a story that made me sigh with karmic relief when I heard about this, not that long ago. As a teen, I worried that my family might have done little to nothing to stop Hitler's purge of French Jews and Gypsies. (I knew nothing of homosexuals then.) It seems that at least Mamie stepped up and did the moral right thing.

⎯⌐

Papou also had his brush with the French Resistance. I was told it was a small role, passing information to and from members of the Resistance, probably in Marseille, where he worked. I don't know if he was already Lloyd's man in France then. But I wish I did. Marseille was a stronghold of Vichy activities, of later Vichy purges of Jews. All we know is that Papou later claimed some kind of medal for his service to the Resistance.

It's from this story that I developed my admittedly romantic childhood image of Papou. Too well can I see him sitting in a café, smoking, playing the spy, loving the risk, and proud of his minor political role in history. But I do wonder what he knew about the prior eviction of Jews in Marseille. Right after the war he became a real estate developer and helped build many big, beautiful buildings along Avenue Cannebière, a main artery that dead-ends with the port. From my research into Vichy, I think it's the site of the former Old Port, the Jewish ghetto area that was razed after its residents were sent to the gas camps.

Did he even know? Is that why that area was up for grabs, open to new developers? What about those insurance policies? Did they belong to Jews now killed?

I'll have to check the timeline now, see how many years exist between the mass deportations from the Old Port and the breaking of new ground for the returnees of Algeria. And more importantly, what Marseille officials were involved. *How many are still around, maybe friends of Monsieur Le Pen?* Again, more questions than answers, when one begins barking up the family tree.

~ 10

It was near the end of the war, my mother told me, that she and several others narrowly escaped being shot by a German firing squad. Here is Maman's version—well, what I recall, since she's now long dead too.

One day when she was in the countryside—visiting her mother at Megève? Living with family friends in the Free Zone south?—a group of German soldiers arrived in the village, shouting and menacing. They were demanding information about the whereabouts of the Resistance, about anyone hiding or helping Jews. Here's where I'm speculating: I figure someone had denounced my grandmother Mamie and her best friend, running the boardinghouse. That's the story I was told not that long ago by a cousin. It was a small community. They said Mamie had a neighbor who was a Nazi collaborator, someone jealous of Mamie, who'd informed the Germans that my Mamie was hiding a Jewish woman and her daughter.

What Maman told me is that the German soldiers quickly lined her up with her mother, Mamie, and other village adults. They were blindfolded. Like many French children, my mother had learned German in school and understood what the soldiers were saying. Seconds before the order came to fire, another jeep rolled up, tires screeching and more German soldiers shouting. Members of the Resistance had been spotted in the hills. Off went the soldiers in the jeeps, never to return. That appeared to be the end of the story. No firing squad, no massacre, my family, my mother, spared. *Super dramatique.*

How did you feel, Maman? What were you thinking? I asked her once.

I was thinking that I was the only who understood we'd be shot. Like rats.

The few rare times she spoke about the war, she would shake her head, just a little. She didn't want to relive it, apart from telling stories of how much she'd missed chocolate, how she used to ride her bike for kilometers to trade eggs for chocolate. I'd remember this story when I'd go buy dark-chocolate-covered orange peels at a local specialty shop in Daytona, during the few short months when she was dying at home. I was twenty-one, just graduated from college, still trying to get childhood and war stories out of her. *I dreamed of this,* she would tell me, trying to suck on the chocolate with the awful taste of chemo on her tongue and nausea roiling her stomach. *Enjoy it while you can. Enjoy it for me.*

And what of Mamie's Jewish friend in Switzerland? She survived the war, and her children have stayed in touch with one of my cousins. The Steens, or Steins. There are ways to learn more about this chapter of history, and I may try. I'd like to know details of that time. Because the mother, father, and grandparents I grew up to know did not strike me as hero types—not the kind to risk their own necks to hide Jewish neighbors in an attic, or to volunteer their lives for a patriot cause. Though they did love children, in the way the French love children (even when they don't love or even like them very much). Children are to be taken care of, is what I'm saying. The children must be fed and clothed and given naps and taught to greet visitors. And to stay quiet while the adults are talking. The French know how to do this well. They have good manners and they are taught the concept of social duty, even though it feels like a pressure to socially conform to me. So I can understand Mamie might have felt an impulse to help Jewish children that overcame her fear of arrest or getting shot. Probably her love for her childhood best friend trumped the terror.

But I'm honestly not sure. I only know it happened and it was intense. I also know that my mother hated Hitler. I understood that as a child by the way she refused to say his name, calling him simply *un homme terrible*. A really, very bad guy. I understood she and her friends, all teens, had suffered from privation, from hunger, from exile, from fear of bombs and fighting, just like everyone. Except she never said a word about the Jews whose suffering and fate was of another category altogether. About what Mamie had done. Why? I still wonder. *Why not talk about such an important thing?*

It was only when we were at the dinner table at times, complaining about something, that my mother would sharply remind us of how lucky we were. About the distance she rode to bargain for those single bars of *chocolat*. How she'd had to hold the eggs she would trade in one hand, while steering the handlebar of the bike with her other hand. Over bumpy roads. Over long distances. How she never broke an egg, and so on. Stories of sacrifice. Stories that to me, a certain-to-be-spoiled American child of francophone immigrant parents growing up in suburban Florida, sounded terribly brave and glamorous. I never questioned any of the rare wartime narratives. But I now wish I had.

⌒

The point of this long, personal aside is that my parents were not *engagés*—as in politically engaged—individuals. *Leave that to someone else*: that's the message I got growing up, when I later watched the Vietnam war protests with them on television, or when I was out of college and first got arrested for protesting nuclear missiles on U.S. soil. They were democrats with a small *d*. As in rather *désengagés*.

My mother was also a Catholic with the smallest *c*, not quite convinced by the whole promise of heavenly reward. She made sure to attend Mass on Easter and at Christmas, and occasionally in between, if only to secure her entry into heaven, should God really exist. It was a safer bet. (Like Mamie la comtesse, she also favored a view that Catholic nuns would be safer teachers for her children than long-haired, young, male teachers in the local Daytona public schools.) That was the extent of her religious belief. Skeptical but pragmatic.

For his part, my father is an agnostic or an atheist—he never quite decides. He's not a God guy though. Politically, he's become a rather rabid political conservative as he's aged, embracing Ronald Reagan, a man whose AIDS policies I deplored. But when I was younger he wasn't engaged in politics, as far as I knew.

What I understood most clearly from the stories my parents told us children was that they were war survivors who had witnessed firsthand, as children and teenagers, the cruelties men can impose on one another. As first-generation immigrants to America, they wanted a quiet place to raise children, and to stay away from anyone's guns or politics. They were passively apolitical. They believed in helping one other but primarily reserved that help, that social duty, for family and close friends. My father was very generous in helping his patients, including poor patients without insurance. But he wasn't the protest type.

All of this serves as a (very deep) background of sorts for why I began talking about my French grand-père and jail earlier. It was related to war—the next big one for France: Algeria. It was after 1960, during Algeria's liberation from France, that Papou's real troubles began. It was then that the government began repatriating more than one million French citizens from Algeria—the pied-noir generation. Often, these were wealthy families with reams of servants and they were used to great comfort in Algeria compared to France. Later, having been booted out of Algeria, they were given a government subsidy too small to purchase a home—at least in the luxury apartments that Papou was then developing in Marseille. The returnees didn't want to live in the designated low-cost houses in popular (read: poor immigrant) neighborhoods. And there, Papou could sympathize. He liked living well; who didn't?

Enter my grand-père to help them readjust. I had always heard that his legal problems stemmed from a false accusation that had been made against a business partner in his real estate business, for which Papou innocently took the fall. But perhaps that was a small, smooth *mensonge* we grandchildren were told so that we wouldn't look badly upon Papou, whom we adored. Just a little lie.

It seems Papou (or his partners in his agency) decided to help the returning colonists from Algeria—but might have helped himself (themselves?) at the same time. He sharply reduced the prices on the high-rise apartments so Algeria's returnees could use their national subsidies—in addition to some off-the-books cash—to buy into his luxe condos. His clients were very happy, but the government wasn't, when it discovered that Papou's firm had pocketed extra cash without reporting it.

One day, then, the taxman came calling, and Papou found himself an accused tax cheat. So was his partner, who, Papou always claimed, set up the deal for which he took the fall. The mayor of Marseille was particularly unhappy with him because the whole affair made the government's housing policy look bad. He made sure my grandfather served time. It was all politics, Papou stressed, when I asked him if it was true he had gone to jail. After the war, he said, it was nothing but *politiques*.

Papou spent a year in jail and lost everything, or very nearly: his many houses, his cars, his reputation, and his license as a builder. That's when his life really changed—in a good way, he told me once. In prison, he slept better than he ever had before. He finally had a chance to read books. He made good friends and learned to work with his hands a bit. And, he said with clear pride, he became a much nicer person. A better father too.

Before prison, he was arrogant and elitist, materialistic, distant, hard, and judgmental. Not someone I would admire, he felt. But, postprison, he became the sweet, affectionate Papou I knew as a girl; one who was forced to rebuild his reputation, career, and personal life from scratch. And, to his credit, he did just that.

After prison, he and Nita settled quite happily in a small apartment in Versailles, just a stone's throw from the gilded chambers of Marie Antoinette. He had his children, especially his youngest daughter, Florence, to dote on, along with my two uncles: his talented artist son, Christian, my mother's brother; and his stepson, Gaston. The family shared a love of golf and television documentaries. Florence became a junior golf champion.

Gaston is the uncle I viewed as a true character. When I later watched *Mona Lisa*, a stylish British noir film by director Neil Jordan, I was reminded of Gaston. In it, Bob Hoskins plays George, a tough but tender-hearted ex-con who falls for a gorgeous call girl who turns out to be transgender. Gaston was a French Hoskins, a bit tough looking but secretly a total pussycat. A *dragueur*, an impossible flirt, Nita used to complain, affectionately, about her son Gaston. He drove an old Deux Chevaux, like a funky Volkswagen made by Citroën that he loved and I coveted, it was so old-school cool. When I visited he would drive me from Versailles back to Paris like Hoskins in the movie, alert to the action on the street, on the lookout for girls, including the streetwalkers. I got a huge kick out of him.

Whenever he could, Papou visited my mother—his oldest daughter, Viviane, now married and living in America—stuffing his suitcase with smelly cheeses and foie gras. What he cared most about now was making his family happy. That, and his cigarettes, his glass of wine, and his newspaper. He was a changed man, grateful for everything. And as stylish as ever.

⟋⟍

Papou and I were always quite close. He used to say we were alike: that I was a younger, American, female version of him. I'm not sure exactly what he was referring to—my physical appearance, my style, my adventurous spirit, my love of coffee and cafés, or maybe some combination thereof. Or maybe it was simply that I look a lot like my mother, and he adored her and missed her when she left France to marry my father. Whenever he visited us in Florida, where my parents permanently settled after freezing Michigan, he always looked at her with enormous affection, the way he looked at me.

I only mention his story in such detail because while I was at the library, running my fingers through the call cards on Fascism and being referred to V—Vichy, I kept thinking that it would be fun, now that I'm becoming such a pro at this archive digging, to see if I could find any references to my grandfather's trial, or maybe his prison record; see what other kernels I could turn up. Find out if the mayor of Marseille who hounded him was a good guy or a bad one; if, for example, he had (or maybe has?) any links to Le Pen's party, which has a stronghold in Marseille. Wonder how old he would be now?

Maybe my grand-père could even make an appearance in Sel's story—why not? I can imagine a role for him: a minor character who strolls along the Seine every night, Le Figaro in hand, looking every part the handsome, well-dressed, elderly Parisian out for a bit of fresh air. Having helped the Resistance, he could be a source within the French bureaucracy, a real estate contact or insurance broker who helps Sel and her buddies find out which buildings that house refugees are slated for demolition or takeover by the pampered son and daughter of a conservative politician. A posh apartment on the Île de la Cité that, not so long ago, after all, housed les juifs deportés.

I think he'd like that. To be immortalized in some way. He learned to appreciate literature in jail: the role of writers and intellectuals, the culture makers. Two of his children, my mother and her older brother Christian, were very talented artists. Papou was open minded and politically liberal and, as I said, he enjoyed his small adventures. For example, although he disapproved of male homosexuals, he didn't mind my budding androgyny at all. He would say he thought men were inferior to women, and, as he put it, he could see the beauty of two women together. I know this is chauvinist—something heterosexual men typically say about lesbians without realizing it's offensive. What mattered to me, as a child and as a young woman, though, was the unconditional approval and delight he expressed toward me, his granddaughter. I felt understood and loved, as a *garçon manqué*. A tomboy.

⌒

Will you indulge me in another family tale? One more story about Papou that I always loved? More than once, he recounted to me how, as a young man, he would go out to nightclubs in Pigalle, the red-light district, with a girlfriend of his who was a lesbian and, together, they would cruise women. Since Papou wasn't shy and usually had money, he would invite a woman over, light her cigarette, buy her a drink, and introduce her to his friend. Then, depending on her personal tastes, he might leave the two women alone to enjoy themselves. So, you see, Papou had a gallant side, even for an old-fashioned *petit* chauvinist.

Of course I'm playing now, playing with my thoughts. Wondering if he ever went to hang out with his lesbian girlfriends at Le Monocle, a famous lesbian bar in the 1920s that stayed open through the war. After the Nazi Occupation, it closed. The club had a reputation for the handsome butch women who wore monocles and carnations in the buttonholes of their tuxedos. (Compare that to the lesbian uniform of plaid shirts and mullet hairdos in the 1970s and '80s. Of course the Paris dykes had excellent fashion. Should we be surprised?)

Anyway, before I commit Sel's story to paper, separate the wheat from the chaff, I think I'm entitled to have a little fun. Something Papou would approve of, highly. *Amuse-toi*, he always reminded me. *Soie gentille et amuse-toi*. Be good and have fun. *Ça passe vite*. It all goes by quickly.

III

New York

~ 11

I'm back in Manhattan, on the Lower East Side. Home sweet home. Avenue C and Seventh Street, across from the Latin bodega and a stone's throw from the little Puerto Rican lunch place where I can get my favorite drink, a *morir soñando*. To die dreaming. (That's a phrase I think of getting tattooed on my body too, a final-wish reminder to myself.)

I feel a little bit rested, albeit more emotionally than physically. I'm hoping I can get back to Paris soon, even for just a week. I already miss Belle, but we left things in a good place, I think. Nothing settled, nothing committed, but a lot of love and affection. I have a lot of catching up at work. Plus I've missed Jersey—quite a bit.

Paris lies across an ocean, but the Seine pulses inside me like a faint vein. At night I stare out my window, looking upon the ruin of abandoned buildings and shuttered storefronts. I see double, superimposing cobbled streets and fluted lampposts onto the graffitied brick of Avenue C. I watch as images of Paris surface and stubbornly graft themselves onto the patina of my daily life here. I only have to close my eyes, gently, to relive the moments. I'm carrying another city inside me, another life, an ongoing conversation with out-of-sight friends and companions who distract me, who make me talk to myself out loud.

Occasionally, I look up and catch people staring at me—the muttering, preoccupied one. I'm taking on Sel's characteristics, content to spend the night on a bench, huddled in a layer of sweaters, watching the sky move over the trees in Tompkins Square Park. There are more homeless people than ever. Or maybe I'm just noticing them more now. They all remind me of Sel.

I was afraid I'd lose her—lose my story—without the physical sight of Paris and her ancient streets within reach; without the damp, sulfurous spray of the Seine to send me into reveries of imagining. But I haven't—yet. Just tonight, in fact, I was startled to look into the mirror and—as I was assessing the damage to my own face: the deep wrinkles I inherited from my father, my sun-scarred eyes, the uneven shape of my lips—see a fleshy, pink, wart-covered tongue poking from Sel's dry, brownish mouth. It made me laugh.

Looking more deeply at the clear lumps of tissue that cover the edges of my irises without affecting my vision, I saw her inside the black pool of my pupils, saw a run of broken blood vessels in her eyes too. Passing my hand over the gathering folds of my cheek, when I turned my head at an angle, I felt the soft part of her face, the shadowed but paler underside. Even her tongue, a coarse map of a world, was warm, her breath coming back at me not sour, as I know it can be after a night of her drinking, but slightly sweet.

In that instant, emerging from my internal landscape, she looked back at me like a mother observes a child. A tolerant, frank look that shows me she accepts my daily abandonment of her life and story to the demands of my real life and sick friends. It calms me, knowing that she survived the trip back. I feel patient, feel her presence.

It isn't as hard to stay in touch with the Paris news as I feared it might be either. I buy a copy of *Libération* on my way from work in Soho, skim the headlines, read about Chirac and Mitterrand. It all comes flooding back: Vichy and Marshal Philippe Pétain; the elderly Nazis facing trials like Maurice Papon. And, of course, the Seine, the river I love. The great, brown-green slug of the Seine. All I have to do is spy her flinted surface in my mind's eye, hear the steady lapping of water over algae-smooth steps, and I feel a mental space opening up inside me; a vista.

~ 12

My friend Johnny isn't dead; far from it. He's a bit thinner, but his bitchy sense of humor is intact. *I don't see the beautiful French boy you promised me,* he says with what the French call a *moue*—a little pout—letting me into his apartment. *And what about those postcards you promised to send? Je n'ai pas received nada, honey, not one damn petite one. I hope you brought some pictures at least. You didn't? You are so hopeless. Well, that's it. Next time you go, I'm definitely coming with you.*

His rant goes on for a few minutes, long enough to let me know he's missed me and is glad I called from over there, but that it still doesn't let me off the hook. He's upset that I went without him, that he wasn't feeling well enough to go—that's the gist of it. But I can see he's all right; nothing too serious has taken place in my absence. I've brought over a bottle of red wine—*I guess this isn't from Paris,* he says, noting the California label. It's only 7:00 p.m., so dinner isn't ready. We're eating meat loaf and mashed potatoes—standard fare, comfort food, easy to make, long to bake, and hard to get wrong.

For the past months, Johnny's stopped going out and developed a domestic life that revolves around shopping and cooking. He's a picky, opinionated man; he knows what he likes and doesn't like. He likes fresh-squeezed orange juice and gourmet vegetables from Balducci's. He likes frozen TV dinners that have one meat and lots of gravy. He likes Classic Coke; there are four large bottles of it on top of the refrigerator, which he pours carefully into tall, neon plastic glasses for a full child-of-the-fifties effect.

Johnny's spent a lot of his life watching TV; he knows every sitcom, every late-night cable show. He's a child of popular culture. When he's not sleeping—which he does a lot, because he's always tired—or cooking—which requires some planning—he's in the bathroom, where, like most people with AIDS, he spends far too much time. There's a rack of magazines in the bathroom, some of them quite old, others current. I end up spending too much time outside the bathroom at Johnny's house too, keeping him company, talking through the door.

No one else is home tonight; his roommates are out at the bars or studying. Except for the TV, which is on, but turned down low, the loft is quiet, with the sounds of traffic along Hudson Street punctuating the air in bursts of acceleration. The loft smells of cooking; Johnny has bought a pie from Entenmann's—peach, another favorite.

Handing me the corkscrew, he glides over to his stereo and pops in Chris Isaac, presses the mute button on the TV remote, checks the tricking activity on the street below—*slow tonight*, he comments—then smiles at me.

Johnny's dressed up tonight, another good sign. Too often in the past months he won't bother to get out of his robe and slippers. He pirouettes, takes back the corkscrew, strikes a pose. *Do you like my outfit?* He knows I do. He's a dapper dresser, a clothes horse. We share a similar style, though he's preppier and, he tells me, I'm trashier.

At thirty, Johnny's still a child in many ways, and he doesn't like to be alone. Aside from the physical pain, the discomfort, and the boredom, this is the worst part about having AIDS. That, and not having a lover. Usually, he stays up all night watching television in his pajamas. He has two IV drips to do, which take four hours to complete. He starts at around ten at night, or later, and sleeps until four in the afternoon. If he wants any kind of social life, he has to do it before dripping, or he has to wake much earlier, drip before dinner. It all requires a lot of effort and advance thought; it's hard to think about going out, seeing a play or a movie, or even a friend, when you feel incredibly nauseated or depressed. The TV is Johnny's constant companion; it reassures him. It's a lifeline to the world outside, a reminder that he hasn't left it yet. He looks over at the TV absently.

Did you hear any good music over there? Before I have a chance to answer, he says, *Nah, I bet you didn't. French rock music sucks, doesn't it?* And he laughs. *Le French Rock. C'est very bad. Oui, oui.* Amusing himself.

He's in a good mood, something that's become rare of late. Before coming over, I got an update from Boy Kelly, Johnny's closest friend and the man who Johnny would marry in a heartbeat. Unfortunately, Boy Kelly's not interested in romance, but he's devoted to Johnny and that makes two of us, though Boy Kelly and I are not sure how we got the positions. Necessity, I think.

Necessity and kindness. The love of a friend, sometimes deeper and more consistent than that of a lover. Boy Kelly plays the part gamely. He and Johnny become a bickering but tender couple, Johnny adopting the familiar part of the rejected suitor; Boy Kelly, the patient, ministering—and, lately, abused—object of love. *Johnny's better,* Boy Kelly informed me. *His KS isn't bothering him as much, or at least he hasn't been complaining about it.*

—

Chris Isaak's voice is haunting, full of romantic longing. Johnny mouths the words; he knows all the lyrics. He's still a handsome man, but his hair is thinning so fast from chemo that it's only a matter of time before he shaves it all off. As he hums, he moves around the kitchen, opening the oven door to peek. It used to be that listening to music was his primary enjoyment, followed by television. But now, I see, cooking is inching up the list. He's even bought a cookbook.

Johnny lacks ambition—or, put another way, he lacks confidence. Self-esteem. He's very bright, but something fundamental has been lacking. Something has made him feel less than; made him fear, then retire, from competition, from the possibility of disappointment, and failure, and of course, success. Before AIDS, he was a good-looking former actor, former waiter, former childhood pianist, former fat kid. This last is the telling detail: his inner child remains enormous, a social outcast, a fairy, rejected. Now, with AIDS, all the negatives remain, but now the positives are associated with failure too. Nothing has added up. AIDS has wiped it all away.

—

I met Johnny when he was a waiter, right after he broke up with the one man he still calls the love of his life, a guy called Britt who sounds like a royal asshole to me. The fact is, Johnny can be difficult too; in fact, Johnny isn't always a nice man. He can be a self-admitted bitch. He was rather spoiled all his life, the product of an upper-middle-class Protestant family. Loving, devoted mother;

cold, distant, mean father. The classic male homosexual profile. Now that he's sick and getting sicker, he's become much more of a pain in the ass: prickly, demanding, and self-centered. I find myself wondering what attracted me to him in the first place, before I catch myself, remember his illness is speaking. His illness has changed him. He's not the same man. I have to work to remember that, to review our good times, his gentle, lighter, fun-loving side. I miss my old friend, lost to me forever.

I still love this very sick, cantankerous John, but I like his sour side less and less, the bitterness that erupts, that sometimes makes it hard to stay gentle myself, to stay giving. He's sick, he's going to die, he's sure of it, and he's so depressed about his life now—the limitations presented by the endless schedule of taking pills and shots and eating, only to feel nauseous beyond appetite, then hungry and weak, but too anxious to sleep. He enters the black hole of all his shortcomings. How soon he'll die is the frank topic of our frequent conversations.

⌒

Johnny tells me I'm the only one of his few close friends or family who will talk honestly about dying with him, without sugar-coating anything. Everyone else gets upset, or changes the subject. I tell him I want to talk about it, want to know how it feels to him, physically and mentally. *I'll be there soon enough, whenever it is,* I say, *you're just going through the door earlier. And you may not go now or soon, so stop pushing yourself out the door.* Hearing that makes him feel less alone, gives him strength, makes him feel that he has something to offer me, a lesson in living I'll be able to use. *It's hell,* he says again tonight, several times. *It's hell because it makes me hate myself even more. But it's good in that way, to realize I can let go of that hate.*

One of the reasons we became friends is because I'm an AIDS activist. I was one of the first people Johnny told about having HIV; when we met, he hadn't told his roommates even though he had known for over a year. Though don't hold me to that last detail—remember, I have an atrocious memory (which is why I have to write things down). But I know it's true that he confided in me and Boy Kelly in a way he didn't to anybody else. That's part of why I loved him and still do, even when he's poisonous: because he's so vulnerable and knows he's going to die without having achieved what he hoped, and that acuteness—that sense of mortality and failure—bonds us. We're spirits and our time is short.

I could go on and on about Johnny. At night, alone or talking to Boy Kelly, I sometimes do. But tonight, watching Johnny feel better, I'm content. He's happy I'm back. He's cooked a good meal. He looks good even if he feels shitty.

⌐○

I have a lot to share with Johnny: first and foremost, the news from the Berlin conference; what I thought of the studies and treatments that were discussed. Then he asks me about Paris, starting with Belle: how was it since he and I spoke on the telephone when I was there? *Is she going to visit or not?* He snaps, angry on my behalf, protective. *What is wrong with that damn woman?*

He shakes his head, not happy, listening to me outline all the reasons why it's hard for her to say for sure if and when she can come. Nothing I say makes any sense to him because he knows I want her—or, want it, a chance to have it, and he wants it for me. *It*: the romance, the white picket fence, the future with someone. He doesn't have much chance of having that himself, at least not with Boy Kelly. Underneath his self-centeredness, Johnny loves me deeply, and he wants the best for me. He knows I've been miserable, breaking up with the Aerialist. *Doesn't that woman know how much you want to be with her? I'm going to have to call her up myself and tell her. Jesus Christ, you lesbians are getting to be as bad as gay men!*

Next subject: ACT UP. *What are the French boys like? What kinds of actions are they doing? Are they as cute, as outrageous, as the boys here?* He wants pictures, descriptions, men he can fantasize about.

I'm the one who introduced Johnny to ACT UP, who literally dragged him through the door to his first meeting. For two years, it changed him, gave him a sense of community, a base of support to face his own diagnosis—even a temporary sense of purpose. Like all the boys there, it gave him a place to cruise, outside of the bars, a place where HIV was small talk, a way to say hello. That lasted while he was feeling well. Now with his KS lesions, Johnny feels like a pariah, even at ACT UP. He feels too ugly to pick up anyone. *I'm a lousy activist,* he says. *I'm lazy.* Or: *This is all too depressing.* Or: *Everyone's hiding.*

He's complaining, but it's all true. His KS is disfiguring; he was never that politically motivated; he was mostly in ACT UP to pick up men; the news is depressing, and there's still a lot of shame. Very few people admit to being HIV positive, even in the meeting rooms of ACT UP. As a group, it is no longer as exciting as it was: fewer people are attending meetings; the discussion is often tedious and rambling. But Johnny is still committed, at least in his heart; he still supports the purpose and efforts of ACT UP. *How do you pronounce ACT UP in French?*

ACT UP.

The same way? Really. That's neat. He means it.

⌐○

I tell Johnny about the French hemophilia blood scandal, the pickets, and our clumsy attempts to make rhymes and chants in French. How ACT UP–Paris meetings are more formal; the group has a hierarchy, with a president and vice president, and so on. Not as unruly as New York, where facilitators have to struggle to keep people from shouting their disagreement with each other at times. About how the social scene is different in Paris, how he would like it, everyone going out after meetings for drinks, to eat. *There's a real camaraderie that's missing in New York,* I tell him.

He listens to all of this, satisfied: he wasn't able to go, but this makes him feel like he was there. He can imagine it. And I've brought him souvenirs: an ACT UP T-shirt, a button from the deaf gays, a safer-sex poster.

What's the French word for condom? He's testing the meat loaf. It's ready. We dig in.

Capote, I reply. *Like a cover, I guess.*

A cap? I get it. Cool.

—⁓

Johnny is WASP stock, Baltimore, New England summers by the bay. He loves French food, but his tastes are strictly American. He's the only one of my friends who actually buys frozen dinners and eats them with relish. He's put little pimentos in the meat loaf and looks delighted with the outcome of this meal. *Pretty fancy, huh? I'm sure you ate well over there, but not like this.* He says this with a straight face, then we laugh. His teeth look unnaturally yellow and large to me, his lips extra red. He's shaved for the occasion, and missed a spot. Johnny has nice teeth, I think, a nice smile. Still quite handsome.

The meatloaf *is* delicious. It makes me feel more French than American, or less American than Johnny, who couldn't be anything else. He pops in another tape—R.E.M.—before serving himself a second course. *What about your book?* he asks, switching subjects abruptly. *What's it all about? Is it a novel?*

Johnny would like to be a writer, or would have liked to have been. That's another part of his relationship to me; he admires me: my ambition, my success. He can't read books anymore, or magazines, really; it tires him. But he likes listening to my stories and what I'm learning about. He's a surprisingly good listener. He really listens, and he has a natural enthusiasm that comes from a basic appreciation of the fact that I'm trying. The fact that I could succeed at my projects is impressive too, but even if I didn't, he would applaud the effort. That's what eluded him as an actor: faith.

This voice, this . . . I guess . . . character, Sel, I tell him, *is very strange. Now I know how actors feel, when they completely inhabit a character. She's like a muse.*

Your inner child, he jokes.

My future self, I joke back. *Anyway, it's been great fun. I'm learning a lot, doing the research too. I have to figure out what it's all about. It's intense to just always have this voice in my head. It's like when you're obsessed.*

Oh I don't know anything about that, he adds tartly, grinning.

He's talking about Boy Kelly. The one he's really wanted as a boyfriend for so long, knowing it's never going to happen. They're best friends now, though; a close second.

~ 13

I've been home a few weeks and I'm still unpacking and reviewing everything that happened here while I was gone. I still haven't read through all the AIDS conference abstracts; there's a lot there. It's been so busy at the magazine too. My Berlin travel piece is done; that was fun to write, to remember being there. I'll send it to Philippe. Which reminds me I have to follow up with CCR, the Center for Constitutional Rights, about the Haiti case. They probably want me to go back to Haiti for more interviews but I can't go right now. I actually have a full-time job now, ha. Maybe early next year.

I just looked back at my calendar and I can't believe how intense the year has been already. Since January the Avengers have had what feels like non-stop actions and street zaps every month. I loved our Bryant Park Valentine's Day action where we reunited Gertrude Stein's statue with her lover Alice Toklas. Lesbian waltzing, it was great. I wasn't so good at it. There's so much fun creativity in the Avengers. So much play. And then the Dyke March, so amazing. I can't even write more about it here because there's too much to say. But twenty thousand women from everywhere in East Jesus. When we started organizing it, we really didn't know who would show up. Clearly lesbians have just been waiting for someone to throw big, street, girl protest parties. I was happy a lot of the boys came to cheer us on too. Robert Hilferty wants to be an Avenger pretty bad. Next year we're going to do the Dyke March here and I bet it's going to be a big deal too. Plus we got a *Newsweek* article that really put us on the map. So a lot of people know about us. Even before the DC march we kept hearing about new groups, and now, it's like mushrooms popping up in all these little corners of the country. Some are just one or two girls, but they're an Avenger chapter. It's fantastic. I don't think we ever anticipated this much success, even if we dreamed of it. I mean maybe Sarah Schulman and Ana Simo did; they always have grand visions for lesbians. But I think we're all pretty happily surprised.

I'd like to go hang with the Austin Avengers; they seem like a really fun group. Fierce ladies. Plus two-stepping. That could be fun to learn. Probably easier then waltzing. And I like the idea of wearing boots and spurs. Takes me back to my childhood. I lived in cowboy boots when I was five.

I'll probably go north first, if I go anywhere with the Avengers. Ana Simo and some other New York Avengers went to Tampa earlier this year; I couldn't.

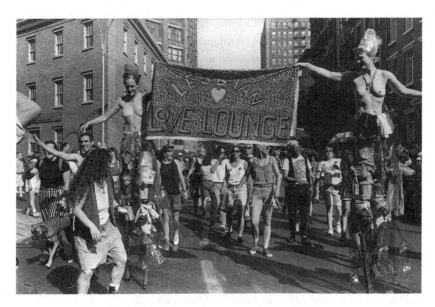

Lori E. Seid's Lesbian Love Lounge, Dyke March, 1993. (Dona Ann McAdams)

It's one of the places where antigay violence is up, some of it linked to Christian activist groups. The same thing is happening in all these places including Maine and Colorado. They have neo-Nazi groups there too. Scary guys.

There's been a boycott of Colorado over antigay Amendment 2. There, the Colorado Avengers have gotten some good press for their actions. Some of them chained themselves up to the gates of the governor's mansion, and I think they were even planning to chain themselves to the governor himself until they realized that might be really serious, like attacking a police officer or something. Real jail time. Certainly sounded rad. I wonder if they ate fire? I wanna see the demo pix.

Now there's Maine. A local group, Equal Protection Lewiston, has asked for help and the Avengers are already up there. There's a gay rights ordinance that's under attack. I think the antigay group Focus on the Family is putting their money behind the attack like they have in Colorado. We need to think of how to go after their leader. He's such a homophobe. That group has so much money. Anyway, Maine. I want to go and hope Jersey will come. *Road trip!*

Before I finish this roundup, I want to mention what ACT UP has done this year too. I feel like I go to the meetings every week and I still miss things that people do, there's just so much, and so many affinity groups and now we're in so many cities too. This year started with the Hoffmann–La Roche action by the Treatment Action Committee; it was a great, successful action. Then a bunch of fax zaps and actions against Jerry Falwell and the Moral Majority and the Christian Right. ACT UP has also been involved in Colorado around Amendment 2. And then all the immigration work before and after Berlin, around Guantánamo. The Haitians who were brought here have been resettled, it's so impressive. Housing Works with Charles King is on fire.

Well okay, we did lose on the HIV immigration policy. Clinton said he wants to lift it and instead he's kept it there. That's a failure to move ahead. No question about that. But we still have had a lot of victories. A huge one is the trifecta around women's HIV issues: the female condom got approved; cervical cancer got added to the definition of AIDS after our fighting about this for so long; and the first Women's Interagency HIV Study, called WIHS, is about to start with some great feminist research docs in charge. I met some of them in DC where we had a meeting with DC health officials over HIV issues for lesbians. It's really interesting research and I'm going to keep track of the project as it develops. We're going to learn a lot about the disease and meds in women, especially black women and women with histories of domestic abuse and IV drug use. Those are some of the categories. So kudos to the women in ACT UP and the research docs. *Chapo*, as we say in Haiti—*hats off*.

There's been other good news too. Our pal Tony Kushner, who's an amazing writer, got a Pulitzer for *Angels in America*, which everyone says is wild and great and I can't wait to see. I bet it's going to open so many eyes and hearts, at least I hope so. Tony's famous now. It's so well deserved. He's such a mensch too.

I almost forgot: WACO happened. That crazy clash between the Branch Dividians sect and the FBI. That has been so dramatic. Wacko Waco. Really, it's been an intense year. And it's not even over. We're still fighting the school board over the Rainbow Curriculum. It already got so badly gutted since our Queens Avenger action and now the city is pushing abstinence, which is insanity in this epidemic. So we can't rest on any of our laurels. Plus Saint Pat's. I forgot to mention that. We still can't freely march and spill our queer green beer with the Irish drunks in that damn parade. I'm sure ILGO and the Avengers will come up with a good action for us to do by March. *Dancing lesbian leprechauns?* I can see it already. Maybe Aldyn will join us. He does such a good Irish brogue. Plus his nice legs in green tights; it'd be *magically delicious*, like in a Lucky Charms ad.

~ 14

I've had a small revelation. A psychological one. I was thinking about my conversation with Johnny about Sel, about this invasion of an inner voice, separate from me and yet not. *What's this all about? Seeing her when I close my eyes, before I'm dreaming. Feeling her present the moment I'm awake. Hearing . . . really hearing her.* It's like I have a parallel soundtrack at all times. It also feels different from conscious daydreaming, which I did madly as a child in school, to the point where teachers noted this problem year after year in my report cards. *Anne has an active fantasy life.* I'm sure I was bored in school. But this is really another level of inner conversation; it's just so . . . unbidden. And I just today realized what's so familiar about the experience.

When I was five, wearing my black cowboy boots with spurs and a hat and being a fast gunslinger, newly living in Fort Lauderdale, Florida, with my parents and two older siblings, I had an imaginary friend. Roy, after my television hero, Roy Rogers. (*I know, this dates me.*) Roy was my constant companion, to the point where my mother would set a place at the dinner table for him, put some extra food on my plate. She'd come into my room and ask: *Who are you talking to, darling? Is it Roy?* Or ask, *Is your friend going to school with you today? Is he here right now?* And I would get annoyed, for she should know. *Of course Roy is here.* And I'd say to Roy—in our silent language—*Can you believe she's asking that? She can't see you. Only I can see you.*

When I was older, of course, I imagined my parents might have felt some mild concern, might have wondered if my overactive imagination was slipping into some worrisome zone of mental health. I have relatives on my mother's side—two of her siblings, both dead now—who suffered from chronic depression. There can be early signs in children. I know, because my parents spent years after my sister's breakdown looking back for them. (*I blame the mescaline.*)

In retrospect, I suspect I was probably depressed and lonely in our new backwater Florida subdivision on a canal with scary water moccasins and rattlesnakes and a new school and my best friend back in Michigan. We had traded cowboy boots; hers were pointed and cool. *Is that why I'm invaded anew?* I've definitely been feeling so blue over the Aerialist and Johnny. Has my sorrow reopened an emotional door? Is that why the childhood memories have flooded me? I wonder. Who is she then, Sel, for me? What alter ego? She's got an edge, no doubt about it. I'm curiouser and curiouser, as Alice said. But I'm not overly worried. I don't think I'll lose myself in any permanent way here. I survived my childhood, didn't I? The question here is the degree of this internal journey. The depth of this rabbit hole and where it leads me. To darker places or some inner wonderland?

~ 15

I'm fully back in my New York life now; back into a bit of personal chaos. The ninth floor of the NYU library—*Science*—has become a refuge from my *other* life, from work, from AIDS, from Manhattan and its intense energy, from the tumult of my personal relationships, from my heart, ever in conflict.

I broke up with the Aerialist, right?—but we *are* lesbians; we don't let go very easily. It's that female tendency, which I don't particularly admire, to hold on. We've upheld the stereotype; acted like a pair of praying mantis—*mantids?*—who get stuck when they couple, then begin to devour each other. In our violent act of separation each of us dies a bit.

So many months have gone by. I've seen her out socially a few times, always in passing. We've moved on; we've both have other amours. Belle's made it clear she wants to remain in an open relationship. Before meeting her, I had a little fling with a roomie of Johnny's too. He has two. A rather adorable, brassy, too young *affairlet*. I have no idea how it even happened, but to be fair to her, she made it happen. Sometimes these young women are very persistent. And why say no to a light affair with someone adorable? *Mais pourquoi?* It was fun, a few weeks of winter affection.

I don't know about the Aerialist. She's been seeing other people, I know. It's what she wanted, why she broke up, in part. But I don't want to know the details. It still hurts. Now I heard she's getting into another intense relationship. It feels quick, but who am I to judge?

When the Aerialist meets me for a catch-up coffee, she says she still feels the old feeling of missing me. Her push-pull feelings. *Pull me in close enough, then push me away. Then disappear.* A drama that kept me stuck for so long. *Why did I stay, then?* I loved her; I wanted it to work. The main reason most people stay in un-satisfying relationships. And it felt more painful to let go. The classic lie we tell ourselves to avoid the loss we already feel.

Now, silence dominates our attempts at conversation—long pauses, not much to say. Moments that remind me of why we couldn't make it work, why, from the beginning, the odds were stacked against us. If we have a hard time talking now, it's not a new problem. We always had a hard time communicating; that's why our physical relationship was so important and so strong. Whenever language broke down, we could touch, we could come together anyway. We would throw each other around like rag dolls, like two beasts in the forest tussling, we would joke—testing our strength, holding nothing back. Rough and tender. I felt met in that place of force. When our physical connection broke down, the bridge finally collapsed. *Yuck,* I think, leaving her each time. *Yuck, yuck, yuck. She has nothing to say to me.*

The last time we went out, I tried to talk to her about my book, about Sel, and the evenings I'm spending in the library; my research into the guillotine and the French who collaborated with the Nazis. She began by being supportive, curious, even enthusiastic, and I felt heartened—*she still wants to be a part of my life, of whatever it is I'm doing without her.* I felt her genuine love for me in that moment. She was smiling, gently, and nodding, as she read some early pages of my Paris diary. I felt the old love flow back.

Then, without warning, a mask replaced her open face and the lover I could never talk to was chewing her cheek, familiarly critical. *Why are you writing about this? Why did you leave that out?* Her expression was ambivalent; her questions sharp and stinging as darts. Something wasn't sitting right with her. An old familiar feeling. *Push-pull. Old stuff.*

I stare down at the first floor of the NYU library, its lovely maze of black, white, and gray geometry. I imagine myself a human rat, trying to navigate it from one corner of the floor to another. The maze is my relationship to the Aerialist: here we are, taking a wrong turn, turning right instead of left; now we're backtracking, but it's no use, we're headed down a blind alley again. *Still in the fog*, I think.

~ 16

When is it that love blooms? The exact moment when the heart begins to beat a bit faster, the senses become alert to the presence of another? With Jersey, as with other lovers I've had, the first moment passed unnoticed by both of us, though Jersey easily recalls our first meeting. In her version, it was after the first Avengers action in Queens last November, at the start of the new school season. In mine, it was a bit later, but definitely before Halloween. That's when we built an Avengers shrine to Hattie Mae Cohens and Brian Mock, victims of a murderous hate crime in Oregon, and slept for a few nights on the sidewalk in a makeshift encampment in the West Village. Jersey was beautiful, a looker. If I had a type, which I sort of do (at least one type if not more), she was it: Jewish, dark hair, smart, fun, and a little feisty. Not a femme, but a sort of tomboy femme, one with good fashion. She was sexy and she knew it, and that was part of her considerable charm.

Jersey was new to activism, graduated from the University of Michigan, my birth state. She would arrive at the meetings a little late, sit in the back. She didn't talk much. She smiled. I smiled but we both played it cool. Later I realized she was in no good position to be flirting with me or anyone because she had two girlfriends, not one, and both weren't that happy with her. And I was in lust-to-love with Belle already and in a postbreakup dance with the Aerialist, who came to Avenger meetings too. We tried to be friendly-to-neutral, as ex-girlfriends, but we had so much history, it was tricky. It wasn't bad drama, but we would sometimes end up making out, at the end of a good-bye, to our mutual surprise. *Oh my God what are we doing?* At other times we would feel the distance, the detachment. *How were we ever lovers? Who is this person? Does she even remember me?* But it really was over and both of us were moving on. She knew I had fallen for Belle and now she could see I was hot for Jersey. I think she was happy for me to not be unhappy about her, but still sad about us. That too is the lesbian breakup way.

I was one of the founders of the group, so I was a cheerleader, helping to get things going in those first days. But I had also learned a critical lesson of activism: to shut up, to let others talk, to talk last if you're a talker like me who has a lot to say and could fill the whole meeting with my opinions. I opted to facilitate the meetings at times, assuring I couldn't talk too much myself, though I probably did and I still do. But I try to give others space. I want to know their opinions. So I paid attention to Jersey, and when she hadn't said much, if I was facilitating, I would look her way, invite her to respond.

I looked forward to seeing her at our weekly Avenger meetings at the Gay and Lesbian Community Center, where I feel like I've been living part-time for a while now. It's like I have three homes: my apartment on Seventh Street, the *Out* office at 50 Greene Street in Soho, and the center. I move constantly between them during the week. Johnny's house is pretty near the center, in the meat-packing district, so that makes a fourth stop. It's easy to run over from the center and take a quick nap.

In the fall of '92, the Avengers were exploding. Every day was an adventure with more girls turning up. I say girls because we think of ourselves that way though we're grown women and some of us have children and we're serious about our politics. I remember the fall air was already crisp and the big, ochre autumn moon hung low between the buildings like a surreal vision at the end of the street. The days blended into nights. And at some point, by the spring, Jersey became the place I was headed.

If Philippe thinks my love life is complicated, he should spend time with Jersey. She's the queen of triangles, and she's always the one in the middle, juggling lovers. Or so she led to believe. I've never heard what her past lovers have to say about it. Maybe they were juggling lovers too. Clearly we're all a bunch of fire-eating, lover jugglers, us modern sapphists. I'm making light of this, because I was laughing about it, laughing at Jersey when first I met her and realized her predicament. It was like an Italian farce, like the lover who is slipping out of one lover's house at night to wake up in another lover's bed in the morning. Jersey felt bad about her predicament too, like all guilty lovers. I was sympathetic because I had done that, at a much younger age. But I couldn't handle the drama, for one. I didn't want to be so pulled. It was hard enough to want Belle and recognize Belle loved me but was not ready for the relationship I was, and that we lived in different countries and that she accepted our bond as an open one, but not the priority. *Just save a little for me.* But I am monogamous, or at least monogamish—I wanted to have a girlfriend who was available.

I can hear you, reader, hear you say: *So that's why you got involved with someone with two lovers already. Because she was so available?*

I don't claim to walk my talk, only talk it. I try to walk it though. I do. And I didn't get involved with Jersey until she was already free of one relationship and ending the other. I believed her when she said those relationships were really over for her, and they seem to be. She's had some processing, but she's not in them anymore. She's with me. We're not saying we're monogamous, but we're girlfriends. She knows I love Belle and want our bond to continue if I can make it work and keep it drama-free.

<hr>

Our aha moment happened in a millisecond, an instant of, *Yes, I see you . . . Well, hello!* I was driving, on the way to an action. In DC, though I'll have to ask Jersey. For some reason I think we were driving her car, but I was driving and she was in the back seat. We were excited; whenever the Avengers are together we're excited. We're energized by protest. So I was driving, and another girl was in the front, and there was Jersey, who somehow, by some miracle, had ended up in my car, or I was driving her car. And I moved to adjust the rear-view mirror, and I looked back and I caught her looking back at me. And I smiled. We both agree that was the moment. *Hello. You're super hot. I like you.*

Except it wasn't simple, because of her two lovers. She needed to break up with both of them, as she explained to me later that same day, before we could have a date. And I think she managed to break the news to one before our first date, then the other soon after, and then it got harder before things settled into a new reality. She kept sleeping with both lovers for a while, crying and letting each other go. She had loved both of them and both had loved her. Someone always loses, or often does. Their triangle had been hard for months by the time she had met me. So she was in the doghouse with her exes. It was a little messy for her. But I didn't pressure her and she didn't pressure me. She didn't ask me to stop seeing Belle or loving her. She knew I had been dating other people and didn't expect me to end anything for her—or vice versa. We just liked each other—a lot—and the chemistry was mad, and there was time now to just enjoy getting to know each other, however fast or slow. So we took our time, and very soon, we were girlfriends.

Welcome to the lesbian way.

~ 17

I've met one of Sel's friends, Henri. No last name, no introduction, not much of a smile. Henri simply appeared recently, much as Sel did, lurking on the edges of my waking day. A name, a face, a body, a personality. A set of issues, though what they are isn't exactly clear. But Henri has them—issues, I mean—in spades. He won't be easy to sort out. Even now, he resists coming closer so that I can get a better look at a tattoo I just spied on his arm. But I've been able to observe a lot.

The first time I spied Henri, he was leaning against a pillar near the Pont Alexandre. Far in the distance was Sel. They weren't talking to each other, but I could tell they were friends, familiar acquaintances. Like two actors frozen on the stage until the curtain rises for them to speak. Henri was lounging, a favorite activity of his, casually but with purpose, eyeing all that passed with a cool, impassive regard. Sel was fishing.

Henri's a former street kid, a survivor, a tough young man who's seen a lot. He lives by his own rules and habits, superstitions and rituals. That's what appeals to Sel about Henri: he's an original, an outsider like she is. But he's loyal—a true friend to a chosen few, including Sel. He calls her *la vielle*: the old lady.

Physically, Henri is also attractive in a rough way. He's quite small—almost a dwarf. Henri might have posed for Picasso, or my favorite artist, Max Beckmann; he's all flat planes and angles, sharp black lines. He has a gymnast's body, with a big chest in proportion to narrow hips. He's muscular, with strong arms and legs. His short stature contrasts sharply with the sense of power and energy he exudes—a contained, explosive energy. He has dirty-blond hair and flinty-gray eyes; his skin is almost leathery from living outdoors so long. His brow juts; his eyebrows are thick and run together above a flat, crooked nose, the result of a childhood fight. He has a thick neck and several tattoos. His teeth are small and stained gray, the top molars sharp, like a vampire's. He has a generous, moist mouth. His hands, like his feet, are large for his body.

He's also pigeon-toed, slightly bow-legged, and flat-footed, which has earned him a popular street name: Pigeon. He walks like one. And he has a bad habit of loudly and compulsively cracking his knuckles against any surface: the wall, his cheek, his knee. Which he's doing right now, waiting for someone. A john, I think. He's a hustler, Henri. A half-gypsy, half-French bastard pigeon man. Few people know about the gypsy connection. It's Henri's hidden side. The buried, still-tender wound. *His shame-pride.*

Henri also has an unusual reputation—it's something of a joke in his circle, but there's a bit of truth to it—as the smallest male whore in Paris and a big top. For the latter reason, he rarely lacks for admirers or tricks; he's an object of fascination and obsession for women as well as men who desire other men. His own taste runs to older, working-class men—truckers, construction workers. He finds married men easiest to handle. He likes darker men, darker boys too, but not young ones. He doesn't have patience for youth, for silly boys. He's a man's man.

Emotionally, he's wound very tight and doesn't share himself quickly with friends. He's choosy. But, like Sel, he enjoys a good joke, and pranks, and knows how to have fun. Drinking, playing soccer, taking physical risks. He loves thrills. In the evening, after dusk, he climbs buildings, using his bare hands and feet, a budding urban alpinist. Sel is convinced he'll take it all too far one day.

Henri claims it relaxes him. Getting away from everyone, above the fray, away from it all. Helps with his jitters, as he calls his Tourette's, a condition he inherited from his mother. Over the years, he's learned to control the symptoms, to predict an attack. But not always. When he gets angry, or very excited— watching his favorite team losing a soccer match, for example—he sometimes loses control a bit: little tics that his closest friends notice. His eyes twitch. When he's upset, he bites down on his tongue to keep it still, to avoid an inappropriate verbal outburst. Swearing, admonishments, noises like grunts that deeply embarrassed him and his family when he was a child. Now it amuses him, to see how uncomfortable people become, how alarmed. *Frightening the horses*, he jokes to Sel.

With his condition, Henri managed to avoided military service. He dropped out of school early but learned to love books, helping a book vendor with a stall along the Seine near the Sorbonne. He also works odd jobs: loading and unloading furniture at the flea market in Saint-Ouen, light construction, occasional security gigs for a friend who hosts outdoor concerts.

Given his unusual reputation, Henri rarely lacks for interested clients and can afford to be selective. He also rarely tricks with the same john twice, regardless of the money. He doesn't want them getting too familiar. More often than not, he'll turn down a trick. Above all, he likes to climb. Go find a spot far above the city with the rest of the pigeons to smoke or take a sitting nap, undisturbed.

Salut, Henri.

~ 18

Hours past midnight. It's raining. Outside, the late fall air is turning crisper. The drafty windows in the living room are rattling, but otherwise all is quiet. The sky is the color of a church mouse, and the fat, yellowish moon that hung so close to the rooftops last night is nowhere to be found. I look at the rectangular streets, the ugly buildings of Manhattan. I'm feeling a little down tonight, missing Belle a bit. Jersey is out with a friend. I miss her too. I was so inspired when I was in Paris. Here, there's no sense of history in the buildings or the landscape. Everything in New York conspires to make you live in the present; whatever exists today gets forgotten, and then physically erased.

Few of my friends here, native-born or recent arrivals, know much about the history of this city: who built the buildings and parks, what famous club was located down the street, what great musician or actor once transformed their sublet into a soirée. That's the charm and downside of urban America in general: everything is for immediate consumption, including people, ideas, and culture. Few bother to take a look back, to see where it all might be going.

In the few short years I've lived on this block of Avenue C, a dozen stores have opened and closed in the neighborhood, tenements have been razed and others refurbished. Neighbors move out before you have had a chance to introduce yourself. To be a New Yorker is to be a flexible pragmatist, a realist; to accept the high price of living and the conspiracy of short-lived trends; to be mobile and accept the transient nature of friendships, apartments, jobs.

What's happening in and around Tompkins Square Park is a case in point. It's still half taken over by a homeless encampment, and the police just keep arresting and moving people out. I don't know where they're going. And they're not fixing up the buildings that they've shuttered around the park. I just feel like the city is changing and not in a good way. I mean, it was bad years ago with all the drugs. I was definitely a little scared when I came down here for the first time, way back when. So much heroin. And there are still a lot of shooting galleries here, toward Avenue D. But they're closing the little mom and pop stores right and left and opening fancier grocery stores, and we're losing the barrio flavor just like we're losing the old Jewish stores below Houston Street. I'm glad we still have all the bodegas but I wonder for how long. It's depressing. Or maybe I'm just feeling low.

———

Back in bed, I listen to the occasional hush of passing cars, the same sound they make as they cross the Pont Alexandre, where Henri is leaning, still waiting for a trick or some excitement; maybe a friend. He hasn't developed his potential as a character, as an independent actor. I close my eyes, spy him, focus to get a closer look. He's hustling, waiting for something, or someone.

Henri gives me his familiar shy scowl. Seconds later, a balding middle-aged man approaches. He walks past Henri, barely acknowledging him. Then hesitates, looks quickly back. A second later, Henri is following him, keeping a steady distance.

When I wake, confused for a minute by my surroundings, the sun is blazing through my bedroom window; the restaurant below and across the way is open. I'm exhausted. Time for a café and a smashed sandwich Cubano with extra pickles and maybe a *morir soñando*. Whatever I've scribbled onto the legal pad by my pillow is nearly an illegible scrawl. I've written it blindly, not daring to open my eyes, to leave the half-dream state I was in when I wrote it, when I spied Henri turning down a street with the older man following him.

Now, as I struggle to decipher the words, the fragments of description and conversation, it all comes back: *the temperature of the night; the man's shiny pate, nervous as he follows Henri; the winding backstreets Henri takes, over and across the bridge onto the Île de la Cité, where he finds a spot on a bench out of sight of the tourists. Where he kills time waiting for the man, whom he knows without asking is probably married, with a wife and children at home, a commuter from the suburbs who'll claim he missed the train, then got hungry.*

Henri saw it in his eyes right away: an expression of tortured hope from a man desperately trapped in a lie. He feels sympathy for men like this, closeted men who are sometimes content just to run their hands over Henri's tiny, massive chest, his muscular back. *Pay me first*, Henri growled. *No talking.*

It's all still here, his voice, his character, his possible story. Just behind my eyes, just under the veil of an ordinary day. I feel like weeping with gratitude. I don't hear it as constantly or without searching as Sel's. But I can find him if I

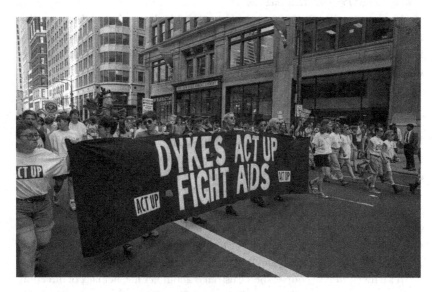

Where the Girls Are . . . Dyke March, NYC, July 1994. (Diane Gabrysiak)

go deeper, try for a dreaming state, work to stay in the liminal zone between sleep and consciousness.

Vivir soñando.

⌒

I was born a nocturnal creature, it seems. I feel most alive at night, when everyone else is sleeping. Night after night, I sit in the kitchen in total darkness, sipping a glass of wine, an insomniac with my eyes wide open. I think about my life, about my friends, the books that are being written, the ideas and ideals that still mean something, the people who interest me. I think about what it means to be alive, right now, in this period of history; what it means to be a lesbian in late twentieth-century America, New York, the East Village; a woman who gets mistaken for a man much of the time; a woman of thirty-five who still feels young. I could never have predicted the social changes that have happened just in the span of my adult life. Rapid, radical changes.

I look down on my own life from a great distance, through the lens of the future. *How will all this, including my small life, be viewed in a hundred years? This time? This epidemic? In a thousand? What should I be doing with my precious allotment of life? Am I doing enough?*

I've thought these same thoughts all my life. For years, looking out on quiet streets in the dead of night, happy to be awake at least.

No desire to sleep. I want to suck everything there is out of every moment. My mind is on fire as always, a mental fever. My eyes itch. I sleep poorly. *It's night again and I'm alive. How lucky am I?*

I know you may feel this way too, reader. Maybe you're reading past the hour of sleep right now, chasing the tail end of a long day, refusing tomorrow. Stealing time from your own precious life; expanding it from within. You too would choose to *vivir y morir soñando.*

~ 19

I've started cutting away blocks of time from my day job at *Out* to sneak into the great stone-and-glass library at New York University. I feel like Sel, an imposter, gaining access to state secrets with an out-of-date ID, this one from the University of Michigan, where Jersey wasted her college years, so she says, skiing. She wanted to be an Olympic skier, might have had the talent, didn't have the drive. Skiing represents ultimate freedom to her; truest happiness. For years, now, she's had a recurring dream: she's at the ski lift, ready to go, and she can't get up the mountain. There's always a different reason why.

It's a metaphor, of course: she's frustrated about her life, her lack of direction and career. Other times she'll wake up and describe it to me, the feeling of a pure rush greater than sex, or as great, with no one and nothing to stop her, just her and the snow, her and nature, her and being, moving, vaulting, flying over moguls—free.

⌒

The minute I enter the library I'm giddy with anticipation. Whole worlds await; the entire universe. I'm like a child in a candy shop: I can't get enough, can't read fast enough, can't absorb enough. I work feverishly, combing the card catalogs and computer files randomly, jotting down or printing out any-thing that might be relevant to what I'm now thinking of as a kind of false novel. I'm a fake student posing as a scholar researching a bogus historical novel from a first-person journalistic perspective that's closer to a memoir by someone with a bad memory. And I feel high as a kite. I don't need anything but this, I think: words, books, lives, ideas, knowledge. I can go for hours like this, ignoring my hunger, my thirst, even my need to pee, until it's so urgent I silently race to the bathroom.

I'll never catch up, of course, but it doesn't bother me. I'll never know enough French history, never mind world history, to write the kind of story I want. I'm too poorly educated from the start to catch up, for starters. No, Sel's story will have to be brought to life through random forays and mental leaps, odd associations, things I connect that nobody else would. A personalized approach to historical redress.

⌒

Once again I have a short but ambitious list of subjects to research. It's easier for me to read in English than French but that's not a problem here; Americans are Francophiles; there are a lot of English-language books on the subject of modern French history, several rows just on the river Seine itself. I'm beginning to realize the benefits of academia: to be able to lose oneself in absolutely arcane corners of knowledge, and get paid for it.

I've also stumbled on a field of scholarly research new to me, one I could get a PhD in at Yale: the history of medicine. I never even knew it existed as a subcategory of history until recently. Had I known, I might have pursued a degree, become a proper scholar. Ah, well, another life not lived. Meandering through the library stacks, I trail my hand from subject to subject—*herbs, astron-omy, physics*—and my mind takes off on another narrative tangent. I'm deter-mined to rein myself in. I'm culling and sifting today, like a miner, panning for the nuggets of gold that have true value to this story. That build a narrative arc, as my book agent likes to say.

I pull out the old-fashioned card catalog. I want to brush up on medieval science, the early alchemists, review the basics. Sel, I sense, knows about metals and their properties, so I must too. I may brush up on my chemistry. Reread Primo Levi's *The Periodic Table*. I've become curious about all the waste going into the Seine: what can it do to the body? What kind of cancers, mutations can it cause?

My hand stops at the row of books labeled *S*. Just here, alone, I have enough to keep me reading for months: *Salt, Sanson, Seine, Space, Syphilis* . . .

I could live in this library; I could set up a little bed over there in the corner. There's no better view in Manhattan. The dying sun casts a burnt-orange glow over the trees in Washington Square Park. I see a squirrel jumping from tree to tree. *Who are all these people, spending their day indoors, like me?* I'm especially interested in the older ones, the scholars. I'm envious of the physics graduate students, the Japanese girl I sat behind today who silently and absently unwrapped a huge chocolate bar as she worked out complex math equations. I want to be that smart. I want to be a Stephen Hawking. I want to understand everything I might about our mysterious universe, whatever we are and what we are becoming. My hand is deep in the candy jar, surrounded by all this knowledge and information. An infinite rabbit hole.

I'm thumbing through the French cahiers with their nice paper that I filled with quickly scribbled notes all those weeks in Paris. My notes and drawings looks like a surrealist's, something that demands considerable interpretation. I see Sel's name everywhere, and arrows, wild snaking arrows. I've highlighted words in my notes: *mud, pillage, war lust, radiation, buboes*. My lousy sketches of things I was fascinated with in the medical museum: hand-forged obstetric tools, syringes with bulbs as big as onions to help push the medicine down through the needle.

My eyes stop. I love this word, *buboes*. I take a random stab at deciphering the page. It's not easy. *Le mal français*. Ah yes, I was taking notes about syphilis, the concubine's favorite friend. Considering it as a possible historical source of Sel's hybrid pox, one that spawned and flowered in the *misfeasance*—another favorite word—of the bacterial dumping grounds at Montfaucon. The poxed sailor, Columbus the Portuguese, carried the buboes of the Old World to the new. When Charles VIII retreated to Italy, his mercenaries were marked also with the scourge. They called it *Le Mal de Naples*. *Of course the French blamed it on the Italians*, I think. *When it comes to disease and blame, it's always someone else's fault.* The painful chancre first appeared in Lyon, then in Paris, in the autumn of 1496, and in ten years all of Europe was infected.

What's this? Another bad sketch I've attempted. *La chute du nez*—the classic signs of tertiary syphilis. A face with a falling nose, like a pig's rotting snout. Which reminds me of poor Michael Jackson, his destroyed nose, and of all the Jewish girls pressured to go under the knife to look more like a shiksa. Of course, these days the boys and men get nose jobs too.

Il n'y a pas de cure sans mercure. There is no cure without mercury. For decades, mercury was used to treat the chancres of syphilis, in combination with the bark of a tree from Hispaniola, the island now called Haiti where my own Papa was born. The tree was called guaiac and was taken back to the Old World by Columbus's men. But the treatment was hardly effective, and mercury left its own marks: trembling muscles, injury to the kidneys, and other internal organs.

I can see Sel in my mind's eye right now: trembling, delirious. Mistaken for an old wino with the shakes.

Sel falls down in the gutter. She can smell the Seine in the trickle of dirty water used to clean the sidewalks. She can barely see the river, but when she looks up, she sees Columbus, riding high, sitting astride the prow like a figurehead. The Portuguese sailor is a beast; what was once a nose flaps like a truffle in the wind. His men look just as bad. Some of them grip the side of the tall ship to steady themselves, their muscles weak. They've adorned their bodies with plunder, with gold, and bright beads, and velvet. They recall the women they bedded with the reverie of virginal boys. And their eyes continue to burn bright with folly and madness.

In my mind's eye, it's like a scene from Werner Herzog's epic film *Aguirre, the Wrath of God*, about the obsessed early world adventurer whose men became poxed and died.

Sel's face is pocked and so are her arms and legs—pocked and scarred from her childhood experiments in cutting off some offending pustules—some buboes—to let the blood and water flow from her swollen legs, to release the fever of fire in her bones. She suffers from blinding headaches that make her cry out and allow others to dismiss her as insane.

I close my eyes to inspect her pitted face, the scars. Like Vito with KS, she's disfigured from her chronic journey with a regiment of warring poxes. What did she look like, as a child?

~ 20

This afternoon when I woke up I had been dreaming about Sebastien. A good man, with a learned aversion to risk. He lives what I consider a quietly exemplary life, with a level of personal moral clarity and self-discipline, and still he suffers. It's just life, and how unfair it can be; how we don't get to choose, not every hand, not every play. Nor can we give the cards back. So I woke sad about him today, and let some tears come, though there is nothing tragic about his life, per se, just fear of a disease that's haunting him, making everything difficult, frightening, unsafe.

Death is all around him, closer than it is to me because he's more physically vulnerable to it, given his sexual life, his age. Like Johnny he's living in the age of the gay pox. And he's terrified of it. Something of that vulnerability and how much I'd like to protect Sebastien and give him strength will be a part of my narrative. Something about how, like so many of his generation, he's been robbed of sexual joy, of sexual exploration, how sex and his essential identity have become one with fear—his deepest fears about his sexuality, what others deem an uncontrollable sexual nature: homosexuality. One that makes him sexually vulnerable yet sexually desiring, and one, he fears, that may one day lead him to a premature death.

Though, I have to stress, Sebastien's fine and independent and doing well for himself in all the material ways, is a success in his family's eyes, I want to mother him right now as I do Johnny. I want to line the narrow box he's drawn for himself with cotton and soften the fearful interactions he has with the world that revolve around being gay and being sexual. He's come a long way to over-come his family's homophobia. But it's still in there, deep. In my dream, I directed my words to his parents, his friends: *Protect him. All of you, love and protect him.*

~ 21

Victory! After quite a bit of searching and making sense of the NYU card catalog, I've found one of the books I was looking for in Paris. I'm very pleased. The small, private pleasures of the twentieth-century, amateur history sleuth. This book wasn't written that long ago. I put it on my head with two other books about execution, trying to tiptoe back to my little hiding place in the stacks without dropping them. Walking like I practiced as a young girl in Haiti with my cousins, perfecting what I felt would lead to good posture, the way a princess might make an entrance to a ball. Slowly, carefully, neck straight, eyes ahead, smiling.

I open it with true pleasure, just as delicious as unwrapping a chocolate. *Legacy of Death*, a book about the Sanson executioners, by Barbara Levy, an aca-demic living in New Jersey. From 1635 to 1889, the Sansons were more feared and revered by the populace than the kings they served. I read for hours, then stop. The Sansons were—are—fascinating. *A family tree of outcasts.* It was all a forced labor assignment: if they refused to serve the king, they would be killed.

Two hours later, I've fallen asleep; there's drool on my notes. I try to make sense of my notes on the history of the Sansons, monsters of France. But I'm not alone; Sel's joined me. I pick up my pen, listening, as she tells me what she thinks about Charles-Henri Sanson—the Great Sanson, a royal executioner. A man she considers a historical soul brother of sorts, whose true legacy, she feels, is misunderstood by historians. Charles-Henri was promoted to the job of bourreau, or royal butcher, on Boxing Day in 1779, having served a twenty-year apprenticeship by his father's side. *Sanson was a slave,* Sel tells me, the rasp in her voice like a child with croup. *You can't think of him any other way. Born to slave parents and grandparents. Seven generations of royal slaves. Put your pen in his hand and let him tell you his story, from his perspective. How much of a monster is he now?*

It's tempting—as with so much of this history—to reconsider, revise. To step into the shoes of the monstrous man and consider his suffering. And it makes make me think: *What if I did that here, for Le Pen and his far right populist movement?* What if I approached them with compassion instead of rejection and a bit of fear? What if I looked at Jean-Marie Le Pen as an ordinary man, one with a real talent for politics, a true intelligence, and one with frailties: a father loved by his daughters; a zealous patriot? What then? If I stepped out of my own box, my own assumptions?

Sel's looking at me with curiosity, as if I've surprised her, for once. As if she's reconsidering me, her scribe.

Are you sure you're willing, child? It's not as easy as you imagine. You might become tarnished yourself. Viewed as a collaborator by others. Anyone who's willing to see the soul of a beast must be somewhat beastly too. Look how they view me. Like the insane one.

Then, like a sprite, she's gone. Leaving me stuck with the idea, this unexpected twist. *Rewrite the story of the Great Sanson? No.* It would take too much time, and it's too far away, historically, from our contemporary life. *Reconsider Le Pen, write his secret diaries?*

The idea compels me, intrigues me, makes me swoon a bit inside. *Would I dare?* I don't know. Somehow, I think it would be even harder than letting myself listen to Sel, my salty tart. But definitely an interesting exercise in historical redress. After Le Pen, I could choose so many others. Dizzying possibilities. Joan of Arc, for a start. She deserves historical reconsideration.

But Sel's right. I might be questioned, criticized, threatened even, for giving a man like Le Pen any measure of humanity that could make his own hatred more acceptable or comprehensible to the average citizen. Still, it's the right path, surely. Why? Because it makes me uncomfortable, for starters, unsure of what I'd find and feel myself. And it leaves me intrigued. Something Sel, *agent provocateur,* has stirred up. Well, she promised me unexpected turns, didn't she? This is certainly one.

10

Paris, de nouveau

~ 22

Winter 1993

It's almost six o'clock. I've gotten back to Paris sooner than expected and happily slipped into my earlier routine: *the Seine at dusk, the Seine at dawn.* It's colder but less so than in New York. I'm feeling fresh after another nap, this one on a bench that faces the entrance to Châtelet-Les Halles. This is where the marketplace used to be, extending all the way to the river. Les Halles, a market of odors, possibilities, and, of course, illegal activities. Now it's a gay, bohemian district leading to the Marais, a former swampland area that housed the original city of Paris. The shopping plaza is a kind of capitalist bunker with so many entrances and exits I think the architect who designed it simply couldn't stop once he got started. His vision—I'm assuming it was a him—is a gleaming, steel-tubed medusa, connecting every metro line, every underground tunnel, every long-lost sewer branch with some shop, or something or someone, to buy or sell. Perhaps he felt it was in keeping with the grandiose spirit of earlier French architects like Eiffel or Baron Haussmann, who built the broad Boulevard Haussmann that runs near here.

Whatever his motive, I always feel like I'm seeing the future of Paris—circa 2050, or 2080: an antiseptic, technological sci-fi wonder operated entirely by robot-computers that see no need for the local butcher, baker, or concierge. Except as consumers. A shopping megalopolis utterly lacking in soul. But gleaming. So shiny and new. Maybe even the robots that operate it will be forced to become consumers.

I'm raving a bit because I just got lost in its tentacles, having some time to kill before meeting Belle. And I couldn't find anyone inside who could point me in the right direction. All the humans seemed dwarfed, their sole attention on shopping and eating. I got lost because ever since Sel came on the scene (it seems so long ago already) my attention has been divided, though I haven't revealed even to Belle the extent to which I'm distracted.

96

Belle has been volunteering at the gay and lesbian center on the Rue de Turenne. It's a short walk along the Rue des Blancs Manteaux — the street of white coats. Every street name in Paris means something, tells a story. Who were the white coats? A battalion of waiters? I like the idea. Johnny would fit right in.

This street has become a principal gay artery, housing a number of bars and restaurants. I spot one where the ACT UP gang likes to go: Le Piano Zinc. It is owned by Jürgen, a German friend of Belle's who acts as paterfamilias and matchmaker to the AIDS activists, helping this one with a job, that one with a broken heart. He offers me drinks on the house whenever I'm in town.

The streets smell of cooking, bread, fish, garbage. It makes me happy. I'm walking not with Sel today but with Henri — that is, I'm looking through Henri's eyes at the young men standing at the bars, those who walk too slowly down the street.

There's a new French type — a gay type — that affects a look taken from French action comic books: men with hard jawlines and the aquiline French nose; men who look like their names should be Marc; good-looking men who have muscles and swear in English and wear white sneakers. They're the new French gay clones who have adopted the mania of the Americans and started working out at the gym during their lunch hours but also dine twice a week, on Wednesday afternoon and Sunday lunch, with their mothers. Mama's boys, posing as gigolos. This is a hustler's street; it's clear from the body language.

Belle is late. She's always late! I find my way to an unmarked door and knock, then ring the buzzer, which is broken. Behind another entrance, I find a winding inner stairwell. It's covered with graffiti, none of it legible. I take a seat on the cool stairs across from the door of the center and wait. It's close to 7:00 p.m.; the light I have clicked on automatically shuts off. I'm sitting in the semidarkness, enjoying the old, musty smell of the building and wondering if I'll come back to Paris to live for a while when I hear giggling. The door across from me opens and two heads peek out then disappear again. A minute later, they're back, a duo of dark-headed boys, one about five and the other maybe seven. I hear a rapid staccato of an Asian language and, a second later, a young woman comes out holding another infant in her arms. She smiles, surprised to see me, and then fires off something to her boys. *Va!* She's shooing them with her arm. Go!

They're beauties, with longish silky hair, plump bodies, and huge, shy smiles. The younger one edges past me, heading downstairs, his eyes never leaving my face. The older one is bolder. He stares at me, at my clothes, my pack, my very short hair, and my shoes. He makes a move for my sunglasses, which are in my shirt pocket, before his mother interferes, threatening a slap. Go!

He hurries downstairs and she smiles at me, shrugging apologetically, as if to say, *Boys will be boys.* Then she goes back inside, leaving the door open a crack. I take the opportunity to peek through and see the woman, still holding her baby, cooking over a hotplate. The apartment is a small room, very narrow and cramped. There's only a dim lightbulb and not much furniture. I imagine she's a recent immigrant who's raising her children alone or with a husband who works killer hours and is hardly ever home. I want to join them for dinner, to learn about their life, but I've caught the sound of a giggle and then I feel hands on my leg. The youngest boy has me. He's taken off his pants and is holding his diaper in his hands. Mama makes a face when she sees her naked son, but then laughs, seeing my own smile. *Il fait pipi*, she tells me, motioning downstairs to the toilet.

Yes, I see. You have to go downstairs to use the bathroom. Yes, I understand. Poverty, lack of facilities, poor maintenance of the building; you dare not make a complaint because they would try to evict you. We both shake our heads in understanding.

Bonsoir, she says, and pulls her boys in, bowing slightly.

⁓

Belle arrives breathing hard, apologizing. The time got away from her. She only has to give the keys to her colleague; he'll be up in a minute. We enter a small, well-lit room, one with a small desk and fax machine, and a small archive of magazines, including many from the United States. She's already explained to me how a group of French activists have fought the authorities to open this center, how they've had to get the approval of many different groups, and how the gay community is slowly beginning to come here to get help, referrals, support.

Compared to New York, or San Francisco—big cities where gay liberation and gay pride marches are well established; where there are a hundred different institutions and services for the gay community—the gay movement in Paris is still newish and those affected by AIDS are keeping quiet. They'll have a drink at a gay bar but they can't come out to their parents or their colleagues at work. Especially about AIDS. They won't go to an ACT UP meeting because it's too militant. And they're mostly white. There's been little ACT UP outreach to gays of color in the banlieues. All this Belle recounts to me in a litany of daily frustrations. She loves the movement and ACT UP–Paris, but, like me, she's critical of the group's shortcomings.

Her friend arrives. He's invited us to join another group of friends for dinner, then to have a drink, then to go to another bar and, after that, a party. It's a weekday night, but no matter. The night starts late in Paris and ends in the early morning or simply goes on. Some people work but many don't; they've been living on some form of the dole for years, and not too unhappily. They're looking for work, but the economy is so bad, it's not worth going off unemployment. The only thing that confuses me is how they still manage to go out. Everything is so outrageously expensive in Paris. If none of them have jobs, how do they manage to drink, eat, take taxis at dawn because the metro is closed? Whenever I ask someone this, they shrug and laugh. *We manage* is the best answer I get.

Before we leave, Belle listens to the answering machine. One message is from a mother in the provinces who is calling because she thinks her son is gay. She's worried about AIDS. He's fourteen. Could she bring him to the center?

It's a touching message. One that prompts Belle and her colleague to exchange a knowing smile. They know why they are doing this work. For women like this; for mothers and their gay sons. And it's a nice change from the crank calls and obscene threats.

Before we depart, Belle slips an AIDS information pamphlet under the door of the Asian family.

~ 23

Tonight we're hurrying to meet Gilles, who we're picking up for dinner before continuing on in a social evening in which Belle has promised to introduce me to nearly everyone who is important to her in Paris. As Belle describes him, Gilles is an original. A new friend who designs shoes. He intrigues her.

The first time we met, Gilles struck me as an overgrown child, which is a look he affects. He's a small man, delicate, but he has a brusqueness about him that makes him look thicker and stronger than he really is. He's got a rather large, egg-shaped, shaved head, which adds to his look of tough delicacy. And he likes wearing large shorts with small T-shirts that make his boyishly muscular body appear a bit at sea in a man's outfit. Gilles, the child-man.

Like Henri, Gilles wears clothes that mimic the hard men he is attracted to: sailors, soldiers, construction workers. But he's not doing it as a pose, or as a fashion statement, the way many gay men do. There's something of the genuine article in Gilles, in his toughness. An extreme hardness, an edge that contrasts with his childish vulnerability. That's what makes him appealing and what I've obviously transferred to Henri. I only realized it tonight.

It's an irony to me that Gilles is so involved in fashion, in women's feet, because he seems so much a man's man, one who has little connection to the

world of women, apart from friends like Belle—a man whose identity and eros
appear chiseled from everything that is not female. Gilles has the traits that I
often dislike in men—emotions, behaviors, and responses that I consider quint-
essentially male, even when a woman displays them: a level of emotional detachment and a certain self-regard that reads as egoism. On the flip side are the
positive qualities one can ascribe to these same attitudes: liberation from the need
to please people, independence, a spirit of abandonment, pursuit and enjoyment
of personal desires.

Gilles's fetish, besides male costumes, is pain. He likes a hard man—*un mec
dur*—who can take a lot of pain and give it too. A hard man who appears physically invulnerable and remote; who doesn't give himself easily, so that when he
does it is all the more precious. To hurt and love such a man: that's it for Gilles.
That's what I've observed in the short time we've seen each other. Enough
time for me to sketch a portrait of Henri.

Henri is not Gilles; I may end up disliking Henri. But I like Gilles and I
can't deny he remains a source of inspiration. Without trying to, I note small
details about him: the large pocket knife tucked invisibly into the big black
boots that he wears with thin socks; his little T-shirts tucked into his shorts, the
sleeves rolled up to his shoulders to emphasize his small, well-defined biceps;
his way of smoking, coolly, pensively; his ability to take up space without saying
anything; his habit of running his hand over his skull, absently, feeling for uneven bumps as he looks around the room, surveys the boys, the pickings. Belle's
right: he's a complex, charismatic guy, like Henri; a true original.

Gilles lives in a remarkable apartment, the kind of apartment that should have
disappeared in a Paris hell-bent on becoming a technological wonderland; an
apartment that could house a dozen families like the Asian mother with her
three young children. It's huge, with rooms giving into rooms, each one covered
with ancient fleur-de-lis wallpaper and high ceilings, replete with chandeliers
and grand mirrors and golden molding, and doorways that fold open and close
perfectly into the wall—all of it evidence of careful craftsmanship and wealth;
the bounty and taste of an earlier century.

I'm not a student of architecture; all I can think of is Marie Antoinette and
the kings of France and their extreme decadence and wealth. This apartment is
beautiful, unbelievable, and I can't help it: I feel slightly appalled that Gilles
lives here alone; that he's received this apartment from his employer as a free
sublet for a year in lieu of getting a raise. How do young Parisians who don't

make that much money live like royalty? Through a system of ongoing patronage, of lunchtime vouchers they've retained from past jobs, of small exchanges,
or simply unbelievable luck like this.

To his credit, Gilles is rather overwhelmed by his good fortune. And, being
the man he is, he doesn't feel guilty about it. At all. Quite the contrary. Rather
than share this apartment with a friend or several, he's relishing his Napoleon
fantasy and has furnished only one room with nothing more than a futon and
a tall, heavy candleholder in order to emphasize the vast splendor of his surroundings. We are invited to sit on the floor or the futon. And, instead of going
out to eat, Gilles has invited other friends over for an impromptu potluck.

This, too, is how the working French economize. While we wait, we open a
bottle of French wine, tour the apartment again to take in all the details, and
listen to Gilles tell us about his vacation in Normandy and about the boy he's
met. The man, to clarify. An older man. For the first time, Gilles says, he's
found someone who's come close. Someone who, to his great surprise, he has
wanted to spend night after night with, in a real bed. Not in a park or against a
nightclub wall. Since Gilles has made it one of his little rules not to bring home
the boys he tricks with, this revelation seems significant, based on how Belle
reacts, emitting a long, low whistle of appreciation. *You must really like him*, she
says. *I'm jealous already.*

Gilles tells us about the man's apartment, about his work, about his opinions,
which are strong, conservative, and apolitical when it comes to activism or
AIDS. *We're so different.* Gilles grins. *It's perfect.* The image he provides of his new
partner is of an emotionally reserved, closeted gay man, a social and political
libertarian, a capitalist, an elitist. *I've never met anyone like him.* Gilles laughs. *He's a
bit of a freak.*

I make a mental note of this: how Gilles likes extremity, inside-outsiders.
It's the same thing I've sensed in Henri. Will Henri also go for men whom he
can't possibly be like? A fascist man, maybe? Another intriguing mental side
note I make to myself. *Henri: will he go to the other side, get sucked in by Le Pen?*

Gilles's new love is a tough nut to crack, and he couldn't be happier. Yet
the more he describes him to us, the less enchanting his new paramour sounds;
the more he seems to me to be a man I'd want to kick in the balls.

Gilles does a little dance around the apartment. He's wearing another pair
of oversized shorts today and his head's freshly shaven—then, for no reason, he
suddenly makes me think of Sartre. Something about his egg-headed vulnerability, his dominating opinions, his enjoyment of an ideological battle with his
partner. He's equally delighted to be the bad boy—bad in that he's flirting with
the politically incorrect. For a second I see Henri entering the apartment, looking
around the rooms, seeing Gilles's small body stretched out naked on the futon

next to his hard-bodied older lover who is fully dressed in a business suit. Henri gives a little grunt and has a satisfied expression that says, *I see what this is all about. Power. Wealth. A rich Daddy-o.*

⌒

Our group tonight is a mixed bag: there are a few young boys from ACT UP; Christophe Martet, a journalist who started *Gai Pied*, the now-defunct monthly gay magazine (note *Gai*, not Gai *et Lesbienne*—a complaint Belle brings up to me later); one of Belle's former roommates and his new boyfriend. The conversation centers on the same topics that occupy most gay men and lesbians who don't know each other that well: sex, relationships, AIDS, and—because they're all planning to go away in July or August—their future holiday plans.

I retire to a corner to talk about the state of French journalism with Christophe, who I like a lot. He's a man like Aldyn who listens before talking, who's interested in opinions beyond his own, who has educated himself politically, who's not afraid to reveal his own ignorance. Christophe is well read, speaks other languages as well as English, and has traveled a lot. He loves a lot of things about the United States, especially the gay meccas of San Francisco and New York, but wouldn't necessarily want to live there.

American culture, he tells me, smiling, *is like candy: great to snack on for a while; a treat, but not necessarily a balanced diet. The Americans I usually meet*—he says, not wanting to overgeneralize, but doing it anyway—*are ignorant of history, of events outside of their own time and hemisphere. Their only point of reference is their own, and it's limited.*

Hmm. I tend to agree with him, to a point. *If you're talking about the mass of Americans—the broad masses—that's true, I counter. But my friends, the people I grew up with, the people I went to school with, the people who live in New York: they're well traveled, and pretty well educated. Not just book educated. They've learned about the world; they've gone places. I know the French get a much better education, but Americans are catching up.*

He smiles politely, willing to concede my point.

We compare the media of France and the United States, also agreeing that the French newspapers are interesting because they take a pointed editorial view while the U.S. papers strive for the canard of objectivity, and fail. He finds the gay press in the United States to be ahead of Europe, with the exception of Britain, where the magazines are well designed, with sharp content and a humor he finds lacking in American publications. There's only one lesbian magazine in France, and while it's strong on analysis, it's a visual and literary snore: dense, without surprises, with narrow politics, he says. Lately it's been improving, due to the involvement of younger lesbians, including some of the ACT UP women. His hope is for a mixed publication, one that will mimic the best of the U.S. press, but will have, he hopes, taking a little dig, better fashion. *A real gai et lesbienne publication.*

～

Almost midnight. We've done nothing but lie on the futon, laugh, smoke a hundred cigarettes, and polish off several good bottles of red wine. I'm feeling relaxed, less critical of the boys and Little Lord Gilles Fauntleroy. Gilles, I find, is quite funny, and very well educated, but he doesn't boast about that. He's also a very generous host, with good manners. And he's as passionate about AIDS activism as he is about his new *un peu facho* boyfriend. Not a quick study for Henri after all, I'm finding.

Suddenly, it's like last call; we realize the subway is closing and everyone wants a nightcap. And nightcap, I soon learn, is a misnomer. A nightcap at midnight in Paris is an aperitif, the first of many courses. And so off we run— and we do run: fast, laughing, slightly drunk—to catch a ride back to the neighborhood where I was earlier. We're headed for Le Piano Zinc.

Jürgen, the owner of Le Piano Zinc, leads us. He's an older activist, a transplant from Berlin who, from the moment we met, struck me as another rare, interesting French gay man like Christophe; one with a lot of emotional depth. I'm starting to really appreciate these men, the serious fun-loving French AIDS activists.

Along the way, Jürgen tells me he bought the bar he owns with his then lover, who died of AIDS a few years ago. It was a real marriage, a good relationship that has now left him newly single at age fifty. Since he's a handsome and rather burly man, with a wonderful personality and an open, generous soul, he's not hurting for partners. And he's not in any hurry. This in itself attracts people. He's not, as so many older gay men become, lonely or getting desperate, worried he won't attract a younger partner. He knows himself and, best of all, he likes himself.

He's also had what eludes many gay men—many people: real love and partnership; marriage; a long, intimate relationship that made Jürgen very happy for many years. He knows it won't be easy to repeat that and he isn't preoccupied with trying. He's embraced a new chapter of life. He's living the life of a mature single man. One who's young at heart—still playful and sexy— but has survived the death of a mate; who's lost everything but still has himself and a lot of life left to enjoy, to try to live happily.

～

Jürgen, I discover, is a very, very popular man. *I have too many friends.* He laughs. *I can't walk down the street anymore.* After so many years, he's a pillar in the gay

•

community here, a minor celebrity. At least, that's how it feels, walking next to him as we pass a string of bars and everybody—young and older gay men alike—offer him their greetings: their tarty, pouty gay air kisses and dirty, sexy catcalls. *Go, baby! Oooh, regarde ça!* To which Jürgen, more a man's man than a swish, is happy to respond. *Alors, look. C'est beau, non?*

At the doorway of Le Piano Zinc, he pauses and executes a perfect curtsy, like a southern belle before her gentlemen callers. *Bonsoir tous les garçons!* Jürgen shouts out.

I feel like I'm in a musical.

⁓

Le Piano Zinc is an old-fashioned cabaret bar, Weimar Berlin–style; a place where anything can happen; a bar where you will lose your heart and regain it an hour later. Inside the atmosphere is cozy, cruisy. There are shy, older men here; flaming queens; heterosexual couples; old-timers; drag femmes; hustlers; tourists drawn in by the activity in the street, amused, not really shocked, but definitely intrigued. Downstairs, the cabaret is about to begin. Jürgen prepares to take over as mistress of ceremonies, introducing the next chanteuse.

He gives everyone a warm greeting, introducing me to one and all. *Hello, darling. How are you tonight? What have you been doing? What will you have to drink? This is our friend from New York. Be nice to her, won't you? She's a sexy girl from New York City. That's it, give her your seat. But stop staring at her; she's not interested in you!*

Jürgen laughs loudly as he pushes us farther inside, past a crush of bodies, downstairs to where the crush is even denser. In every corner, someone's straining to hear the piano, to see the singer.

The singers are talented. This is a drag karaoke cabaret for the cognoscenti, a kitschy talent night with an emphasis on talent where no one would dare to sing if he couldn't. Everyone mouths the words, but here the songs aren't old Broadway tunes but French classics: Edith Piaf, Jacques Brel. We're quickly enveloped in smoke and songs that lasts for hours. Papou would be right at home, I think.

This is the life of gay Paris, or, at least, one of its heartbeats. Night after night ends like this, with a chorus of high trilling notes as everyone chimes in to sing "L'hymne du Piano Zinc," a gay anthem that does for a select generation of Parisian gay men what the songs of the Village People do for American gays: lifts them up, makes them shout and laugh, makes them feel the rightness of their love and their right to love.

I turn my head. Belle has her hands in the air, mouths the words, smiles sweetly at me. This is her world, her family, her life. She's having a great time.

•

We close the bar, still singing, and walk the streets randomly, like a large, noisy pack. Hands wave at us, friends invite us to have another drink, to stay up so that we can all have breakfast. Somewhere along the way, we've picked up Antoine, a former roommate of Belle's, but lost Gilles. At my suggestion, we head for the river to watch the last of the night pull its dark veil over the water, the bridges, the trees lining the banks.

That's where Sel spots us. I'm a little drunk, but I sense her presence in the distant fog. She's heard us approach, a boisterous, tired group. She can hear everything we're saying. She watches me walk quietly, hand in hand with Belle. She smiles at Antoine, tête-à-tête with a cute boy he's just met. By the time we reach the next large avenue to hail a taxi, the others have all left us.

Sel is a distance behind us, receding in my mind, an old woman dressed in a man's coat this morning, one who has left her shoes on the pavement next to the bench where she's been keeping watch tonight, where she was cleaning her toenails with a pocketknife. A mental spy who's missed nothing of the evening, and who, as I lean against the taxi window to watch the street cleaners converge on a corner, is humming the closing refrain of the night's song: *Moi, je suis dingue, dingue, dingue du Piano Zinc . . . Me, I'm crazy, crazy, crazy for the Piano Zinc . . .*

~ 24

The day dawns gray and I'm groggy. I tiptoe around the apartment, leave a note for Belle and another for Aldyn. I've scheduled a busy day. My destinations are Pigalle and Montmartre, the northern quadrant of the city, and, hopefully, a glimpse of Montfaucon, the human gallows.

It's a quick metro ride from Nation to Pigalle, a subway ride I always enjoy because of how the composition of the city changes. At Nation, all of Paris is hurrying to get to work. Workaday Paris, the toiling classes: secretaries, day laborers, students. Today is Thursday. It's almost 9:00 a.m. and the train is crowded. I study faces, watch the well-dressed French read their newspapers, and the German tourists who fill the aisles with their bags. A young man jumps the turnstile and slips into this car, glances around for a transit cop, then takes a seat. Instantly, he's bored and dozing in a corner, a portrait of urban disaffection.

Half the car empties out at République; more passengers embark. There are more Africans, more Arab men and women, many in traditional dress. I smile at a middle-aged couple who I guess are from West Africa, based on their accents and their brilliant, matching tie-dyed tunics and dress. He sports a knitted skull-cap; she, a scarf made of the same material. Both wear sandals. They're silent, don't even speak to each other. But their fingers touch.

I work to avoid the probing eyes of an Arab man sitting directly across from me. His teeth are stained. He works a toothpick with his tongue. His very being screams loneliness. He's left his entire family back home in Tunisia or some-where else; he wants a girlfriend, or just a girl to talk to. Even a girl like me, looking so uninviting, eyes deliberately averted. All over the city I keep encoun-tering men like him, men who, like me, troll the Paris streets and subways alone. Lonely immigrant men with dark complexions and shabby, formal clothing who have no idea how to approach me, a strange woman who looks more like a man, or to the attractive white French woman sitting next to them at an outdoor café.

In France, racism is in the air, in the soil, mixed with class divisions; it's like the perfume on these same women: ineffable, inevitable. How can they approach this white foreign girl who, they are convinced in advance, will want nothing of them, is prejudiced and afraid of dark men, of the Arab, the Maghreb? They can't; not easily. Not without risking social rejection that lurks under the polite French veneer. Is that what he's thinking?

This man's eyes are angry under his intense gaze. I try to ignore him, think it best. He's staring hard at me, meaningfully, still whispering. He hasn't had a lover or sex in too long. He must fuck. He doesn't say this but it's clear to me. *Madame*, he says in thick French, *Ça va? Quel est votre nom?*

The other passengers ignore us, ignore the growing drama. He shifts closer to me, persistent, trying out a broken English. *Psst! Madame! Mademoiselle! Where are from? United States? No? Allemagne. English, you English. No French? Oui, madame. What name? You very beautiful. What wrong? I am very nice man . . .*

I don't give him the chance to act or say anything else. My expression is neutral but closed.

A second later, he jumps up, then sits down again, right next to me. His accented English is perfectly clear, his knowledge of French too: *Well, go hell American woman! Conasse! Merde!*

I move away. His furious breath has left spray on my ear. From the corner of my eye, he is still staring at me, his eyes angry pools. I sense he's not mentally all there. Moments later, he's standing up, facing me, facing the others, talking to himself, reciting some diatribe. I can't meet his eyes. He's freaking me out even if he may be harmless.

When I stand up to get off at the Barbès-Rochechouart station, he moves too. He's going to follow me; he's determined. I quickly step outside, and so does he. Then, as the doors close, I duck back inside. As the train passes, he keeps staring at my face, his expression hard to read.

⁓

Looking back, I begin to write his story in my head. This lonely man is emotionally adrift in Paris, socially and sexually frustrated. He's alone and has no French friends. At home, in his country, women are taught to respect him; a woman doesn't ignore a man when he pays her a compliment or sits next to her. When he tries to sit closely to let her know he's noticed her. What is wrong with wanting a woman these days anyway? What is wrong with these French women, these American and German and Italian girls? These foreign girls? They're all rude, they're crazy and racist, they dress like whores; they've forgotten how to be good women. Why won't one of them even give him a chance? Talk to him. Just talk. Do they think he's some terrorist? He, a most devout son of Mohammed? They know nothing about him.

⁓

The little exchange has clearly unnerved me. I get off at the next stop, Anvers, and walk toward the Boulevard de Clichy. The morning pedestrian traffic is thick. African women and their children are knee-deep in bins of discount clothing and fabric, hawking plastic tablecloths, children's knapsacks, used radios. Inside bars, African men with skullcaps stand in quiet groups having their coffee, staring openly at every woman who passes.

This is where the action is: the sex clubs, the topless revues, the daytime cabarets and peepshows. But, like the rest of the city, the neighborhood has fallen on economic bad times, and many have closed. The tourists still come to the Moulin Rouge and to climb up to Montmartre and to buy a sex toy to laugh about back home, but there's less money in the skin trade and the competition is stiff. I pass young women standing on corners, talking with friends, glancing at the men—the johns standing at the bars. This is Sel's territory, and Henri's. They know the narcos, the madams, the strippers, the businessmen with fetishes. I walk up the picturesque streets, stopping at a butcher shop to examine pigs' heads dyed red and hung on hooks (grotesque, comic), thick loops of sausages, and inviting tins of products from other lands. There are many new restaurants, small and dark. Beyond a dim restaurant corridor, a group of what appear to be Vietnamese women clean turnips and snap peas, squatting over red plastic buckets.

I browse the windows of tourist shops, buy small, silly gifts for friends. It's too early for the new antique stores to have opened, but I note the trend: a younger, hip generation of entrepreneurs is gentrifying the neighborhood, selling bootleg cassette tapes, used clothing, art. Montmartre, long the haven of poor artists and musicians and writers, is becoming popular again. The rents are cheap and the view can't be beat.

I take the *funiculaire*—the tram—up to the Sacré-Coeur basilica, recalling the days in my childhood when I went to the Place du Tertre with my parents. The square is a kitschy postcard, I think: artists border the many cafés, drawing portraits, landscapes, caricatures. Some are mediocre, but several are excellent.

~ 25

I have a scrap of paper on which I've scrawled Théodore's address. I find the building a few blocks from the basilica, among the quieter residential streets. It's lunchtime, and he's expecting me. *La voici*, he says, smiling, excited, drawing me into a small apartment where two other Haitian men are seated. I don't know them, but I assume they're recent émigrés too, possibly activists like Théodore. A woman pokes her head in from the kitchen; she's the wife of the owner of the house, Théodore explains to me; they were the ones who were kind enough to put him up here.

I know Théodore from Haiti, from the days just after the fall of Duvalier, when a younger generation of military officers tried to oust the generals who remained loyal to the ex-dictator. Théodore was jailed and tortured, along with several other activists. After he was released, his tormentors still at large, he filed for political amnesty and arrived one day in France with his suitcase, a small amount of money, and little else. Now he's here, in France and safety, and he wants revenge.

Along with the others, he's filed an international lawsuit against the regime that tortured them and that's where I've come in to the picture. I'm assisting his lawyers . . . sort of. Acting as an unofficial courier for the legal firm, carrying documents for them to sign. In my capacity as a journalist, I interviewed the former officers in Haiti accused of the crimes; corroborated their stories. I took the testimony of several who identified the officer who beat Théodore around the ears, permanently damaging his hearing. That's sealed my friendship with Théodore, who, like other survivors of horror, cares above all that someone believes his story.

There is no dearth of witnesses in his case, but still, the case is weak. Not all of the others involved who have also been given political asylum can come today, so Théodore will give them their papers. He is so happy and relieved I'm here that he squeezes my hand twice, almost hurting me. This case has become his life and his lifeline; his ticket out of the nightmare, but also into a future that is foreign and frightening.

⌒⌐

We sit in the drawing room, the shades drawn, a stone's throw from the Sacré-Coeur basilica. In Port-au-Prince, there's a Sacré-Coeur too, around the block from my grandmother's house. There, just recently, several gunmen opened fire during the funeral of a man killed by paramilitary groups. We talk about the incident. Théodore knew the dead man, his wife, his four children. Every day, he borrows a radio from his friend and listens to the news from Haiti. But he feels far away, and worries about his wife and children whom he had to leave behind. He's asked for them to come, applied for the visas from the embassies there and here. But no one can tell him when or if they'll be allowed to join him. His enemies want to kill them because they failed to kill him. He's losing sleep thinking about it. His wife can't work; she doesn't dare go out.

All of this comes out in a steady stream. He needs to talk, I think; he needs to get out of his head. After a few more minutes he's finished the update and looks at me pensively. *What's going to happen? You. What do you think?*

He doesn't like my answer: *I honestly don't know.*

Théodore sighs, then brightens. *Let's not talk about these things anymore right now. There's time for that later. Let's have a drink.* He opens a bottle of Martini & Rossi, and we drink a toast. To him, to his family, to Haiti, to his new life, to the success of the lawsuit. Soon the others arrive and, in no time, we're getting drunk. It's midday and the political exiles of Haiti in Paris are sitting down to eat: rice and beans, fried plantains, spicy meat. Théodore seems happier now, happy to see and talk with others from his world, his past life.

I ask about his new friends, his search for work. He doesn't have many, and he's too busy looking for work to go out at night even if it weren't too expensive. And, anyway, he can't enjoy himself, knowing his wife is under threat.

That's not true; not completely. I can see he's eating well; he's gained weight, is even a bit overweight. I know he has friends in the Haitian community here and doesn't spend much time alone. He's not the type to stay alone. He likes to be surrounded, to be the center of attention. He's a jovial man, energetic underneath his current agony. And compared to the many Haitians and other exiles who are here illegally, he's well off. He has the blessing of the French state, which gives him a small monthly pension until he can find a job, access to other services and benefits, enough food to fatten his belly.

Life is hard, yes, but not as hard as it became in Haiti.

Relatively, given the political state of affairs in Haiti, he's gotten very lucky. He's survived the generals and their coups d'état, and he's getting help, free of charge, from a talented team of international lawyers. Still, I can't help but feel for him. He's dying, somewhere inside; his natural ebullience is a shadow. He looks pale too, like a tropical flower in winter.

After lunch, we review the case. I ask Théodore about his health. He still suffers from bad headaches, blinding migraines, shooting pains in his ears. His eardrum is perforated and won't heal, says the doctor. And now, months after his release from jail, he's having problems with his long-term memory, things about his childhood. It upsets him. *Will this be a problem if he has to appear before the judge?*

I instruct him to provide the lawyers with a medical record, signed by the Paris physician who's treating him. They'll need a complete update about each separate injury: his hearing, his memory, his broken hand, his cracked ribs, his damaged kidney. When we're done, I do the same with the others. They weren't tortured as badly as Théodore, but they're also badly traumatized. They've become collectively paranoid—more than usual, I think—worried that the ex-Duvalierists plan to send minions to assassinate them. They're especially worried because they can't find work. They're feeling pessimistic about their prospects.

Can't you help us find jobs? You have friends in Paris. Théodore nudges me. *Ask someone for us,* he demands. *You know people. You've got friends.*

Like Théodore, the others are dreaming big about this international lawsuit, placing too much hope on a victory and a financial settlement as compensation for their suffering. It's my task today to gently lower these expectations, to explain how hard it is to collect the money even after a judge rules in your favor—should that happen.

They listen quietly, taking in this reality check. I step outside the room to get some air, to let them privately confer. Through the doorway I can hear them debating, disagreeing, whispering. I step back inside the room. They pull back from their huddle, smile at me.

Alors? I ask. *Ça va?*

With a shrug of his shoulders, Théodore replies, *Il faut gagner. C'est tout. Il faut la justice.* We have to win. That's all. We must have justice.

They're among the newest generation of exiles to France. They've heard me, I can see that. The case is a long shot. But they prefer to focus on the prospect of victory, of one day returning to Haiti, to a sunnier future. If they lose the case, then what? Are they destined to spend the rest of their lives—another thirty or forty years—away from home, family, country? In a city where it snows in winter and people notice their French has an accent? No. They'll put such thoughts away. Théodore's wife will come here; his children too. Somehow, he'll get a job; enough money to live on, and save, and bring the others over if he must.

Everything will be all right, somehow. He has faith. He's Catholic and believes God must have a plan for him. The alternative is despair, depression, poverty, and the constant memory playback of how they beat him, how they threatened to starve him, how they promised to kill his children. He can't let them torture him further. It must stop. He must refuse to let them win.

Théodore accompanies me back to the church. I leave him at the top of the steps leading down from the basilica. He's a man open to miracles, having lived one already. He's alive and should be dead. He got out. *Without faith*, he tells me as we embrace, *I'm a dead man. I wouldn't be able to live like this, on a friend's couch, all alone, living on the charity of people. I have to have faith. Faith, my family, and good friends like you. I have nothing else. Thank you.*

Walking back, I pull out my trusty outdated guidebook, curious about the origin of the name of the district, Montmartre. Ah, here it is. It derives from the Mount of Martyrs, a theory I assume was put forth by Christians ever in need of a new martyr. They proposed that Saint Denis and his companions, Rusticus and Eleutherius, were beheaded at a base of the mountain, and that Saint Denis, no slouch, walked to the site of the basilica at Saint-Denis with his head in his hands. I wonder if this tale has anything to do with the modern expression *keep your head up*? As in, *Look now! Life's not so bad. No one's cut off your head. So stop walking with your head in your hands!*

Below my feet, the *butte sacrée*, the sacred mount, rises 423 feet above sea level and 335 feet above the level of the Seine. Sounds like a lot of stairs. I need the exercise; I should walk down. I'll just keep my head up. No walking with my head in my hands for me. *Non, non.*

I head for the west side of the tram to begin my descent of 235 stairs. There, beside the main portal of the church, is a statue by Armand Bloch of the Chevalier de la Barre, a young lad of nineteen who was executed for refusing to salute a religious procession. A secular rebel. I smile at the chevalier, one who was not deemed worthy to carry his head in his hands and be enshrined as a martyr. But one whom Bloch nevertheless found fit to commemorate. *Right on.* I nod to the chevalier as I head down the mount. *Fight religious orthodoxy.*

My little guidebook is full of tidbits. This hill was once the key military center of Paris, providing, as it does, a panoramic view of the entire city and suburbs. It's here that Henry of Navarre, another Protestant rebel and one of my favorite French kings, held court in 1589, and here that the Communards, more rebels, took control for two months. It was here too, at a spot close to where I take a breather, looking at the city through a bolted telescope, that the Germans made Montmartre the target of long-range bombing in 1918.

Scenes pass before my eyes. I imagine watching the bombers come, hearing the whir as they drop their cargo. I envisage my mother, a young girl, listening terrified as the German firing squad prepares to shoot her, her mother, her grandmother.

Unbelievable, such real stories; such true events. Hard to believe that things happen as they do, and to people we know and love. These terrible things happened today or yesterday, or many years ago, and they become words, stories, too easily forgotten. But here, now, is Théodore, another survivor of dark politics, or a dark period, a dark history, and this is his life; a modern exile's life with a new chapter unfolding in France. He awaits victory, and justice, and a miracle. But he's not going to count on it. As he's reminded me, *We Haitians don't forget that the French locked Toussaint in prison and threw away the key. We're not innocents.*

Toussaint L'Ouverture. The brilliant Haitian general who spoke perfect French and had impeccable manners and taught a slave army in the swamps how to defeat the better-armed French. Who was still tricked and captured and starved to death in a French tower to grow gray and cold like the good king in a fairy tale. A tragic history lesson that Haitians consider practical advice still today, for all the obvious reasons. *The children of slaves remember the master.*

~ 26

I want to play hooky today. I've scheduled myself to go back to Monmartre because I ran out of time the other day with Théodore. I'm looking for Tomb 27. I know, from my library research, that it holds the remains of the darkest family tree—the Sansons—all buried together there. Seven generations of royal executioners and their offspring, vilified and feared as the servants of the devil by the superstitious citizens of France from 1635 to1889. My library friend has looked in vain for the first-person diaries of the royal butcher and his son and promises to keep looking. I've left her my address and fax in New York to send whatever she finds.

I did note that the last direct ancestor of the Sansons died in 1920, but that in May 1971 and May 1972 two red geranium pots were placed in front of the tomb, which immediately set my imagination on fire. *Who is mourning the Sansons?*

When I got home from the library the other day, I flipped through the phone book but hesitated and decided not to call the few Sansons listed to see if they are related to the First Butcher. Apparently, there were twenty-three Sansons listed as recently as the early 1970s, when one of them, I assume, decorated the family plot. Without knowing more, I've decided that Sel may somehow be connected to the Sansons. Or she may know one of the descendants. Sel could narrate the fuller story of the Sansons too, one that presents their version of history. *The unexpurgated diary of the First Butcher.*

But my feet hurt today. I don't have the energy to go all the way to Tomb 27. I want to put my tired feet in the water, cool them off. When I do, minutes later, I feel a shock. The water is so much colder then I'd expected; my feet feel pain, then pleasure. I feel instantly better.

I'm by the Pont Alexandre III. An unceasing flow of tourists is heading for the Bateaux Mouches and cocktails and the romance of the river. Sel, close by me now, has taken a nearby seat on a slimy step lapped by the water, her feet more swollen than mine, like a diabetic. She grins at the tourists who can't see her. She's missing several teeth in back. A dental catastrophe. *Is she planning to take a dip?*

Sel slips in the water with as much grace as a walrus, and slips off the dusty tent dress, lets it pool up and over the messy nest of her knotted hair. In a second she and the dress and the vision have slipped below the surface water, lost from my mind's view.

I'm so tempted to jump in. Then I remember all the lovely details of anthrax and prurigo I've read about, the constant number of bloated river rats that I've seen along some of the quais and think better of it. *Leave that one to the muse.*

~ 27

Another day, another long walk, another nap, more dreams and visions. I've been trying to sketch Sel. Watercolor paints would be better than a pencil or Sharpie. She remains mysterious to me, this internal image I have of a rough woman who looks far older than seventy, who carries sickness but is strong as a mule, with fat calves and hard thighs under her bulk. Sitting beside a bucket full of mud in my mind now, holding a battered wooden spoon found on one of her sorties. Beside her is a length of torn plastic tarp, stolen from the booksellers across the way. She's digging for mollusks. She's on a dig, an archaeologist with her tools of historical excavation.

I try for a portrait. My muse, posing. A smile closer to a grimace; her mouth a garish display of broken teeth like the best of the royalist queens, a rotten crown. Her matted hair full of mites, worn up in a loose bun today. I should draw the body map of her markings, her pox scars, like an acupuncturist's chart. Her journeys with infirmity.

The soil here in the gypsum base of Paris is so thick with clay it sticks to my fingers when I dig at it, wondering how far down the mollusks might be. Sticky

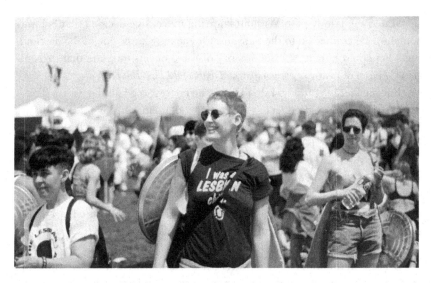

Author in Avenger drag at inaugural Dyke March, Washington, DC, April 25, 1993. (Caroline Buckler)

stuff. I work on a quick sketch: Sel, giving herself a beauty bath, a mud clay facial.

I study my new sketch. My rough muse appears covered in shit, if I'm honest. Not a good look.

The sketch makes me think about where Sel lives. Below the ground, at least in winter. Before I leave this trip, I'll try to revisit the Catacombs, this time with the eyes and needs of a night crawler, a thief, a revolutionary, a Resistance fighter, a wino, a drug addict. I plan to go as far underground as I can, to see where Sel may venture, where the homeless sleep in Paris's caves. It's a miracle how anyone besides a rat can survive so far below ground with so little light or fresh air. But many here do, just as they do in New York. Human warrens far below where I'm sitting, and in the unused arteries of the metro.

Of course there's as much safety in darkness as there is danger, though Johnny doesn't feel that way about going blind. We know that it's a possibility, because we've had friends who have CMV, cytomegalovirus, in their eyes. CMV, part of the unleashed world of poxes that shadow HIV. I can't imagine what that world looks like—to have seen and known a visible world, then inhabit only its memory. What does one see? Is it shadows, or at a distance, as Sel often is in my mind; an image I see best with my eyes closed, without any other visuals to distract me? I can't imagine it would feel friendly, that dimming world. But maybe I'm just uneducated, as I have been about the deaf. Probably.

~ 28

Early morning. Week two. I've gone out, slipped outside of the apartment at the first sign of dawn. I've left Belle, left Sel, left Henri, left my life in Paris for a moment, left the present and the future. I've woken up in the past, in the space of my emotions, in old memories of the Aerialist. I'm missing her today, this morning. Badly. I find a corner of a building, slink down against it. Feel it slipping up again. The sense of loss. The tide.

We were together for around five years but the last two were rocky. She was ambivalent about being in a relationship, and that translated to ambivalence about me. Not at first of course, but gradually. A steady retreat, I felt.

We had such an intense connection. She was my introduction to the PS122 performance crowd. We went to so many great shows there, so many performances, so many parties. Karen Finley, John Leguizamo, Holly Hughes, Reno, Annie Iobst and Lucy Sexton of Dancenoise, Carmelita Tropicana, Split Britches, Charles Atlas, Ishmael Houston-Jones, Eileen Myles, John Kelly . . . there are just too many to name. Every week was like a feast of talent. The Aerialist would tell me about her friend John Bernd, a talented dancer who had died of AIDS in 1987. She misses him a lot, would dedicate her dances to him. He had been her role model.

The Aerialist isn't a talker, not a stereotypical lesbian process queen—quite the opposite. With me she had trouble putting into words what wasn't adding up. Instead, she would take her space, withdraw, go dance it off. When our troubles began, we would jump on the subway to Coney Island and ride the old wooden roller coaster again and again. It was our form of therapy: *shake it out.* And it worked for us, for a while. It would put us back into the land of fun.

We traveled. I had joined her on dance trips to Tanzania and to Venezuela. So many adventures. But so much drama too, so much not feeling good—at least for me, in the end. We started in such a connected place but got stuck somewhere, a groove of draining conversations. I was worn out. Five years of my life, the last one a constant loop of conversation: *Should we break up? Take a break? Sleep with other people? Are you in or out?* Part of our problem was timing. The Aerialist hadn't had many relationships; she still needed to sow her lesbian oats, so she said. I had done that.

I know it doesn't make sense. I've moved on. I love Belle. I met Jersey and that's happening. But you know what? I miss her, I do. I'm talking to myself, to my mother, so long dead now, to Papou, who was always so kind to me. *I hope we can be in each other's life. But I'm not sure. It may just be gone for good. That's what makes me sad.*

I never grieve on time. That's what others tell me. I grieve when I'm no longer supposed to, when it no longer seems appropriate. I miss my mother, keenly, to this day. With lovers, I grieve before the relationship is over and even after, when I've moved on, grief roots me. *It feels like another death,* I tell them.

I think of Johnny, who dreams of having the long-term lover like Jürgen did, never had a solid live-in partner—only his Britt, never had a mate in the ways I have, more than once. I'm spoiled; I've loved with passion and the fullest heart and I was loved in return. It's the end that hurts.

Of course we'll become friends, I assure myself. *Something else will blossom. It has to, right? Eventually. Things take time.*

I say a small secular prayer. For peace: between us, and in myself. She had another journey to take. *That's all.* There will always be a bridge between us, I think later, walking slowly toward the river, a solid bridge made up of the history of our relationship. *Soul meets soul and they unite. A great energy is created, flows up and into the ether. It's never lost. She's not dead. She's just not in your life anymore.*

~ 29

I'm back in Montmartre today. I had to get Théodore to sign some more documents. He met me earlier but couldn't stay for coffee. Now I'm standing outside a bookshop, one of those that makes Paris a reader's paradise, with huge bins of books in no real order—accounting, botany, and medical texts, cheap detective novels, comics; books in as many languages as you might speak, and, best of all, no shopkeeper eyeing you with a keen awareness of how long you've been standing there, looking at the pictures of early Paris without buying a thing.

Like a child, I sit on the sidewalk with my oversized picture book and my notebook and pen and mentally recite the names of the suburbs and municipalities: *Villejuif, Montrouge, Saint-Cloud, Meudon, Gennevilliers, Saint-Germain-en-Laye, Pontoise, Montmorency, Montreuil, Vaujours, Champigny* . . . I've been coming to Paris since I was an infant, but I've never ventured far out to the suburbs. They remain as foreign to me as another country.

I wonder about the origin of their names. Villejuif is obvious: it's the old Jewish district. Montrouge, I take a stab, was so named because the dawning sun reddened its hilltop. Or maybe because it was a communist enclave, or attracted Russian exiles? I know there are colorful dramas behind the names. Was Villejuif once a ghetto, like the one I visited in Prague? Did it develop before or after the Vichy government agreed to begin deporting Jews? The next time I come to Paris (I've decided to come back soon), I'll borrow a friend's car and drive around the suburbs. Ask Philippe and Marina to be my guides. They'll point out different things and bicker about politics, and I'll end up with a lively, biased view of history.

I put the book aside and spot another gem: a 1982 copy of *National Geographic*, with an article titled "The Civilizing Seine." I devour it, scribbling randomly as always. *The civilizing Seine, my ass.*

I pick up a few key facts. Today the Seine is fed by the tributaries of the rivers Yonne, Aube, Oise, Marne, and Eure. Between Châtillon and Troyes, its waters flow through quiet villages then to the regions of Burgundy and Champagne. As the main route for commerce into Europe for centuries, it earned the name *fleuve civilisateur*, the civilizing river.

I snort aloud, startling a man reading at the next bin. *The civilizing river*, I think, *one used by every invading army to pillage and rape the locals and dump their bodies into its waters.* I'm tempted to write my comments in the margin of the magazine for the next reader. Every book should have blank pages left at the end for a reader's comments like this; it would provide a necessary balance and put the historian or journalist on alert. *Stop glossing over the facts!*

Of course, that includes my own story here. So don't hesitate, reader. Take notes, add your comments. Do your own research and feel free to correct my interpretation of historical events. I'll be all the happier.

⁓

I study the paintings of the Seine in the Middle Ages in the magazine. I look at the pictures of Rouen, where the citizens celebrate the festival of Joan of Arc wearing Norman costumes: lace shawls and odd high, lace hats for the women, black coats and tall, black hats for the men. No question what Joan would have worn (*Uhm, butch cross-dresser?*). It makes me want to visit cities like Rouen and Troyes, where, the author—clearly a romantic—writes, *Half-timbered houses in the Old Quarter have been inching toward a kiss above narrow streets since the sixteenth century. The most famous street is the cobbled Rue des Chats, where the houses nearly touch.*

I want more time here in France. I could travel the length of the Seine by slow boat. I bet Philippe knows someone who knows someone who would take me for a reduced fee. We could organize a group and spend a week; Belle, Gilles, and his manly boyfriend could all come along. The boys could visit the Napoleon museum at Fontainebleau to admire the uniforms and the sabers of the monarchy. We could sleep on deck and I could learn more about the stars, which are hard to see above Paris because of the lights of the city but can easily be spotted if you climb the Eiffel Tower, another thing I've done in the past but won't have time to do. Something Henri does for fun, I've learned.

A thought occurs to me: *How many people have jumped off the Eiffel Tower?* It seems such a spectacular suicide. I know it's a morbid thought, but I won't be surprised if some French civil servant has deemed it worth documenting. *Les suicidés de la Tour Eiffel? Oui, madame, right this way. Of course we don't know that much about them. They jumped without anything in their pockets to identify them and from such a height, you understand, there wasn't much left of them. . . .*

I'm silly, I know. But a girl has to have her fun, as Papou has advised. I'll research the Right and Le Pen and my family's roots, such as any may exist to be found. But I will have my fun.

⌐⌐⌐

I hear a little chuckle. *Sel. Pest, flea—always underfoot.* Pilfering used books again. Sel uses them as tinder to light the fires she makes in trash cans to keep warm during the winter, fires that leave her dark overcoat smelling thickly of woodsmoke. Did I tell you that she has a sly sense of humor; a penchant for playing tricks? Whenever a new book comes out about a French politician she dislikes, she visits the bookstores. This winter, she plans to stay warm burning the newest offering about François Mitterrand, written by Pierre Péan.

The elegant president's hagiography is in this bookshop window. It's clearly a revisionist tale, titled, in French, *A French Youth: François Mitterrand, 1934–1947.* In it, the French president, who long trumpeted his cultured, humanitarian side, reveals that all the sniping journalists who have been dogging him lately are right, *après tout.* He was, in fact, a youthful member of an ultraconservative French nationalist paramilitary group, the League of National Volunteers. He did later distinguish himself by assisting the Nazi-allied government of Marshal Pétain in Vichy as a minor official of its commission for repatriated prisoners of war.

And that's not all. After the war, our cultural man of letters befriended René Bousquet—the man accused of sending thousands of French Jews in Marseille to Germany's gas chambers. It was a long friendship, he admits, that lasted until 1986, when Bousquet came under fresh investigation by the great Nazi hunter, Serge Klarsfeld, for crimes against humanity.

Side note: I wonder if Papou knew Bousquet? If Bousquet worked with the mayor of Marseille, Papou's nemesis?

I'll never know now. It's a pity of sorts that Bousquet was assassinated not long ago by Christian Didier, a writer who everyone said was crazy to do such a thing. The press deemed Didier bizarre for his obsession with modern-day evil, with men like the imprisoned German war criminal Klaus Barbie, the Butcher of Lyon, whom Didier had plotted and failed to kill in 1987. Didier was arrested and jailed for four months for that.

In my files back in New York, I have a copy of an article I clipped some time ago about the Bousquet assassination. I remember the salient facts: the

Jewish leaders in France regretted Didier's actions; they wanted justice, they said, not revenge. The killing reminded the French about the Vichy government's involvement in deporting its Jewish population to death camps. Didier justified his action as necessary, given the obvious reluctance of French officials to peer into the not-so-distant past.

I'll write a note-to-self to see what more I can learn about Bousquet's boss, Pierre Laval, who, with Marshal Philippe Pétain—the *grand homme* of Vichy, showed the Germans how efficient the French can be, when pushed. Their decimation of Marseille's Jewish population was done quickly and brutally.

As with Mitterrand, there are still hot debates in France over whether or not Laval was a good man forced to make hard decisions in bad times; a hero and not a villain. Laval's supporters continue to claim his prewar record shows he was a patriot. During the war, they claim, it was Laval who suggested to the American chargé d'affaires, Pinkney Tuck, that the United States send ships to save Jewish children in Marseille. Obviously, the French who survived the war have had a clear and different opinion on this matter. Laval was found guilty of high treason for his role and executed by a firing squad in 1945. They felt he was still making excuses for murder and hadn't changed; he hadn't truly accepted responsibility for his actions.

This last detail I recall from my quick skim-reading of a book I looked at in New York. Laval tried to kill himself just before being shot, but the vial of poison he had long since hidden, stitched into his jacket lining, was too old and didn't work, so the French executioners pumped his stomach repeatedly, in order for him to be properly awake before they shot him dead. That, I believe, is the act of *the civilizing nation*.

Throughout his career, President Mitterrand has argued that France has little need to apologize for the collaborationist Vichy government he served, however briefly. He had even less to say about why, every year since 1981, he's arranged for an official wreath to be placed at the tomb of Marshal Pétain on Armistice Day. I just learned about that, by the way. That singular act alone has convinced me of Mitterrand's obviously mixed feelings about his Vichy colleagues and what they did. As the expression goes, the devil is in the details.

Well, that's a detail one really can't ignore. *The devil may be in Mitterrand too.* Mitterrand could easily downplay his links with Vichy, but instead, he's almost flaunted his connections, invited his critics to scrutinize him more closely. Is this misplaced Gallic arrogance? Or the actions of an unrepentant Vichyite?

Two other former Vichy officials now face trials for crimes against humanity: Maurice Papon, the wartime chief of police in Bordeaux, is over eighty; Paul

Touvier, a militia leader and aide to Klaus Barbie, the Butcher of Lyon, is in his late seventies. Barbie died recently, in 1991. Papon is well known to the French; he served under de Gaulle and was budget minister in the early seventies.

Would it surprise me to learn that Papon was an associate of Mitterrand's? Not at all. But I don't expect to read the intimacies in the new Mitterrand biography. Even I can tell it's what the staunchest historian would call a whitewash.

I'm tempted to turn to the man nearest me, who's been watching my unusually animated interest in the bookstore window, and ask: *Have you heard of Christian Didier? The one who shot René Bousquet? He served only ten months in prison for that so I think the judge must have agreed with his approach to summary justice. Someone should send him a copy of Mitterrand's new book, don't you think? I'm sure he'd find it quite amusing.*

⁓

Like Christian Didier, I'm feeling a bit like fate's child today, an obsessed writer borne along by a sense of missing history, by what's been deliberately ignored — the holes in the national biography. One whose muse, Sel, can see the lines connecting a man like Charles-Henri Sanson, the Royal Executioner, to Klaus Barbie, the Butcher of Lyon, and his *confrère*, René Bousquet, the Butcher of Marseille, to François Mitterrand, Royal Apologist. Like Sanson, she also thinks a man like Didier deserves more fame than ignominy, deserves a royal pardon, some royal understanding, for his *actus gravitas*.

I do find it interesting that the French press declared Didier a madman for his obsessions and actions yet jailed him for only ten months for murdering Bousquet. I suppose they couldn't declare him sane. Because if he was, what does that make them or everyone else? Mad? Or just madly complicit?

⁓

I have to take an aside, reader, to share what I learned today. Again, I'm struck by what I don't know and should have. Again learning the less glorious side of the golden story, this one about the liberating Allies and the United States, both during and long, long after Vichy. Up to just a few years ago, really.

I'm sure you're familiar with Klaus Barbie. I paid attention to his case when it was in the newspapers about five years ago. It was actually 1987; he was convicted of crimes against humanity on Independence Day, July 4. Wonder what I was doing that day? Celebrating our vaunted freedom with fireworks that make me jump? Probably. I wish I'd known. Then I would have broken open the champagne.

Barbie was one of the last really notorious Nazis still living large in South America when he was finally captured. What I haven't known until now is how much we—my U.S. government—helped him do so. He was found by the Klarsfelds, who remain France's most famous Nazi hunters. I think they may be my new long-distance role models. But about Barbie: his family's name comes from a French Catholic family named Barbier (perhaps a family of barbers?). They left France for Germany at the time of the French Revolution, which is when his ancestors might have run into my ancestors jumping from the king's ranks to join the revolutionaries. Barbie wanted to study theology, but his father died; he instead joined the military. In 1942, Barbie, a rising star in the Nazi ranks, was assigned to Lyon, where he set up a torture center for the Gestapo at Hôtel Terminus. He personally oversaw tortures of French Jews and Resistance members too egregious to detail here; I'll spare you. Except to say they included skinning people alive, one of many testimonies that emerged in the trial that began in 1984.

What pushes someone to do this, to go so far in their desire to extinguish a life? The question must always be asked. Like his idol, Hitler, Barbie suffered a lot of abuse at his violent, alcoholic father's hands, until at least age ten. One imagines a child beaten constantly, and toughed up to become a seething adult. The tortured becomes the torturer, a familiar story. All the rage of his life finds a target. Instead of God, he worships a devil. Barbie is said to be responsible for fourteen thousand deaths: women, men, and a lot of children. He's especially remembered for sending forty-four kids from an orphanage in Izieu to the camps to die.

(Such details make me feel suddenly closer to my maternal grandmother, Mamie. If she did anything to help even one Jewish child survive, she's a great woman whose actions deserve my gratitude and our family's respect.)

What happened after Vichy, after the closing of the camps, is the part that also sickens me. The poison that continues to rot, all the way up to the present. In 1947, instead of being locked up and tried, U.S. intelligence agents (presumed to be the CIA) recruited Barbie and a lot of other Nazis to help spy against suspected Communists in Europe. When the French ordered Barbie to be tried for crimes against humanity, the CIA helped him escape prosecution. He was one of the Nazis who slipped out via the now infamous ratlines to South America set up by the CIA, in league with other intelligence agencies.

Barbie ended up in Bolivia, where his talents were put to use by military strongmen there and in Argentina. He purportedly helped the CIA capture the leftist hero *guerillero* Che Guevara. He remained a right-hand man to the worst dictators, and helped the brutal Luis García Meza Tejada take power in Bolivia in a 1980 coup.

That was *not very long ago, right?* The start of AIDS. The year that followed my mother's death, on New Year's Eve 1979, when I was fresh out of Barnard

College. That's what throws me off so much when I do this research: to feel the past yanked forward, put within arm's reach of my own life, our present day. It can feel shocking.

Now here's the part that makes my heart skip a little beat, the part that makes it feel so much more personal. I just read this week that Barbie's lawyer in the 1987 trial was none other than Jacques Vergès. I think he turned up to help the lawyers in France whom Baby Doc hired after he got to France. Have to check with Philippe. The name rings a bell. Under Vergès's advice, Barbie told the court in 1987 he had *nothing to say.*

Now I think maybe I should see if I can interview Vergès, if his office is here in Paris. I wonder if I'd get an appointment. That would be a true encounter with another kind of devil. The lawyers for the wolves, the smoothest talking devils around. I don't even know where I would start. I might not be able to do it; I think I would just want to get violent myself, throttle him. I have none of the sangfroid of the Klarsfelds, whose massive book about hunting the Nazis is now in my possession. It's a thick, paper brick of detailed, almost forensic evidence, of Vichy crimes, incredible in scope and depth. The Klarsfelds are amazing, like Primo Levi. Flushing the rats from their caves of historical amnesia.

And I get it now; I see how this internal journey with Sel is forcing me to reeducate myself.

A final little note: Barbie had wanted to study theology, before he became a model soldier for the Reich. He suffered from leukemia, cancer of the spine, and prostrate cancer before he died, in prison, at the age of seventy-seven. Just two years ago. *Two years ago!* A few years of suffering a slow death is hardly equivalent to fourteen thousand lives lost. It's a crumb. But at least he was caught, and judged.

His case has left me with more questions, as always. *Who was in the courtroom, in 1984, when Barbie's trial started? Who else has been helping Vergès protect the other wolves still hiding around here? Maybe smaller ones, no less vicious then Barbie? Who is François Genoud, the French financier who supported Barbie in his trial? What possible stripe of terrible person is he? Is he helping Le Pen? What lawyers are defending the deniers of the Holocaust?*

And Barbie: What did he think about all those months? Did he secretly beg his gassed dead for forgiveness? Did he pray to seventy-six thousand saints? Did he regret anything?

I'll add these questions to the growing list in a little notebook I've devoted entirely to Vichy and the cabal supporting Le Pen. I'm no Klarsfeld, but I want to do something with this research. The Klarsfelds are up high on my moral shelf now too, I have to say, right next to Primo Levi and the man I've most admired for years: Claude Lanzmann, the director of *Shoah.* He and his multipart documentary on the Holocaust set the bar for me in terms of witness art. What an incredible film and man and testament. I would be thrilled to do even a fraction of what any of them have done to expose and right history, to bring some justice to the crimes of the Holocaust and Vichy. For now, I just need to educate myself, and look for any connection that leads to the wolf who's not afraid to show himself, Le Pen.

~ 30

I took a detour this morning, missed the visitor's tour of the Hôtel de Ville. Stopped by Pont Saint-Michel, had some coffee, took a moment to be a tourist. Now I'll have to choose between another session at the library or a visit to the sewers. There are books waiting for me at the library that I barely glanced at last visit; it's an easy choice.

The librarian greets me conspiratorially then reports in a whisper, *Still no luck with the Sanson diaries*. Never mind. I've found another book about executions that drew crowds who camped by the guillotine for days, fighting for a spot close to the basket where the head would fall. If Sel wants me to get tough, I've got to learn about the executioner's trade and how to give orders like one. The historical killers and the contemporary ones. I skim the book, jotting down the details that strike me.

The list of executions is long and diverse: royal dissidents, common prisoners, temptresses. Many executions due to infidelity. *A Madame Tiquet conspires to kill her husband by enlisting the services of her porter, Moura, who is hung as Madame Tiquet watches.*

There are enough details here to visualize the scene. There's a big storm. Madame Tiquet is dressed in white; her chariot is black and pulled by her horses. After the execution, her body will be put back into the chariot and taken away. But the rain is heavy; the executioner's hands will slip or the crowd won't stay to watch.

I'm guessing, because all I know from this book is that she waits half an hour for the storm to pass before facing the gallows. Climbing the steps, she kisses the frame of the gallows before placing her head in the groove of the wood. She is then executed by Chevalier Charles-Henri Sanson de Longval, royal butcher, who needs three blows of his axe to complete the job. By then, the rapacious crowd has seen enough. They cry out: *Pity!*

I look around the library. Who here voted for François Mitterrand? Who supports Le Pen? Who cried out *Pity!* when their neighbors, the Jews, were led away by the Butcher of Lyon and his cronies? Who's now protesting the eviction of citizen Arabs by the antiterrorist police unit?

There's definitely something in this archival research for me, and I'm struggling to figure out what it should be. Will I have to go inside the heads of Papon or Touvier, the men who ordered the torture? Is that where all of this is headed?

On March 28, 1757, a man named Damiens was slated to be torn apart by four horses, a popular form of punishment called écartèlement—pulling apart. Men and women stood on rooftops to watch; they were hurt falling to view the spectacle. Damiens arrived. His eyes opened and closed convulsively. La journée sera rude, he remarked. The day will be rough.

Like Madame Tiquet, he waited half an hour before his public torture began at five o'clock. He looked on the crowd with singular curiosity, wrote an eyewitness. Then he was held down and covered in molten lead, before four horses split him apart, each horse being pulled toward a different corner by the executioner's men. The extension of his limbs was incredible; those in charge ordered his principal muscles to be cut. Damiens finally expired at 6:15 p.m.

How far did Papon go? Did he personally oversee torture? What about François Mitterrand, fine representative of the civilizing nation? What did he really do and think as a young man in 1945? And what do his children think about him? What about the children of Le Pen, the aspirant successors like Marine Le Pen, dutiful daughter? Her name keeps turning up in the press. She's being groomed; groomed to become a wolf.

What do Papon's children say when journalists confront them with the evidence that their father helped chase two hundred Algerian freedom protesters to death by drowning in the Seine? The Massacre of 1961. Papon was the prefect of police at the time, given carte blanche to shut down a freedom protest by thirty thousand Algerians in the heart of Paris. I knew nothing about this event until a few minutes ago. They died right where I was just having a morning croissant, over at the Pont Saint-Michel. A watery cemetery, cloaking a crime that's still shrouded in denials.

I was only five years old. But later? No; I don't remember anyone in my family talking about Algeria, except as somewhere pretty to go maybe; visit a souk, ride a camel, buy a handwoven carpet. I don't remember a single word about this ignominious chapter of still-recent French history. I haven't gotten that far into the Klarsfeld's massive book. Maybe they talk about it. It's related to Vichy, another thing I didn't realize until this very minute. The Algerian war of independence started exactly as Vichy ended—literally: on May 8, 1945, the official end of World War II. That's the day that French local forces fired on anti-French protesters in the Algerian market town of Sétif, west of Constantine.

Where is that, Constantine? Why don't I know these things? I should know. I went to college. Why didn't I hear about the crimes of Vichy in Algeria? I have so much to learn.

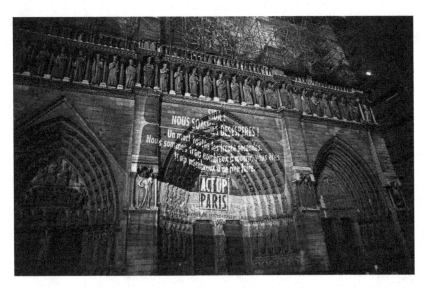

ACT UP, slide projection on Notre Dame Cathedral, 1994. (Diane Gabrysiak and Anne Maniglier)

Then what? What am I gonna do with this damning information? Use it, I know, but how exactly? Through Sel's story? My dubious muse, guiding me through the history of French executions here today? I have to keep faith, I suppose. A writer's faith, whacking down the thicket of my own flowering imagination to forge a proper trail.

One thing I have relearned from today's research: the common man is capable of anything, of such monstrous acts, watching a man pulled apart by four horses and still strain to live and then applaud, even push people off roof-tops in order to witness the torture. How many people watched the Algerians being chased into the Seine? Did they clap? And the Jews? Did they clap or stay silent? Sel wants me to enter the mind of the silent ones, all these people in this library who say little about what's happening in France now. They're the greater target, aren't they? The too-quiet public. Same as in NYC, America. Amerikkka, right? Our great racist nation.

I have to stop now. My mind is just rolling off the rails. Two hundred Algerians. Right over there. Jesus!

⁓

Time for a mental break. Outside, sitting on the library steps, I watch French people smoking. I want a cigarette, a *filtre*. A *loosey*, as they still sell single cigarettes at the newspaper stall on Saint Mark's Place in New York. When I'm in France, I become a smoker too. Everybody in ACT UP smokes, though here and there a few people have quit. France is slowly becoming American in this way too. Creating smoke-free zones in a country long covered with a haze of tobacco.

Back inside, I feel someone looking at me. It's Henri. As always, he's an observer, quiet, judgmental, coolly reserved. He's standing behind the librarian, watching me read. His head reaches the librarian's shoulders. He's tiny and more brutal, I realize, than I thought. He once choked a man and almost killed him with his bare hands. He possesses a blinding violence that erupts, one he unleashed on himself when he was young. Beat himself in the head with his fists. Frustrated. A young juvenile delinquent. Henri is interested in the case I'm reading about.

In May 1726, the regent Étienne-Benjamin Deschauffours came before the Bourreau (executioner) of Paris, the son of the First Butcher, Charles Sanson. His crime: Homosexuality. Before Deschauffours was killed, two hundred other men were identified as suspected pederasts, but they were spared.

Why was Deschauffours singled out? I wonder. Hmm. Leaving that question to someone else.

Henri's slipped away. He's poking around behind the library stacks. He's a small, pale shadow, dressed in white jeans and a drab T-shirt so worn it would be almost useless as a rag. He's looking out the window now.

At what? The spot where Deschauffours was killed?

I crane my neck to look at the courtyard outside the library, the buildings beyond.

Henri's climbing now, in my mind's eye, climbing the stacks like a monkey. Walking like a trapeze artist along a narrow banister that curves above our heads. He's entered the forbidden zone: the locked archives.

Is that where I'll find the real truth about the Nazis still hiding down south? Those who may know more of what happened on the Pont Saint-Michel that day, to the drowned Algerians. It's still a crime seeking answers. But that would probably take too long, too many years. I'd need an insider.

The librarian.

She looks up at me in this instant, smiles, gives me a polite nod.

⌒

Where did Henri go? He's gone. He's outside walking along a window ledge. Taking a little stroll with his friends, the pigeons. Leaving a message for me that I can't read from here. Tagging the building, maybe.

I get up from my chair, look through a tall window. I can't see a thing; have no idea what it looks onto. The street behind the library, I guess. And, from there, the rest of the Marais, the rat maze where I walked the other night with George and the gang en route to Le Piano Zinc. The ex-Jewish quarter. The

Arab market quarter. The modern homo quarter where drunken soccer hooligans who support Le Pen come to get drunk and later assault gays. I've read about that too.

I just notice Henri's right hand is badly scarred. A bottle fight? And he has a scar on the back of his neck, a faint hook-shaped scar. He's survived these streets, but he's a small man, one who's paid a price for his vaunted freedom. A victim of gay bashing? I make a note in my pad: Henri, a child boxer, like my Haitian grand-père.

~ 31

The Catacombs of Paris represent the ultimate in French vanity; display their penchant for order. Who else would store millions of unidentified bones and place them in neat, sometimes artistic, piles? Only a nation obsessed with cataloging its existence and making anyone who bothered to die there a kind of hero. The Catacombs make me laugh. You can't descend into the dark tunnels and look at the intricate designs of long and short bones and skulls—the circles and great Xs—without appreciating their droll, morbid humor. The French like to laugh at death, I will grant them that; the more grim the circumstance, the greater the joke. Yet they fear it so much that they have to erect dubious citadels like this one.

I've entered the main entrance at Denfert-Rochereau where Colonel Roi-Tanguy, leader of the Forces Françaises de L'Intérieur, established the headquarters of the Resistance, first located under the sewer facilities at the Rue Schoelcher. I wonder if they were forced to move because of the stench or for fear that a German bomb would release a river of moving shit upon them.

The Catacombs look cleaner and more spacious than I recall. When I was young, I remember rats slinking away into the deeper, dead-end tunnels. The lighting has improved and, while there's a limit to what one can do with a pile of bones and skulls, it seems that the director has made an artistic effort here as well. Like a shop window, there's more variety on display now; more emphasis on presentation.

I'm looking for the bones that were moved here from the Cimetière des Innocents in 1785. The cemetery was created for plague victims, those who died at Hôtel-Dieu, those who drowned in the Seine, and others, and by the time it was closed, in 1870, there were three thousand burials there. In 1861, one could visit a pathologic and geologic collection, which included samples of all the soil in which Parisian bones had been buried, as well as examples of all the bones disfigured by disease. That's the kind of specialty collection that would interest Sel, who can easily trace these bones to neighborhoods where certain illnesses remain endemic and occasionally burst into epidemics.

A hundred years ago, activity at cemeteries was much more interesting than it is today. Back then, there were people like Dr. Nicolas and Dr. Guillotin. And Madame Tussaud. She used to follow the horses carrying the guillotined back from the Place de L'Hôtel de Ville to where they were to be buried and, as the undertakers waited, she would make a wax cast of the severed head, studying it carefully for eye color, lash length, and skin tone so that she could make an exact replica. *What a woman!*

~

Time flies when you're talking to the dead, but not when you're paid to watch them sleep. I catch the eye of the guard, a thin fellow of around fifty who, I've noticed, has been checking his watch. I ask him about the Catacombs, his job, how he got it and why. His story comes out in an alcoholic breath and it's a sad one. Our friend is a drunk, a man of the state who worked for a dozen of France's museums before landing here. The pay is good but the job, he grins unhappily, is as boring as you'll find. He likes meeting people, especially foreigners, and has learned what he knows of the world from tourists. He's become a connoisseur of global travelers, and boasts that he can tell I'm from New York or San Francisco.

Wonder what gave it away? Boots, short hair, stinky armpits?

He's got his eye on his watch now. Fifteen minutes left. There are a few visitors behind us and, as he waits to let them pass, I ask him about himself, the job. He's happy to share.

The son of working-class parents, he had a bit of school and didn't want to do hard labor like his father. His first job was working as a security guard; his best job—the one he is still proudest of having achieved—guarding one of the principal galleries of the Louvre. It is clearly the most glam of museum-guard jobs, and one he regrets losing.

The problem, of course, was drink. He started drinking when he was a teenager, then more when he did his military service. There he spent most of his time standing at the entrance to a military station, checking the passes of visitors. He's always had a lot of friends; everybody drank a lot. He was almost always drunk on the job, but he held his liquor well. He didn't drink in the mornings, but you know how it is. He gives me his rueful, unhappy nod again. It gets cold in the winter when you don't move around.

Now that I look at him closely, I see he's a classic rummy. He walks somewhat stiffly and the tip of his nose is graced by the telltale network of exploded blood vessels. I wonder what his poison is—if he's a mixer who starts with a good full-bodied claret at lunch, followed by several whiskeys, and, to polish it off, a half-dozen chasers, each a potent dose of 100-proof something that would light my stomach on fire.

France is a generous welfare state; it rewards its loyal servants and looks kindly, if pityingly, on those who turn out to be failures. The Catacombs is clearly a hardship post; the only place for a man who needs to drink but can stay on his feet without swaying too much and is, after all, still an honest, hardworking fellow. I feel sorry for this man, though, because he deserves better; it's dim and damp and achingly lonely in the Catacombs, and the stairs, as I've mentioned, are a killer. He gets two breaks on the job: one to eat, the other to get some air.

I see his life stretching before him and behind us: he must live for these breaks, for his half hour standing in the bar, chatting as loudly as he wants with his good friend the barman and whatever regulars are there, not forced to whisper, happily eating a toasted ham-and-cheese sandwich with his first glass of wine. And then it's time to go back down, *Down There*, to these infernal dark rooms and their piles of dry bones and the rats and mice that make their nests among them, no matter how hard you try to prevent it.

⁓

Closing time. The guard's stiff step quickens. He's got to make doubly sure no one is lingering behind us, and takes polite leave of me. We're almost friends, I feel, in the space of one short, sobering conversation. I tell him I'll be back to visit in a few months and that, by then, I'll know a lot more about his guarded possessions.

I take the stairs slowly, the way he must, feeling the lassitude and the resignation of the day, of his routine. He's employed and, as he repeated to me three times, it's honest work and someone has to do it; and, besides, it's not that bad, spending some time with the dead. It gives you time to think.

I bet.

Daylight. Pre-dusk. A return to the world and the living. I give a final look back, knowing what's *down there*: the empire that has existed under this city since the Romans built the first caves to honor their dead. The sky has a charcoal edge to it, like a graphite pencil being lightly rubbed onto airmail-blue paper. I head for a bar and a short drink. A toast to the guard: another day and it's not over yet. *À la votre.*

⁓ 32

Every night in her apartment, Belle is hunkered over the Minitel, a computer machine that's smaller than a typewriter pad and has become the premier means of getting information and gossiping to friends for everyone in France. It is a kind of national Internet, linking homes, but instead of talking, you type. But not everyone can get this version of the Minitel; it's especially made for the deaf, and that's how Belle has gotten hers: through her contact with the school for the deaf, where she studies.

It's Tuesday night, time for ACT UP. Belle's going to translate tonight's meeting for a few of her deaf friends. The meeting is businesslike, with a long, structured agenda and reports from various committees. I see right away that the AIDS activists here remain essentially French in their bureaucratic, top-down approach to organizing. There's a president, a vice president, and as many minor posts as any French company. ACT UP–Paris may be a vanguard direct action group but it's not anarchist; it's corporate dissent.

A few of the deaf boys point to Belle. One draws his fingers together at the corner of his eye; that's the signed name they've given Belle, who has large, almond-shaped eyes. They look at me with little knowing smiles; there are no secrets here. I'm the one who's visiting Belle, who's become her lover. They're friendly, shaking my hand, saying things to Belle and to the others that, without understanding the specifics, I can make out. Such as, *Oh, so this is Anne-christine. We've been waiting to meet you. Belle was so excited you were coming.*

At night, Belle has been talking to me about her journey into the world of the deaf; an incredible journey for her, and one that is forcing her to reevaluate her own position as a member of the mainstream speaking world. Like her deaf friends, she's begun to shun the spoken.

The deaf are specialists at communication, nimble nonverbal linguists who've developed their own codes to chat on the Minitel. It's the visual aspect of the deaf—a picture says a thousand words. I watch the conversation fly around me in quick, simple gestures. These deaf activists are newer recruits to ACT UP but not to AIDS. For years, they've been dealing with the French government's unwillingness to provide education and resources to at-risk, deaf gays. I watch Belle translate the meeting; compared to them, I know, she's slow, spelling out words with her fingers while they nod, wishing she would speed up. But I'm impressed she's learned so much.

Sign is a constantly evolving language, like slang, a visual argot. It's flexible and designed to get to the point. One can spell out safe sex, combine the known signs for *safe* and *sex*, or come up with a single sign that would express it. While Belle struggles to string together long phrases, the others make up words and expressions on the spot, and in a second, the others have adopted it.

The sign for ACT UP is a triangle made by placing both hands in front of the chest. *Gay* is a short pull on the ear; *lesbian* an *L* made with finger and thumb, placed at the base of the chin. Sign is not a universal language; after all, French is French. The few words I know in American Sign Language are met with curiosity.

What is Anne trying to say? They turn to Belle for help. She laughs. *She has no idea what I am trying to say either.* The deaf laugh at me, but their eyes are kind. At least I'm trying.

———

The two most handsome boys are Belle's close friends, Grand B and Petit B. Both were born totally deaf. Grand B is tall and lean, with smoldering good looks: dark hair; smooth, pale skin; an aquiline nose; and pretty lips—classic, chiseled French features. He's an ardent deaf activist, currently engaged in a one-man war against the French medical establishment, which is actively promoting the use of a hearing implant that he considers a vicious, medieval tool; an unnecessary operation that, to drive his point home to his hearing gay brothers, he compares to sex aversion shock therapy used to quash homosexual desire. All this I learn rather quickly, within minutes of our being introduced.

Petit B is smaller; a sweet, well-muscled, Moroccan boy with full lips and curling lashes over dancing eyes, and a natural pout that knocks the boys out. He's a huge flirt and immediately flashes me an enormous grin that takes over his whole face. Something in him reminds me of Henri. The way he knows that other boys are fascinated by him. The ACT UP boys can't talk to Petit B, but they want to; they want to flirt back, he's so adorable. *Too bad for them*, Petit B suggests, giving me a sly, knowing look, then laughs, a series of mild, high-pitched grunts. *If they want me, they're going to have to work harder. Learn to speak my language, if you know what I mean.* He's wicked; a temptress.

I immediately imagine Petit B as a young rascal; a small, olive-skinned boy with a head of fuzzy, black hair who takes his mother's kohl pencil to line his eyes, then wraps her veil around his head, leaving only his flashing doe eyes to seduce the neighborhood children.

Petit B is having a hard time being serious during the meeting, making faces every time I catch his eye, pointing not very discreetly to Belle, drawing a valentine over his heart, telling me, *She's got a crush on you.* I see that he's a brilliant mime and a natural comic, with a plastic, expressive face.

Will Henri be deaf? Have a deaf lover? The thought skips through my mind, momentarily distracting me. I write a thought down on the flier I've picked up that describes an upcoming dance, adding, *Humor is a survival tool for the deaf, their play at the expense of the hearing. I can imagine all the terrible words they use to describe us.*

I understand Belle's attraction to the deaf world. To me, up to now, the notion of not hearing is like being underwater, a silent world that I've always thought would be lonely. That is a stereotypical and biased view of the deaf: as lacking. My assumptions have been so quickly challenged and just as quickly fallen away, seeing how engaged these activists are, how in control of their world, how complete they feel without verbal speech. I am the fool: deaf is not silence but another way of speaking, encompassing many languages and cultures. A people maligned, institutionalized, pitied, put aside, treated as stupid, deprived of education and resources, of parental love, of society's admiration. And, like other historically maligned groups, a triumphant people, survivors, aware of all those who still remain locked inside silence, inside depression and despair, those who have been abandoned or killed themselves trying to fit in. Only now, slowly, are the deaf reclaiming their heritage, their history, their pioneers, their struggle.

I look over at Grand B, whose hand is up. As Belle translates for the room, he launches into a diatribe about the ministry of health, their failure to do HIV outreach and education to the deaf community. He mentions the demonstration I've attended, chiding ACT UP for its own failure to reach out about the action; to inform the deaf about the state's HIV policies. He's on a roll, a proud spokesman for his community, which is, he says, *deaf and gay and proud, but tired of the ignorance of hearing people who call themselves activists and haven't the first clue about his life!*

His spirit is fiery and there is generous applause—fingers waved in the air by the deaf contingent, which is picked up by the rest of the room. *Watch out ACT UP! The deaf are here, they're queer, they're not waiting for you to hear!* I like my chant, write it down, and pass it to Grand B, who reads English. He laughs, giving me a thumbs-up.

The meeting is long and, to me, tedious, because I'm not involved in the internecine details of ACT UP's small, daily battles: education, materials, the ignorance of this or that public official, the money that's needed to promote the upcoming dance, the response to the scant media coverage of the blood-scandal protest.

There's a break midway and everyone is outside on the sidewalk, smoking and arguing. I'm thrilled to see that the spirit of defiance is alive and growing here in Paris, while in New York so many AIDS activists are burned out. There are around three hundred people at this meeting and, tonight, in addition to several of the deaf who are attending for the first time, there are a dozen other newcomers, including several lesbians and straight women, who introduce themselves to me.

One of them, a new friend of Belle's, tells me that ACT UP is beginning to attract feminist women who have long battled the state over issues in women's health. I can tell that these women here will soon be among the most outspoken and daring when it comes to actions. They have an analysis that comes from their experiences of being female; a history of being disempowered by institutions, of being ignored by the health care system. The boys of ACT UP are lucky, having them here.

By now, I'm familiar with rituals of organized protest: after the meeting, we'll eat and drink. It's 11:00 p.m. and not yet the weekend, yet no one complains. We take over a restaurant, connect tables, spill out onto the sidewalk like an exaggerated tableau of the Last Supper. It takes a long time to get our food and even longer to pay, but the night is hardly over. Once again, I'm crowding into a taxi, convincing the driver to let the boys sit on each other's laps with the promise of an extra tip—*Oh, bien, pourquoi pas? Hein?*—and soon we're riding along the lip of the Seine, heading again for Le Piano Zinc, where Jürgen, who is riding in the car ahead of us, hops out and stands at the doorway of his kingdom, demanding a kiss from each of us as the price of admission.

> *C*'est quoi ce pays de merde?
> *Christophe Martet,*
> *ACT UP–Paris*

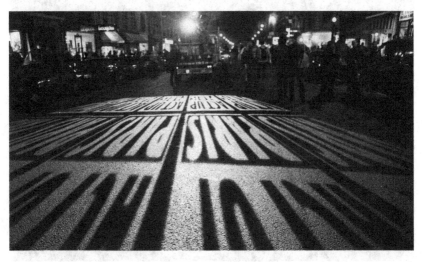

ACT UP, slide projection on the streets of Paris, World Aids Day, 1994. (Diane Gabrysiak and Anne Maniglier)

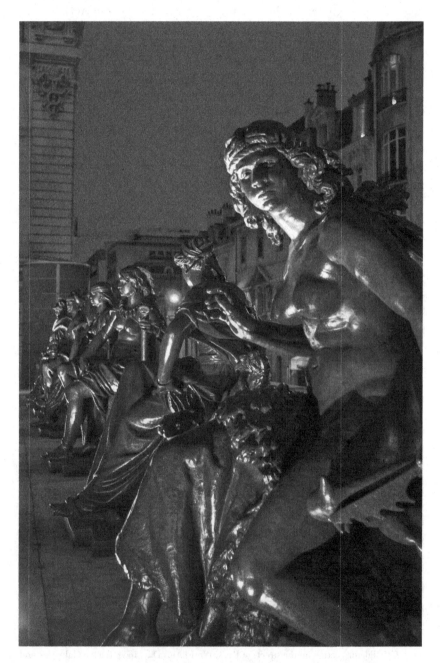

Statues in front of the Musée d'Orsay, Paris. (tomcraig@directphoto.org)

~ 33

The sun is so bright, dappling the river. I'm back at the gay beach, having visual delusions. Small daydreams, quite pleasant. Right now the Seine is covered with marigolds. Millions of them. A golden loom crossed and dotted with black lines and spots—a swarm of blue-backed dragonflies and other darting insects pollinating the riverbank, reseeding a transgenic bloom. In 150 years, the flowers will lose their petals or gain extra sexual parts, turn dimorphic, breed with inorganic species. Fistfuls of poxed flowers will sprout along the shore.

Now the picture is changing: the river is clogged with fur balls vomited up by all the cats of France who have been bred into gentility. Shoeless, Henri dives from a tall building onto this soft carpet, removes a small pair of waterproof binoculars from his pocket, trains his eyes on the heavens. The sky darkens like a black cow, the symbol of dusk in India.

A lavender moon rises, fat and solemn. It illuminates the fascists, advancing behind a low cloud front, marching behind a presidential banner. Henri sticks a finger in the water to test its strength. With a ripple of the river's surface, the new moon drops; the invaders fall from the clouds and drown.

Saturday. Only a few days left before I have to fly home. I get up while the sky is still dark, drink coffee, then catch an early subway train, heading north. Again, the composition of the train changes as we hit the poorer districts. At Belleville, I look out to see the police checking the identity cards of two youths who are being frisked against the wall. Without even seeing their faces, I know they're Arabs. They turn around but keep their faces down; their eyes won't meet the riders who keep their distance from the scene. What are they accused of? Jumping the turnstile? Transgressing some greater border?

Both youths are dressed modestly; one wears a tie. The police return their wallets. There's no crime here. But that's not the point. The purpose of this daily exercise is intimidation: to let the immigrant Arab population, like the African, know that terrorism will be met with force, that the metro will not be a free ride, that French women are not to be pursued. The Algerian grandchildren of a generation that overthrew their oppressors, the civilizing French. Has the colonial mentality really changed? Not that much, I feel.

It's pretty evident in the Maastricht Treaty, a document that is taking up ink in today's newspaper. It loftily aims at European unity, but even a casual reading reveals the steely reality: the border of Western Europe is crumbling after the fall of Communism; it's too porous, leaves too many opportunities for the poorer citizens to seek work and residence in a neighboring country. The

Maastricht Treaty poses as a cooperative agreement, an exercise in sovereignty, when all it reflects is an old-fashioned tightening of the belt. Like these Arabs, the old enemy—the East—will not be given a free ride into France, into the Western European capitalist market. The men and women of sixteen nations have found common cause at Maastricht: a unified border, a unified currency, a unified police—Europol, a unified defense strategy, a unified antidrug and antiterrorist policy, a unified media.

As for these two Arab youths, they've been warned like the ghettoized citizens of Lodz were warned: their work permits and limp identity cards risk becoming so much dust if the Maastricht Treaty becomes law.

Sel has gotten a copy of the Maastricht Treaty. She rips it into long strips and uses it to wipe her ass, then discards it into a growing refuse pile. But before doing this, she perches below the Pont Saint-Michel, gravesite of Algeria, and, like the town crier, reads aloud the finer points of the charter to the junkies who congregate there. They're nodding, but few pay much attention; it all sounds like old news. They've been living in the future of Maastricht for some time.

~ 34

Early Sunday, too early. I'm half-asleep on the subway and it's chilly. Past Pigalle, past Blanche . . . I change cars at Place de Clichy. My destination is the great flea market at Saint-Ouen, which is a paradise to me, a veteran thrift-store shopper. It seems everyone is going there on this train; whole families are onboard, the children scrubbed clean, wearing their weekend best, excited for this outing. It's still early; the market has only been open an hour, but already it's packed. I make my way slowly. Here is where I find the human flow that Maastricht would curb.

Everyone with something to sell has taken up a spot on the sidewalk. The more established vendors lay out their wares inside permanent stalls. All around the exits of the subways, there are cars for sale, the owners hovering close by. Women stand, holding shawls, skirts, shoes in their hands, hawking them, pushing them toward passersby. There are so many nationalities here, so many languages. *A Tower of Babel.*

Further along, the flea market becomes a small, labyrinthine city made up of concrete storefronts and makeshift stalls. I snake through the crowd fingering lace undershirts, polyester dresses, cheap oversized vinyl luggage, imitation designer clothes. I've got my eye out for the products of French war: high-laced paratrooper boots, thick belts and socks, mesh shirts that slide on the body like silk.

I comb through stacks of postcards that remind me of my mother: hand-painted, black-and-white pastorals; portraits of anonymous men and women in formal wear; the sights of Paris during the war; people in the cafés; the Folies Bergère in the 1920s. I finger bowls of colorful blown glass, admire huge travel posters with their art deco design: Nice, Cannes, La Côte D'Azur, with palm trees in the foreground, a steam cruiser in the background.

Here are the colonialist objects: bowls, plates, stand-up ashtrays, paintings, many representing Africans with exaggerated features—huge, red lips; they are always saucy women, muscular men—sexual predators. They've come back into fashion as a form of kitsch for a younger generation that confuses racism for nostalgia.

I admire French design, the cultural emphasis on beauty. There are gilded picture frames, exquisite furniture from many periods, stained glass that's been physically pried from some abandoned church, long sofas that make me want to remove my clothing, put on a day robe, and spend the afternoon making love.

After two hours I'm exhausted and the crowd is only growing bigger. I take a strong coffee in a shop behind the market. I'm the only woman in a room of men who look like they make their living doing hard manual labor. I like their natural style: rough pants, tight T-shirts with emblems of football clubs, bright-orange overalls, sandals worn with socks. Henri's kind of men.

The coffee is Turkish, so sweet I have to suck it between pursed lips. Then I indulge myself and have a cold beer, staring back at the men who act as if they don't see women who look like me that often. One of them eventually offers me a cigarette.

⎯⌒

Round Two. Back in the trenches of the market. The crowd is thick. It's getting late; Belle is going to meet me in a little while. I pick up a sweater, a pair of pants, some khaki boots that a French recruit has worn down at the heel, a heavy lighter, postcards, a piece of material from which to make curtains. I feel jubilant. I've spent less than fifteen dollars. *Chouette!*

⎯⌒

Lunchtime. I take mine sitting inside a small restaurant with three large tables in it. One seat isn't taken; I squeeze in next to an old man, his children, his grandchildren. The menu is couscous. I order it with a tall mint tea. The talk is loud, animated. I feel at home here. This is the community that Maastricht fears, the solidarity of the poor, their laughter, their joking, the children roaming freely out into the street and back again, unafraid of strangers. I turn down a sweet pastry made by the owner, but he pushes it into my hands. *Prenez ça, c'est un cadeau.* Take it, it's a present.

He asks me about myself, where I come from, what I'm doing in France, what I've bought. Clothes for my brothers? No? . . . my husband? No . . . Ahhh for myself? . . . He nods, smiling to himself. He understands, winks at me. There's an old sexist saying among Arabs: *A woman for babies, a boy for love.* He pats my hand, adding in rough English, *Take another patisserie, mademoiselle.*

For a while in the afternoon, I'm on my own. I take a long walk through the streets in the district. Most of the blocks are quiet, residential. Belle's warned me that this is a dangerous area—there are daytime hold-ups—so I stay close to the main artery. Eventually I find the block where her friends live. They are both quite active in ACT UP. The apartment is charming, a two-story affair in a quiet corner. A pink triangle on the door greets me.

I'm always curious about gay men who live together and these two are no exception. Physically, they're opposites: one is dark and stocky, with rough features and a brusque quality. His lover is pale and blond and quite thin, a wispy dancing queen. The dark one strikes me as a very angry man. Later, though, I find he's got a tender, vulnerable side under all that toughness. I call them Oui and Non. Oui is the blond whose eyes light up when he says yes to an idea that excites him. *Ah, oui!* His happy energy is infectious. He's got a wicked, seductive side. He wants you in on his confidences, his gossip. He's got secrets that he's ready to share.

Not so his boyfriend. *Non,* with him, really means no when he says it, which he does almost automatically with his body language. Non. He's a resister, a rebel, an iconoclast. I like Non; he's rough-sexy. He's shaking his head at Oui's gigglishness, amused at how daft his boyfriend can be. Meanwhile, Oui pokes fun at Non, pokes him in the ribs, tickles him, whispers coy nothings in his ear. They're total opposites; a perfect match.

Oui and Non are in their late twenties, and have been together for years. The intensity of their love is obvious in the way they tease and provoke each other— a bit, but not too much, coming forward quickly to soothe the ruffled ego.

Later, we're joined by several other activists and spend the evening playing music, talking about the cities we've lived in, our sexual pasts, the books we've read, where we've traveled. Like my gay male friends in New York, these boys have lost count of the ones who have died and are worried about ACT UP's ability to survive, as those with the most knowledge and activist savoir faire fall sick and die. Oui is clearly on his way. It's hard to imagine him getting much skinnier. He's developed two of the infections that most people with HIV develop later and, tragically, he can't access drugs to treat them. They're not available yet in France.

Oui makes light of it all, though, telling me of his various revenge schemes, how he dreams of being an AIDS kamikaze warrior like Aldyn, holding a high government official hostage until someone decides to release the state funds needed to mount an effective educational campaign. It's becoming a shared activist fantasy.

Should I go to the United States? Oui corners me. *Can you get me a bootleg shipment? There needs to be a better pipeline,* he complains as Belle joins us. *We need to do something about this in ACT UP–Paris. What should we do? What are you doing in New York? Do you get arrested? How often? Do they give you good food in jail?* Oui makes me laugh. He has odd questions. He's a bird, in his energy, in his flitting movement, in his old-fashioned gay fairyness. *This boy never passed,* I think, *not for a moment of his life. He's just so . . . gay.*

⌒

We talk about it for hours: how to get past the red tape; how to pressure the international drug companies to begin trials simultaneously in Europe and the United States; how to set up buyers' clubs for alternative therapies. Compared to Johnny, who's in similar straits and paying through the nose for his expensive experimental treatments, the French system offers better health care, and it's subsidized. No one has to go on total disability, or give up a paying job, in order to get care. But it's hardly a party and, compared to New York, many of the doctors in France are ignorant of the latest treatment updates.

I promise to do what I can for Oui, to urge the activists back in New York to take up this cause, to establish a computerized data exchange that will allow the anecdotal information from individuals like Johnny and his doctor to speed across the Atlantic by fax. But all the while we are talking I can't help but feel sad—for him and for Non—knowing that whatever we can manage, it won't be enough. Not fast enough. This boy is too sick. The energy that shines in his face, the light in his eyes, this fervent desire to live, is burning him up. He's ready to burn until the millennium, but he knows he won't make it. So does his lover.

⌒

Oui's skin is pale and covered with a rash. His blood is thin now too; he's anemic. On the way out, he shows me his bathroom cabinet, *his shrine,* as he calls it, *his ritual of worship,* the names on the various pills and bottles unfamiliar in French. And, all the while, Non moves behind us like a bull, like a boy who has had to knock into things all his life. Saying, *Why are you showing her that? What can she do?* I see Henri in Non; he is a boy Henri would like, or would befriend. A boy who's used his fists more than once to resolve his problems. Or wishes he could. On account of his love for another boy.

⁓

I'm well fed, no longer tipsy, but tired. I pause at the entrance to the metro. An old woman is sitting on the steps, midway down, a large sack at her feet. She could be a stand-in for Sel. She's Arab, with tattoos on her face: a pattern of dots on each cheek. She's wearing a colorful head shawl; another one covers her shoulders. Her feet look almost deformed, curling into one another, with thick, yellow toenails. Her pipe lies in her lap, unsmoked. She mutters to no one in particular and doesn't look up when a man drops money into the cup by her sack.

I want to know her life story: how she came to be abandoned here by her family, her children; whether she's begging for herself or her sons or someone else. She catches me staring and fixes me with a dispassionate look before pointing to her cup. Her teeth are ringed in silver, every tooth. *Madame?* Instead of putting my bill in the cup, I hand it to her. *Tiens*, I say: *Here. I hope this helps.* And instead of looking away, she nods at me, a sad look of acknowledgment. *My life is bad. Look at me.* Her gestures tell me everything.

There's something so vulnerable about her—not at all pathetic, but something very wrong that's left her here, a proud, strong woman, forced to beg for money from strangers in a strange land. My heart lurches.

I could stay here and talk to her, but that would take more than a few minutes and I can hear the metro arriving, and now here is Belle waving, holding the door, shouting, *Hurry, dépêche-toi, you'll miss the train!*

Now I'm riding back, but her face stays with me: her thick, dark brows; those placid but searching eyes. Hers is a story to tell: the story of a woman struggling to live as she shakes a cup at the people who pass, their hands full of things they've bought at the flea market at Saint-Ouen. Not exactly like Sel, but with many of the same features.

In the window of the train, I catch my reflection, imagine a pyramid of dark-green marks on each cheek. *Who would I be if I were that woman? When she looked at me, who, what did she see?*

⁓

Her eyes were small, her brow thick. She had a lady mustache. Her fingertips were stained with henna. She wore an undergarment trimmed with lace under her wraps, a surprise. She had a pair of sunglasses. Where did she get them? From the flea market? I try to imagine her wearing them—dark, mod glasses like a spy in a French *roman noir*. A nationalist working for the Algerian secret service, recruited to keep a bead on the enemy of her people, Le Pen. Parking herself outside the gates of the new headquarters of France's intelligence agency. Looking for who comes in and out, for any older men who resemble the police officers who acted under police chief Papon's orders, held their guns steady as they chased the children of Algeria over the lip of the Pont Saint-Michel to their death.

~ 35

My relationship with Belle is a dream of its own, a fine, pure dream, but the reality is sobering: she doesn't seem to want anything more than what we have now; doesn't want to think about tomorrow. Today I'm here, for one more day, but tomorrow we'll be apart, for months, maybe another year. Nothing is certain, nothing can be assumed, except today. And I've learned enough by now to know that I can't change Belle; that, no matter how much I want her, she's clearly not ready for more—not from me.

I've also learned a hard lesson from the Aerialist: beware of ambivalence in love. Ambivalence is a dangerous kind of glue that makes it difficult to move, that has kept me immobilized in the past, unable to break free, estranged from my own happiness. I feel I need to make a decision. All signs point to Jersey. *Where does that leave Belle? What's going to happen with us?* This thought, like all the others, glides across the Seine, which is green black today, with a strong current in the middle, bubbling and rippling around the base of the Pont des Invalides.

Tell me, is this a good thing? My relationship with Belle? I've directed my question at Sel and Henri, who've been listening to my chatter with half an ear each, a bit bored. They've heard this kind of talk a million times, from a million lovers who've stood here before me, and they're not impressed. Not with the depth of my love or sorrow, not with my ardent heart; not with my hopes.

Leave the suffering to someone else. I don't know which one of them has spoken up, Sel or Henri. But I've heard it, clear as a bell. The kind of advice my father might give me. I can't feel too sorry for myself. We're on a journey; we have other things to think about, more important things this week: a battle to fight, a story to narrate if I'll only get on with it.

They're right. I only have a day left and there's so much I haven't done. My mind is already half on New York. Will they survive the journey? The thought worries me. Then I glimpse Sel ahead, rounding a corner in my mind's eye. She's turned back to look at me, seen my hesitation. She gives me that amused, pitying look again, one I can see she reserves for fools. *Stop worrying*, I hear. *We're parasites, remember? And you're our host. It's not going to be easy to get rid of us. Isn't that right, Henri?*

The cackle of geese. Isn't that how I first described Sel's laugh? Like something brittle, glass being stepped on, or a match dragged across the floor—or, even better, fur against glass, her thoughts rubbing against mine, sparking a disturbance. Then, like a faint breeze, she's gone and, with her, Henri. A pair of migrating birds, I think: a ragged lark and her pigeon-toed messenger companion.

ひ

New York, de novo

~ 36

MARCH 1994

How the weeks fly by! Twenty-four-hour New York, mad-rush Manhattan. I'm back and in fast motion. My Haiti book is out. I finished it in mid-1992 and it's been a slow build to this moment, when it's really out of my hands, out in the world now. Getting into libraries I heard, which makes me happy. The first industry reviews were good; I'm encouraged. I decided to throw a big release party in January, use it to raise some funds for Théodore's group, the Haiti torture victims. We invited some fancy folks: Harry Bellafonte and Jonathan Demme and Ramsey Clark—people we work with in the Haiti Refugee Advocacy coalition group. Michael Ratner at CCR has been a sweet support. Susan Sarandon was a no-show. She was Jonathan Demme's celebrity invite; a long shot. I was really hoping Ariel Dorfman could make it; I admire his work. Great moralist. Sadly, he had a prior commitment, sent a sweet note.

I'm hiring Jay Blotcher, who's a PR guru and is an ACT UP pal, to help me set up a book tour. The only catch is that it's on my own nickel, which is a small nickel. Apparently first-time authors at FSG, my book house, aren't given much in the way of publicity budgets; they reserve the bucks and the prime bookstore reading slots for their famous writers who sell a lot of books. Let's hope mine sells some. It's all going to depend on the *New York Times* book review. I'm getting one, I heard; that's already something. But it could be a sink-or-swim something. So say my friends at the Writers Room. Doesn't matter how much other critics love their work; the word of the *Times* critic is God to publishers. Fingers crossed then.

In the meantime, I'll do what I can to toot my little horn. Until the tour, I'll keep myself distracted with Sel and her wild bunch. That's what everyone suggests: start another book.

My mind operates on two tiers: the present day before me and my assigned tasks—editing, researching, writing—and a second, deeper subterranean level where my imagination is keen; a dreamy place I would like to inhabit more of the time. Slice my mind open like a can of tuna and smell the rich scent: the river Seine, the stink of washed-up carp that fill Sel's pail as she gathers her next meal.

I'm perusing a Penguin edition of the *Dictionary of Science* today. Who was Monsieur Penguin? He established a nice series of books. Whenever I see the little Penguin icon, I feel assured that the book will be of quality. If that isn't successful brand recognition, nothing is.

I read dictionaries the way bulimics binge. Like a starving woman; indiscriminately. Everything interests me. I'm a whore for knowledge. I'm tempted to write down everything that might tangentially relate to Sel, to the properties of her metaphoric chemical being, to Henri's celestial musings. I'm like a mental hoarder who's being asked to clean house or lose the house. I'm uncertain at this stage of research how or if I'll need these little tidbits of knowledge in the future, how they directly relate to this larger moral-historical research Sel is pushing me to uncover. But I'm determined to be more selective.

I do admit I got distracted a moment ago when I learned that the moon is steadily moving away from the Earth. This struck me as a bad thing, no? What will that do to the seas, the waves, the tides? Nothing good, I suspect.

For hours I read, I discard. Ideas, sparks and tangents of narrative possibility rise up. I allow myself to consider them, but only for a moment, like the falling stars I am learning about. I'm reading alphabetically, to keep myself in check. My eyes stop on *S. Salt of lemon (chem): potassium quadroxolate. White, soluble, poisonous, crystalline salt. Used for removing ink stains.*

Really? A white salt that might pass for table salt? Something Sel might try to use to poison a fascist on the pretense of removing an ink stain from his shirt? This thought doesn't have the ring of a very realistic narrative tangent, but I may read more about poisonous salts. Poison isn't so original, but it's still so appealing, so nineteenth century, so vengeful.

Heading home, I stop at the drugstore to search for some salts of lemon to see if I can finally get the big, black ink stain out of the pocket of a favorite pair of ruined white jeans. It's nice that research and fiction can be useful in such practical ways.

~ 37

Happiness again. Adventures in research. Blessings.

I've discovered a treasure among a pile of esoteric books being sold at half price outside the NYU library. A book about the history of the guillotine, the great French instrument of royalist-cum-democratic justice for so many decades. In addition to *Guillotine: Its Legend and Lore*, a paperback, I've purchased *The Drug User*, a collection of essays and first-person accounts of drug use dating from the Victorian era to the 1960s. I haven't decided who's addicted to what in Sel's story yet—whether she's sampled the different Victorian drugs herself—but I still want to know how they affect the body. Sel needs a good working knowledge of the poisons in particular—*laudanum, opium, arsenic*—since they're enjoying a renaissance today.

I read about the revival recently in a magazine. *The New Victorians.* A breed of young fashionistas in New York, London, and Berlin, who favor a louche, decadent style: long shirts with French cuffs and high collars for the boys; bustles and cinched waists over a gym-trained derriere for the ladies. Apparently, slugs and frogs and other staples of Victorian medicine are also making a comeback. *The more modern we get, the more we crave nature's pure, coarse touch—especially if it's repellent. Ain't it true, Sel?*

⌐

The guillotine book contains over a hundred drawings, pictures, and newspaper reprints. There are tidbits that amuse me, like a small decapitating device that became a favorite children's toy, then how miniature guillotines were worn, jewel-encrusted and dangling from earrings or set as glistening brooches—*look, don't touch!*—and pinned onto evening gowns. Given the French *amour* for their morning baguette, it makes sense that bread slicers shaped as guillotines sell well in the local markets. It's all interesting but not that relevant to me except as intellectual fodder and historical trivia, until I stumble across a chapter titled *The Nazi Guillotine.* At once I feel my stomach tighten, feel Sel and Henri, reading over my shoulder, take notice too. Why did I think the guillotine was only an instrument of the distant past, a historical artifact? *How did I not know?*

⌐

Between 1933 and 1945, I read, the Nazis beheaded tens of thousands of people in Germany. Some 16,500 people, the author estimates. Hitler had twenty guillotines built to get his killing program off the ground. In a single sweeping ten-month period from 1944 to 1945, over ten thousand people were beheaded; in 1944 alone, four a day were decapitated by an intrepid Nazi executioner—a total of 1,399 victims. How many of them were Jews, homosexuals, Russians, gypsies, abortionists, and anti-Nazis isn't documented here.

It's safe to wager a bet though. They included Hans and Sophie Scholl, the young anti-Nazi brother and sister activists who were members of the underground White Rose movement. They were guillotined at Stadelheim by Johann Baptist Reichhart, a German master executioner who, like the Sansons, came from a family of executioners. Reichhart set a record by killing 2,876 victims, most of them political prisoners, a figure far greater than any Sanson. After the Nazis were defeated, I'm depressed to learn, Reichhart served as an advisor to Sergeant Johnny Woods, the official hangman for the American forces, on how to prepare a gallows for the Nuremberg war criminals. I didn't know we still hanged our enemies in 1945. But then we also helped executioners like Klaus Barbie escape to Bolivia.

The French guillotine was still in operation when the Nazis invaded Paris in 1940. Various communists and resistance fighters were beheaded, including women. The men spat in the executioner's face; the women were dragged, screaming bloody murder and cursing the executioner's name: Desfourneaux. Why isn't this more widely known? Is it? Maybe it is in France? I should ask my cousins.

I make a mental note to go to Kim's video store on Avenue A in Manhattan to see that *White Rose* film about the Scholls too. I'm certain I've seen it there.

I have a morbid thought. About those decapitated heads. Wondering where they went. Were they dutifully counted and shipped off to medical schools around the world or private museums always in the market for a human head in a jar of chloroform to display? It's something the Nazi doctors would do. The French Vichy civil servants? They would keep meticulous files too.

It wasn't that long ago, I think. *A historical blink of an eye. My parents could have watched the executions themselves. They were high school students. My father attended medical school at the Sorbonne. Did he ever wonder about the identity of the cadavers he was cutting up in his classes?*

You see, this is how my mind works. I make so many connections. Here now, I discover the guillotine was set up to cut off the heads of women like my grandmother Mamie.

Remarkably—or is it so remarkable? (*No,* Sel cuts in, *not surprising at all*)— the French executioner and his assistants were cleared of charges of collaboration by the post-Vichy government. Then they resumed their duties in 1946, *beheading ordinary criminals.* I've added those italics here because, honestly, can you believe it? They were still beheading prisoners in the fifties in *la belle,* civilized France?! *For real. Were we too, here in the United States? When did we stop?*

I do a quick mental calculation. Papou did his one-year stint in prison for his troubles after the war. He was an ordinary prisoner. Did he know about the prison guillotine?

Apparently, the executioner went crazy in the last five years of his life. He had terrifying visions and died at the age of seventy-four. I imagine the nightmares: one bloody chopped head after another dropping off the giant blade of the guillotine into a cart to be hauled away. Each one looking forever shocked, with bulging eyes, the way they must have felt.

⌒

The guillotine was officially retired in 1977. *1977!* I was a junior in college, starting Barnard, quitting tennis. Today it collects dust in the Museum of Folk Arts in the Bois de Boulogne, a park on the outskirts of Paris. I may drop by to see it the next time I'm in France, out of curiosity. The Mitterrand government clearly doesn't want to display it more openly. *Wonder why not? Does the sight of it prick the president's conscience?*

The past is not so far away. I could take a taxi ride there to see it for myself, on my way to see where the Rio trannies are flagging down clients in the Bois.

Thank you, Gertrude Stein: a fascist is a fascist is a fascist.

~ 38

ACT UP reinforced an important lesson: don't wait for someone else to fight your battles. Even within ACT UP, we still have to push to become even more visible, to demand more active solidarity from the boys. We being the feminists and sapphists, who, statistically, are still far below the public radar compared to gay men, both with regard to HIV and AIDS and general visibility. Most lesbians I know really don't want to think about a possible risk of exposure to HIV despite all the ways we women get down with each other. So our battle isn't just with the public, or NYC officials, but our own community, our own circles. The conversation is never easy.

It's true that exposure via saliva is nil: so oral, hands, and sex toys are safe. But, there's a *but.* What if a girl or woman has HIV and is on her period? What if the sex is rough, and someone bleeds? How did she get HIV, people ask? Lesbians have sex with men and shoot smack. I have close friends who fall into the category and struggle with addiction. Others do sex work. There are a lot of lapsed Catholic girls out there, making a little extra money, or paying off student loans, working as dancers in strip clubs, offering lap dances that sometimes go further if they like a client, or if the money is just too tempting. If you went to a strip club, you would know this. I didn't myself, until I started having friends who work in the clubs. There's a sex-work sisterhood. The women I know are safe-sex educators; they're S-and-M bondage mamas and daddies, and they're lesbians.

Others grew up fast and hard in high school, were hardcore punk teens who loved Jello Biafra and the Dead Kennedys. Were little dykes early on, then got kicked out of their families, churches, and hometowns, taking refuge on a friend's couch. Or cycled through foster homes that look poorly on gay children and ended up on the streets, or in juvie—juvenile detention centers. So you see the pattern. My point is that lesbians are vulnerable to risk and we need to talk about it.

Then there's poverty and racism. And sexual violence. That's something no one talks about enough. Double or triple that for women of color, especially black women in the United States, who are statistically ten times more likely to have HIV than white women. We're also affected by other diseases that aren't getting enough research or funding: including cancers of the breast and cervix and all the autoimmune diseases like Lyme and MS and lupus that friends we know started having after college. We need more attention to lesbian health issues. That's the message we've been giving to ACT UP, to our communities, and to the scientists and government too. We need research into HIV in women, and in lesbians. We need lesbians in clinical trials.

Who cares about lesbians? We do. The women of ACT UP. The caped crusader Avengers. We're making noise about it.

I'm supposed to go to Maxine Wolfe's house this week for a potluck to talk about the lesbian HIV agenda. We're also planning an action to target Rudy Giuliani, and the Dyke March. I want to go but I want to write too. Is it always going to be like this, such a conflict between activism and art for me? I want to do both, but the week's half over and it's all been work writing, not fun writing, not my journey with Sel. Maybe I'll find time this weekend.

Max is one of the women who put together ACT UP's 1990 book on HIV in women. She's Jewish, a red diaper baby, with great daughters. I think of her as a crone in the most positive sense of the word, with long, gray hair and wise-woman energy. She and I have clashed at times, in ACT UP and the Avengers. She's very fierce in her politics, like Sarah Schulman. I suppose I'm quite opinionated too. There are two other kitchen-table-founding Avengers — Anna Simo, who's an old buddy; and Marie Honan. I include Anne Maguire, because she was at our first meeting even if she didn't get involved right then. The Irish lasses of ILGO, feisty dykes. Truth is we're all opinionated and passionate girls. I know I should say *women*, but with the Avengers, we feel like girls in our girls' club.

We're also Dykes. As in capital *D* lesbians. Dykes are the slur that comes before the blow. Dykes are the unruly stereotypical Angry Lesbian that society fears. We wanted to take the word back, play with it, own it. Now we do. Even me, 'cuz I was never a big dyke.

When we did our first visibility action at a schoolyard in Queens in November '92, I wore a T-shirt that said: *I was a lesbian child.* I thought about it at the time: *was I a lesbian child? I don't think I was.* I came to my sense of sexuality late, in college. But I knew what I was at age five: a boy pirate, a scout, a cowboy. Not much of a girl, though. Not someone who could tolerate dresses. I should have worn a T-shirt that day that said: *I was a lesbian boy.* That would have been more accurate. I was a little tomboy butch, definitely. But I never thought about other girls, or boys, really, except to wonder why I didn't want to kiss the boys. I just felt nothing for them or anyone except my teachers. I had a mad schoolgirl crush on my high school teacher, only a bit older then I was at the time. But it was a fantasy; he was safe, out of reach. I was a late bloomer.

So now I'll embrace the slur: call me a butch dyke. I won't be offended at all. I'll just work to fill those big boots because there are some awesome, gorgeous, handsome, strong women out there.

These days the Avengers are full of younger dykes who don't seem worried in the least about taking on their labels either. They're a sex-positive, gender-fluid bunch, ready to have some fun, to stir things up a bit. We came up with the name Lesbian Avengers—a retro-campy, comic-book, superwoman-hero name—to make people laugh and disarm them. And to scare them—*just a tiny bit.* A name that ensures we won't take ourselves too, too seriously either, which is the stereotype people have of scary lesbians: serious, shrill, sexless, and no fun at all. I look at that picture I showed Philippe of the big DC Dyke March: all of us holding garbage can shields to drum on; sunny, funny noisemakers. Our protests read as theater and fun to those watching. But if they took a flyer, saw the names of women like Hattie Mae Cohens, who was burned alive for being a lesbian, or those who are sick with AIDS, they would have felt our fury and our sorrow and our demands for justice too.

The only thing I was initially uncertain about was the Avenger logo, but it was passed by group consensus. After some debate (*but we don't sanction violence!*), we adopted a little bomb logo—again the campy joke. Only now do we see how much that little bomb scares people. So does our signature action: eating fire, something we've all learned to do. We were taught by one of the Aerialist's best friends, Jenny Miller. She's a bearded lady and a lezzie and has a political circus, Circus Amok.

Eating fire is a little circus trick and what girl doesn't like the circus? Once you get over the hump of putting a kerosene-soaked rag torch, lit on fire, in your mouth, it's easy. (*Tip: don't close your eyes! Your hair can catch on fire.*) You just close your mouth over it; it cuts oxygen off from the flame, which dies instantly. The torch can leave an icky taste in your mouth, but boy, does it impress a crowd. And cops. *Dykes with torches! Watch out!* We did have quite a few straight-girl allies who showed up to march as honorary dykes in DC; they were more then ready to don a supergirl cape and eat some fire too. I guess that song is true, *girls just wanna have fun.*

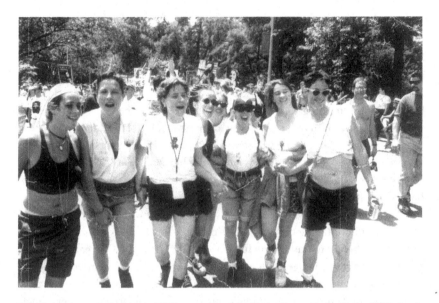

Friends in Protest: Dyke March, NYC, 1994. *From left*: Cindra Feuer, Catherine Saalfield, Sarah
Pettit, Christina Wheeler, Roxane Tynan, Maria Maggenti, Melissa Painter, Anne-christine
d'Adesky. (AC d'Adesky)

~ 39

I'm steadily boning up on the Vichy France collaborators and the link to
Europe's new fascists. There's not much about the Euro skinheads and pro-
Nazi groups in the U.S. newspapers; only tidbits in the *Economist* here and
there, often tied to economic news. The *New York Times* has trained its foreign
coverage on Bosnia and the disintegration of the former Soviet republics. The
only time they focus on modern neofascism is when there's an election. When
Italy's new golden lady, Benito Mussolini's granddaughter Alessandra, makes
another colorful statement to the press.

She's quite the character, I'll admit. One would have trouble writing a
Hollywood script as good, as juicy, as her life: ex-Playboy model (*two magazine
covers—impressive*); niece of Sophia Loren; pop singer of romantic songs (her
album was titled *Amore*; what else?); she's even had a part in a film where she
played a nun. Of course, it was a revisionist story: how the Italian Catholic
Church rescued Jews from the Nazis in 1943. But *still*. She's quite the package.
I'm keeping her in my mind for my story as one of the fascist women that will
turn up at some point; maybe at a party or a fascist meeting that Sel crashes.

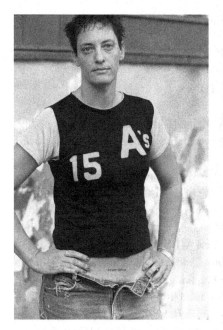

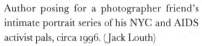

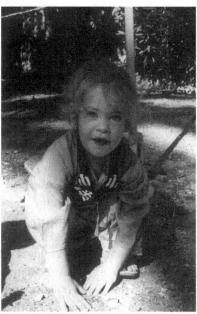

Author posing for a photographer friend's intimate portrait series of his NYC and AIDS activist pals, circa 1996. (Jack Louth)

Author as inner samurai warrior child in Fort Lauderdale, Florida, age three or four. (AC d'Adesky)

Alessandra reminds me of Giorgio Armani's sister, Rossana, for some reason—same look, though not a platinum blonde. A modern Italian type, anyway. Something coarse and sexy at the same time. A tough, opinionated broad who loves high fashion. I wonder what her relationship is with the Vatican.

I'm now adding Alessandra Mussolini to my new top ten list of modern fascists. I've got Milošević and Radović in Bosnia and Serbia. In France we have the Le Pens, *père et filles*, and the Brunos—Bruno Gollnisch, who joined Le Pen's party in 1983, and Bruno Mégret. I have a bunch of names of other National Front party members too, but they're my B-list, lower-level fascists.

Here we have Pat Robertson and Jerry Falwell, the Christian fundamentalist leaders, and their ilk. There are a lot of new faces at the local level. And the white Aryan nation of course. David Duke, leader of our modern KKK. He's a good ole boy from Baton Rouge who used to wear Hitler costumes to celebrate the Fuhrer's birthday, so I've read. Duke's now run twice for the U.S. presidency, as a Democrat in 1988 and two years ago as a GOP candidate. He calls himself a *racial realist*. What a concept. What a guy. I'll have to check on the KKK's website, see what they're up to right now. Probably in tight with the *God-hates-fags* antigay ordinance groups.

Who's at the top of your list, reader?

~ 40

It's already spring. The year is filling with death. Unexpected. Too soon. The kind that leaves you with regrets for everything not said, not done, not known. *The end of the future.*

Our golden boy, charming Aldyn, has slipped away. From one minute to the next, it feels. Not much warning; none of the usual signs. No AIDS in the classic sense, just pneumonia then rapid kidney failure. A sudden crisis, a sudden elevation of enzymes, the expectation of a quick recovery and, instead, death. I don't think he even qualified for the revised AIDS diagnosis.

He was just Aldyn, poster boy of robust health, albeit saddled with a catheter poking out of his abdomen and a urine bag hanging from his belt at one point. Still cruising boys at the hospital with his usual insouciance in those last weeks, and a bit more wit. *I think it's got a certain sexiness*, he'd say, patting his pee bag. *Definitely attracts a certain type.* And it did, but not the S-and-M freaks or those into golden showers. Just the usual nice men drawn to Aldyn's Irish good looks and smart mouth; his refusal to abandon life's pleasure.

After Paris, I'd run into Aldyn in the usual places—ACT UP meetings, mostly. In addition to his usual duties as a cheerful facilitator at our regular Monday night meetings, he was hard at work setting up links between long-term survivors in other countries, post-Berlin. He was full of energy; no one saw it coming. Nor did he right then.

But I told you earlier: he never expected to remain forever healthy; even with high T cells and no sign of immune decline. He never pretended. *I'll die of AIDS*, he'd predicted to me in France. *It just might take me a lot longer.*

At Saint Vincent's, where all the boys go, he was Aldyn, only a bit shaken. *The first cut is the deepest*, he joked with me. He started out with a cold that he couldn't shake, then pneumonia. The first time his kidney rebelled, he had a fever, then chills. His kidneys became weak. Once admitted, he used his time well, interviewing other patients with HIV, documenting services needed, sending out faxes to demand what was promised but denied. A one-man activist machine. He refused to stop. Behind his bed on the wall were petitions, press releases, and a picture of himself at Berlin. He wanted sympathy and he wanted action. *Tell people.* He pressed a petition into my hand. *Tell them my kidney's failing. Tell the reporters.*

How does it feel to have sex with a catheter poking from your belly? How does it feel to go from golden boy to an invalid with the weight of a half-filled bag of urine sloshing at your hip? I admired Aldyn all the more, facing the end with true bravery, in full action.

Under his easy smile, after his many, many friends went home from the bars, Aldyn was like many of the boys I befriended in ACT UP: a bit lonely and privately terrified of dying. He just didn't make a big deal of it. Like Johnny, he didn't have a steady boyfriend right then and longed for one at times to fill a terrible void. He wasn't overly lonely, but he wanted a companion to laugh with, to sing songs with in the shower. He wanted a companion for the dark nights. None of us had a clue. With so many of our friends so much sicker, hanging on to life by a thread, Aldyn was still in the safety zone, still zipping around town on his bicycle. But here he is now, gone forever.

At ACT UP, we've all cried and marched in the streets for him. He's deeply missed. He was loved by so many and admired by more. There's another public funeral event planned for him this summer at the Yokohama AIDS conference, a scattering of his ashes. I may not go. After I heard, I lit a candle by his picture and got a big bottle of good Irish whiskey and toasted him and his amazing life. I've learned even more about him with all the eulogies. He was a soldier, and an antiwar protester. He promoted black studies at Harvard. He really did so much in such a short life. I'm so glad he got to love so many boys. He was a friend, not super close but a trench friend. We felt bonded, especially after Berlin.

Here, now, I see him jumping into bed with Belle and me. I remember my promise to him and his promise to me. He'd proposed himself as a muse, a guiding light, a touchstone for me in moments of writer's doubt. *Lolita, patron of troubled young men with golden futures cut short. His alter ego.* I'll light this candle and think about him, think about his pursuit of pleasure, his selfless, hardworking soul, his good brain, his sense of community, his singing, his Irish smile and twinkling eyes. *Don't forget to dance,* he advised. *Damn I'm gonna miss him.*

$\mathcal{V}I$

$Paris,\ enfin$

~ 41

July 1994

A full thirty-six-hour cycle has passed since the night's tempest. I wake into a blue afternoon and the knocking insistence of the large, wooden-framed windows of Belle's small apartment. Or that's how I feel, upon waking. That the wind, nature, life is calling out to me, pushing away some earlier malaise. A bit of depression fueled by jet lag. I've been back in Paris for several days and my sense of time is still off. I thought it was noon and awoke refreshed, only to note that my watch said eight o'clock.

In the room next door, Belle is listening to a French chanteuse whose singing is old-fashioned and familiar. Barbara, a new discovery for me. Her voice sounds like Marlene Dietrich: guttural dips, prolonged high notes, all plaintive and boozy; songs of love. I'm reminded of my mother, a style queen like Dietrich.

It makes me recall my mother's mothball-scented clothes: the heavy pinch-waist Dior suits she kept under wraps in our Florida house that hinted at a glamorous youth and an exciting nightlife; many pairs of soft leather gloves, each having a single, covered button at the wrist; sheer scarves; palm-sized clip-shut box purses; slim silver cigarette holders; tiny brimless hats to be worn at a rakish angle. I never saw my mother wear any of these, but in the pictures and the few 16 mm movies she and my father shot of their vacations together before my birth, she wore herringbone suits and a dark-green cape I inherited, looking 100 percent *très française, très chic*. She had had a glamourous life before she moved to America to become a doctor's wife. She didn't regret the move at all, but she missed wearing her fancy clothes. They were too warm for the Florida heat.

You can wear them one day, she urged me from time to time, knowing my waist was not small enough, that my arms and thighs were too thickly muscular from

154

years of tennis, that I was her tomboy daughter with Farrah Fawcett hair who struggled to wear dresses. As much as I wanted to please her, I couldn't wear her Paris couture. Even the gloves were too tight. My hands felt like sausages.

Still, we didn't give them away, not until after her death. Throughout my childhood, I would open her drawers and hat and glove boxes, taking in the smell of her exciting life in Paris.

Of course, one of the reasons I'm here researching my family history is because of her. My earliest memories are linked to trips we took to visit relatives on the southern coast—Nice, Cannes—or to Chamonix, for the end-of-summer, annual family gathering. She's been dead more years than I can count and I forget to remember her sometimes. I like to be reminded and the memories are always sharp, tinged with a sense of loss and nostalgia. I always love seeing her face again in my mind and it always hurts. I see her more when I'm here, in France. I imagine I'm looking through her eyes here; looking at the same views and buildings she once saw. It calms me. *Regarde, Maman,* I say now, getting up to peer out Belle's window at the surrounding rooftops. *Look.*

Belle has moved closer to the Eiffel Tower and, just beyond, my river. I've laid personal claim to the Seine. Soon, later tonight, I'll take a walk. There are festivities planned to celebrate France's national holiday.

Wonder where Le Pen will be celebrating? With his family and daughters? His daughter Marine is my age, maybe a year younger. I could try to find out, but I won't. There's a limit to how much I'll mix business and pleasure. Right now, I'm visiting with Belle, who I've missed. I want to enjoy my time with her.

The sounds of explosion begin from somewhere far off in my sleep. I think I'm in Haiti, then I'm half-awake and the French are celebrating their freedom again. Outside my window the Eiffel Tower is again a shining star lit like a Christmas angel. Beyond my view I imagine the Seine smiling as only a river can smile, long and sinewy and generous, licking the taste of sulfur and gun powder that drops into her water from the fireworks that have begun.

When I lean over the apartment banister, I see giant irises moving toward me: green circles inside red; opium poppy visions. I think *virus, virus, virus,* seeing a giant projection of what is happening in my friend Kiki's body back in New York. A boy, Kiki. I call him Joan, a pet name, after Joan Crawford, his idol and muse. Because he tries to live up to her famous ultra-bitch persona.

The giant, white macrophages are getting bigger, too big, and cancerous, the cells falling apart from within, leaving holes in Kiki's blood. His body is being ravaged. In the sky, the drama of his viral battle is being played out, the fireworks exploding, fading, traces of ash.

When I hear the whistle of the dropping fireworks bomb, I imagine Kiki's mind exploding from inside, over and over again, his pain glittering. Another white flower blooms in the sky, trickles down like the falling tail of a kite, and slowly fades. I can barely remember what it looked like.

Will I remember Kiki if he dies? Will I think of Johnny? How often? Will I bring Aldyn with me on my walk later tonight? Will his voice pierce me as the voice of this singer, Barbara, is now doing? She's making me remember Aldyn is dead and the virus won.

Only hours ago, Kiki and I were talking on the phone. He's just started taking the newest experimental drug for cancers linked to AIDS. Daunorubicin. It uses a relatively new technology, liposomes, that encase the drug in a lipid, allowing it to more easily cross membranes, enter cells, and be delivered into a tumor or infected tissue. A little chemical smart bomb. But the drug is still hard to get access to—read: exorbitantly expensive and not covered by his fancy comprehensive health insurance. *Too new*, his insurance company told him; *we'll wait for more data.*

Last month, he threatened to publicly broadcast his own liberation day parade, to go on television and allow close-ups of his ugly body and scarlet Kaposi's sarcoma lesions, to show people how ugly this disease has made him feel, how criminal it is that the drugmaker hasn't rushed this drug out to the market. To become his own one-man Action Jackson media campaign, like Aldyn did.

Truth be told, Kiki's been arm-twisting me to go after them: daunorubicin's manufacturer. He's been putting pressure on them through the media, through his own writing for the gay press. Playing his part; creating a major drama. A Tennessee Williams high-southern-drama moment, full of hysteria and pleading on his part for immediate *compassionate use* access to the cancer smart bomb; not just for himself but for others with KS, like Johnny, who aren't responding to the existing arsenal either.

Smile for the cameras. These are the moments when being a journalist has its advantages. People either seek exposure or want to avoid it. The drug companies have had a hard time ignoring Kiki in his high-southern-bitchy Crawford moments, holding court for the press. He's organizing his own small army of Kikis and plans to dog health officials and their potential allies: the doctors planning clinical trials of the drug. That's the data we need so urgently to get the drug approved by the FDA—the next step before marketing and broader access. It can take months—even years.

Kiki may get into the first trial but not the second, which is already planned. He's organizing others who are ready to be prodded and purged, to be guinea pigs in a trial, to religiously take a chemo-toxic drug that might not work, that has known and clear side effects. The drugs will cause him to lose his lovely, swept-back golden mane; his pride—the last thing a southern belle wants to lose. All this for the chance—the prayer—that it might reduce internal lesions of KS that are pressing on some internal organs, including Kiki's prostate. A painful swelling that makes it urgently necessary to be closely tethered to the bathroom like Johnny has become of late.

But Kiki won't go down without a proper, all-fists-flying fight. I talked to him about how the French right wing and the drag queens both claim Joan of Arc as their heroine. He's channeling two Joans now: himself and Crawford— the moral heroine and the righteous bitch—and charging forward.

And now, I see, he's won. *Score one for Team Kiki.*

For now, he clarified, spelling out a longer war that looms around fast-track access to daunorubicin. He's been given a short-term compassionate dose for himself—enough to see if the drug makes a real difference—but no longer-term commitment from the drug manufacturer or trial. Still, the drugmaker is on the alert, clearly aware that exposure of Kiki's elephantine, blackening legs on national news would be a possible public-relations disaster. It might scare away the important potential investors at a time the company seeks them, at the pre-approval stage, armed with some promising data. Data that spells possible billions in sales and profits in the future. *That's what they really care about,* Kiki told me yesterday. *Who cares about my fucking balls?*

———

I'm distracted from this thought as the entire sky goes deep red pink—*the color of stained tissue under a microscope*—then slowly bleeds and dissipates to the muted pink red that's left when you press fingers on closed eyelids, hard. That gives way to blinking white lights when you open them again. A lingering pale red that now outlines two small white clouds by the Eiffel Tower. More meta-phors come: *The red like a stain of blood seeping through a white shirt. I've seen it, in Haiti; I've held people shot in the stomach, the chest, with blood spurting like a small fountain, or slowly spreading into a wound like that. A pale- to deeper-red stain like a sunset you want to hang on to, that's fading fast now, leaving me with the echo of scattershot explosives in my ears.*

To my right, four big searchlights crisscross the sky and I think, *You're looking in the wrong place for your heroes, you French leaders. Look down; shine your light behind you, over there toward the Place de Clichy and the flea market, where Oui, another dying boy, another of your patriot sons, lives with the knowledge that he probably won't get access to daunorubicin.*

They're even further behind in France. Like Kiki, Oui's pale, thin body is pockmarked like the victims of earlier plagues.

KS, the pox stigmata of our time.

~ 42

I've gotten an update about Oui from Belle. Everyone's afraid he's going to die very soon. The medicines aren't working; he's so far gone. It's something he's not afraid to admit to me or anyone else. At ACT UP–Paris, he's been a

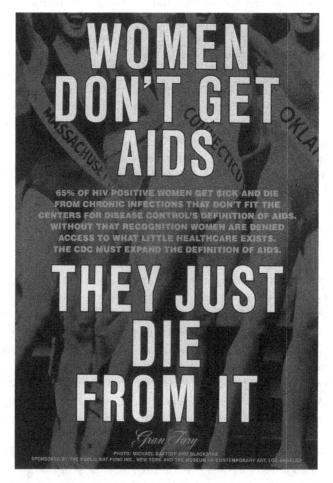

ACT UP's Women and AIDS poster by Gran Fury. (Gran Fury Collection, Manuscripts and Archives Division, New York Public Library)

cheerleader, a leader, a media spokesman for HIV drug access. And, like Kiki, Oui has lost the ability to be polite. He's upset and desperate. But he's gotten so thin and weak that it's not possible for him to make the trip to the United States, to protest-beg for a drug that many of his American gay friends can't access either. I'll have to go and see him this visit; he won't come over here, to Belle's house.

We spoke last night on the phone. *I'm so sick, Anne, and it makes me so sad.* Oui has none of Johnny's bitterness, but I feel it for him: the sharp sense of betrayal, the *pourquoi moi?—why me?*

Pourquoi toi, indeed. Pourquoi Kiki? Life's absolutely not fair. Kiki's balls are aching to explode. He's in pain all the time. He looks grotesque and he knows it. Kiki, a man who loves beauty, who loves drag, who loves what's feminine in himself and in other men. It's not fair and the drug companies have made it crueler. The system of profit that we rely on to heal ourselves is so broken, so craven. We have to take them on. We need affordable, lifesaving drugs for Kiki and Oui. We need them yesterday already.

⁓

I'm overdue to be back in touch with Théodore and the Port-au-Prince exiles. Since my last visit to Paris, Haiti's come flooding back into the global news. The political chaos is ongoing, as are the extrajudicial killings, but elections are being planned. I imagine Théodore is actively involved here, organizing the exiled community. I wonder if his family has been able to join him by now. He's such a pusher, such a doer; I can't imagine the French authorities not relenting, just to get him off their backs.

I'll have to pass on his name to the producers of two American television programs who've called me, asking for an opinion piece on the possibility of a U.S. invasion of Haiti—something that could happen in the coming week. If it does, I'll be ready with my comments. And I'll try to get Théodore a little coverage too—his case, the plight of the Haitian political exiles. But I'm not rushing over to Haiti. I've had enough ambulance coup reporting for the moment, *thank you very much.*

While I was watching the giant-pink-flower fireworks blossom and fade earlier I wondered if Théodore was watching them too, from his amazing view in Montmartre. If he put his fingers in his tortured ears, unwilling to be reminded of what could be happening at home tonight, in Haiti. *We're all veterans of phantom wars, aren't we?*

Inside the apartment, I hear Belle inside, laughing, on the phone with a friend. *Lighten up,* I remind myself. *You're in Paris again. With Belle. Everybody's still celebrating. Go have a glass of champagne. Amuse-toi,* as Papou would say.

~ 43

Days slip into another week. I've decided to stay longer in Paris. There's more research to do. At the same time, I've hit a fresh wave of creative shoals. I'm grappling with the direction of my ongoing writer's adventure and Sel's story: *Novel or secret diary? Her journal or mine? Some combination of genres?* What's most clear, and consistently available to me, is the inner voice—the little rasp of conversation that I've trained my ear to listen for; a constant sharing and commenting, an alter ego with a longer, sharper grasp of French history and a freer tongue.

I've also felt the impulse to push away from fiction, toward some harder or more immediate reality. Wanting to consider a different kind of war diary, one that gives a more immediate voice to my dying friends like Kiki. He's won another round in the drug-access battle but may lose the big one: his life. I'm preoccupied by the effort to get them a weapon that works. Kiki, Johnny, Oui . . . just in ACT UP there are a number of boys on the waiting list for the new KS drug. I check in with my friends, get daily updates. They feel desperate. Each day offers small, fresh horrors.

~ 44

Kiki is a talented columnist with a wicked wit, who fantasizes about writing his gossipy memoir. The colorful life of a high southern sissy who fled to the Big Apple and managed to attend the most fabulous parties, meet the craziest, funniest people, and sleep with all the wrong people and some of the right ones. And who will die tragically, and too young, like so many great rock stars. We've talked about it. He can't write his own memoir, as much as he'd like to. Death has him in its sights. He's going to go, it's clear to him now, and he can't figure out how to make the most of the time ahead; how to stay productive. He's writing his *POZ* columns and he's organized a group: Lesion Liberation—a true tart's corps.

You know what I'd write, don't you? he said to me back in New York. What he says to anyone who happens to be near him, to his readers: *The goddamn truth. I'm not dying; I'm being murdered. I'm being sold down the river by people within this community who claim to be helping people with AIDS.*

So write that, I told him. *Do it. Start today. A little a day, it will add up before you know it. You should do it while you want to, while you feel the pull.*

But he has a million things to do in the present—in the life still to be lived— that compete with documenting his own life, his past, especially since his future is not a given. He's dreaming about his memoir without a plan for the actual writing. *Can't I dictate it to you?* he whines. *I'm lazy.* Plus, he has his doubts. *Who wants to read about another bitter, dying queen? I'm not famous enough.* For now, he's busy doing his columns, or lining up celebrities to interview for *Vanity Fair* or the *New York Times Magazine*—his paid gigs, when he still can get them. He can't travel far now. But he needs the cash and wants the fancy byline too; the brush with star power and the glam life; the parties, even if he feels too ugly and poxed to attend. He faux-complains: *They're gonna have to pay me a goddamn lot of money to make me go to LA to talk to that bitch!*

So . . . we both know his memoir is unlikely. He doesn't have the emotional energy to confront the taunting beasts, *doubt and time,* an enemy duo always ready to waylay our creative efforts, even when we are in perfect health. With death stalking, his faith is also wavering. A holy trinity of writer's block.

~ 45

I've been making the rounds of somewhat specialized museums and libraries, in between some reporting. Each offering morsels of Sel's story to me. I spent a good morning at the historical library, whose archives could keep me here for another decade. They're amazing. I began with the simple desire to see a picture of Barbette, a character famed in the Parisian demimonde: a cross-dressing Texan male named Vander Clyde who wore a blond wig and an ostrich feather costume weighing fifty pounds and who made a name for himself—herself?— doing a remarkably smooth high-wire trapeze act at the Cirque Medrano, among others.

Barbette reminds me of Kiki, reminds me I owe Kiki a call. Just to hear his bitchy, molasses-slow complaint. Kiki wants more media attention to KS in the prostrate. I've passed him a few names to follow up. Not sure what this can do, but anything that makes Kiki feel some forward action is helpful nowadays.

Barbette's name came up in a big picture book I have about the golden period for Americans in Paris because his act vied with the more famous Josephine Baker (who's identified as a naked cabaret dancer) in terms of artistry, coquetry, and *scandal.* As Jean Cocteau, who loved Barbette, once teased Baker: *He conceals everything, you reveal everything.*

Even more revealing is a tidbit about Barbette by the premier French gossip of French nightlife, Maurice Sachs. Sachs was a Jew; he was also a gay man, and later accused of being an informer when in the Nazi camps. He failed to make it out of Europe. He was shot in 1945 during a march by the SS as they retreated from an Allied attack. (Knowing nothing yet of the incident, I automatically presume that Sachs's open homosexuality also played a role in his arrest by the Nazis.) But, during the good years, Sachs made a surprise visit to the circus artist, only to find Barbette reclining backstage naked, de-wigged, his carefully shaved pale face covered in black pomade. Next to him, on a night table, was a book titled *L'Onanisme, seul et à deux (Onanism: Alone and Together)*. Such details make a legend, at least for me, and I was eager to see a picture of the daring Texan drag queen.

⌒

I found very little in the few books on reserve about Paris circuses and nothing salacious or enlightening about high-wire masturbation. Nor was there any mention of Barbette in a signed autobiography by the founder of the Cirque Medrano. *Was it because Barbette was a drag queen?* I eventually found one journalist who wrote that *the most impressive circus act of all time was Barbette with his genius of light movement.* Elsewhere, this same author, who took pains to identify himself as heterosexual, describes Barbette using the feminine pronoun, and stresses, for a public who will regret never seeing them, *Barbette's beautiful legs.* Since I haven't found any pictures of Barbette yet, I've had to content myself with my vision of a coy diva with a pale, graceful, muscular body, whose legs and underarms are shaved, who applies black pomade carefully to avoiding staining his wig.

Why the black pomade? Some blackface minstrel holdover from his Texas past?

'Cuz he's a fuckin' racist fool. I smile, hearing Kiki's voice break into my mind. Kiki never minces words; I have to give him credit for that. If he ever wrote his memoir, he would call it the way he saw it. There are many fools in Kiki's life, including nearly everyone in the south. Right now the journalists at the *New York Times* and *Daily News* and *New York Post* are the biggest fools. *They're missing an important story*, he's told me. *Every single man in America wants to know about what could hurt his balls.*

Quickly now, I'm jotting down the flights of narrative fancy: perhaps Sel will use a tunnel leading to the Cirque Medrano, wanting to see a performance by the famed Barbette. She'll arrive in Barbette's dressing room, having used the basement entrance to the circus office that connects with the cavernous branches of the Catacombs. An entrance that served contraband traffickers and escaped criminals and Sachs's contemporaries—the gay Jews of Paris— who, fleeing for their lives toward the Spanish border and the anonymity of Morocco, met their escorts under the cover of the big tent. Sel brings Barbette a special gift—the rich mud of the river—to use as a facial (better than his pomade). And she listens, crouching, hidden, as Barbette and Jean Cocteau and their coterie of bitchy queens and fag hags gossip about the closeted *Le Monde* theater critic sitting in the front row who isn't fooling anyone with his female escort. They've pegged him as a tranny chaser.

As for me, I too like a man with shapely legs. I try to remember what Kiki's legs looked like before he became the Elephant Man. Now, like Johnny, he prefers to wear a robe over hospital scrubs that are suited for swollen thighs and ginormous cancer balls, as he's taken to calling his condition.

An addendum: not enough has been written about the disappearance of men's legs to the ravages of AIDS, in my opinion. Not enough about the pain felt by gay men who are more attuned to fashion and what's pretty than a lot of women. Such losses matter; they matter hugely. They hurt our vanity and sense of self and these are elements that make us feel human and comfortable in the company of others. No one likes ugliness, not really. Kiki's legs are monstrous and there's no getting around that fact. And that's killing him, as surely as the virus.

~ 46

It's one of the ironies of the cultural war that Saint Joan, Catholic heroine of the National Front, is also the chosen patron saint of cross-dressing homosexuals here too. They bring flowers to Joan's statue every year and feast in her honor. La Fête de la Sainte-Jeanne. I want to call Kiki. He'd appreciate this. *Fools*, he'd say with a laugh. *Fools! Now, how to use this juicy tidbit in my story? A fascists-queens standoff, fighting over the right to claim their icon. Or maybe they'll all show up at a party in period costume? That would be more fun. No one does royal better than a drag queen.*

As I meander the streets of Paris, ducking into an Arab tea shop for a bit of overly sweet mint tea to sugar-shock my system and wake up, I make up a mental party guest list: *Alessandra Mussolini? The Le Pens, of course. Maybe the rising wunderkind student leader of the Front's youth wing, who apparently wears leather; he's so modern and cool? Someone in ACT UP spotted him in the Marais, close to a bar with a spanking night. Spying or slumming, we wonder? I'm sure some of the homophobes in the Front are closet cases, just like in the church. Self-hatred, turned outward. Like the Christian Right evangelists who keep getting arrested for the very sins they preach so loudly against. The ones who keep trying to reprogram gay people to go straight, as if. Instead, they end up as tabloid fodder. I supposed it's a personal issue to them, their struggle to stay closeted.*

I'm going off on a tangent. *The party list—who should come?* Let me think . . . if I really wanted to have fun, I could have Papou make an appearance, and his old lesbian friends from cabarets in Pigalle. Oh, and Barbette.

What about me? Where do I fit into my own narrative? Should I write myself in? Make an appearance, be a journalist covering the party? I could bring Johnny and Kiki and Oui. And Aldyn: he could show up as his little punk tartlet alter ego, Lolita.

It's coming to me, this scene. Very Hieronymus Bosch.

I'll let this scene auger. If it lasts more than a day or so in my mind. Still, I can see Sel there, donning a special frock for the Saint Joan festival; something especially ugly or, conversely, something beautiful that emphasizes her ugliness. Dolling herself up for a personal encounter with the big man himself. Maybe a ladies first dance request just to throw Le Pen, the guest speaker, completely off balance. He wouldn't dare refuse, with an American journalist nearby taking notes? There I could be, maybe.

She does keep me entertained, this salty muse of mine. Or a little unbalanced. Take your pick.

~ 47

Today is Sunday, and though the sky is Impressionistic—a swirl of blue and misty white—I feel a cool current that will bring a storm later-on. I am hyphenating this way because I've absorbed the literary cadences of a famous addict, the Englishman Thomas De Quincey, whose nineteenth-century classic, *Confessions of an English Opium-Eater*, is a dense but engaging read.

For example, De Quincey is fond of the word *way-lay*, and uses it generously to describe the fateful, and eventually fatal, way that opium takes over his life and senses. This, despite the fact that opium produces a remarkable clarity of vision and helps one confront long-held fears, leading to competence and confidence— a point De Quincey takes pains to explain to his Gentle Readers, as he calls his audience.

De Quincey has also reintroduced me to the word *evanesced*—a verb in this case, as well as a state of being, i.e., a way of departing the world by disappearance; as the sage Brit puts it so sweetly, referring to the first druggist who ever sold him opium and later disappeared: *I believe him to have evanesced, or evaporated.* According to seventeenth-century denizens, this was the preferred and more dignified route for kings and blood royals in particular to take leave of the world, especially in moments of high unpopularity.

I'm not merely amusing you with ancient wordplay. But I'm a bit of a mystic like De Quincey, though I'm not an addict in an active sense. He's a transcender, as well as a confessor; a night owl, a wanderer, a dreamer of vivid dreams who enjoys it when daytime reality is turned on its head to reveal a lurking world of strange chance and potential journey. Evanesced is the perfect way to describe what's happened to so many people I know. Like Aldyn. One day, they simply disappear from the place they occupied, from their daily station. They've evanesced, leaving me looking over my shoulder for them at times, even here in Paris, a place I know some of them never set foot in but dreamed about.

Back to De Quincey, though. What may prove useful to me, or to Sel, more accurately, is his detailed account of the use of opium, both in his day and prior to it. Sel is familiar with tincture of opium, a vile-looking brown substance boiled down from large white-brownish turds, round mushroom caps that have been cultivated with black soil still clinging to their surface. I saw a large glass jar of it yesterday at the Museum of Public Assistance.

~

In 1804, when De Quincey was still a hardworking Oxford boy with a weekend drug habit, East Indian opium was three guineas a pound and Turkish opium, or *madjoon*, cost eight guineas, which made it—and, here, again, note the delicacy of De Quincey's language—rather *dear*, as in expensive. There are other important details, such as the seven thousand daily drops De Quincey worked his way up to, and his estimate that twenty-five drops of laudanum, the name for the tincture, is equivalent to one grain of opium. Seven thousand drops is about seventy teaspoons. Being a Gentle Reader, I also felt exquisite pleasure—a squirming up of my insides—taking in the sensual auditory details of his drugged nights at the opera, listening to a certain Grassini sing. Was De Quincey a fag? I'd guess so, based on this last detail.

I have yet to get to the part of the book in which he describes his Pains, but they too will become context for Sel and her ability to provide for those who come to her for assistance. The things I most appreciate about De Quincey already are his earnestness, his curiosity, his precision, his need for ritual, and most importantly his lack of regret for being—as is publicized on the back jacket of the paperback—*a fugitive from respectable society.*

Obviously, I was meant for opium—or, at least, its positive side—which would let me dream and write dozens of books, keep me high, yet clear-headed, in harmony with myself and nature, light in my spirits, perhaps capable of listening to opera, and wouldn't leave me depressed the next day. Had De Quincey been born a bit later, he would have discovered what others have: that a mix-and-match of narcotics might have tempered the nightmarish turn that opium caused his mind to take.

Today, I suspect, De Quincey would be at MIT, doing brain research, following up on Timothy Leary's LSD experiments, turning on and off his opiate receptors at will, listening to opera in the laboratory on his Walkman, his expression always one of curious wonder. *Happily earnest and high as a loon.*

~ 48

The Museum of Public Assistance contains an archive of the Hôtel-Dieu, where, for many centuries, the victims of plagues—syphilis, pox, cholera, et cetera— were isolated and treated. It's the third archive I've combed in two days for documents and objects that might help me reconstruct the setting in which Sel carries out her mission, as I've come to think of our shared story. The other two are the Museum of the History of Medicine and the Museum of the Prefecture of Police, a kind of crime museum.

From these archives of French medicine, I've learned where and how to cut the body in fifty-two places whenever bloodletting is advised; where to procure giant leeches that might be used to treat hemophilia patients; what the doctors of the past favored to give addicts and prostitutes and French housewives with insomnia, or the clap; and finally, how to treat scars left by, say, the surgical removal of cellulite around one's thighs, an issue that preoccupies many women here: a tincture of opium, followed by a good Burgundy.

I appreciate this very civilized approach to the body's ailments. Of course one might welcome a stiff drink in the drawing room before the removal of one's good knee. Of course one should follow a tincture of opium with a claret or a good Bordeaux, after having drained the body of blood via myriad careful incisions to relieve it of one's Pains. I would've enjoyed being a Victorian. The bespoke fashion, the habit of public strolling, the penchant for letter writing, the willingness to poke and cut the flesh to relieve emotional Pains . . . I like it all. Look at all those clever, pocket-sized razors and hand saws and elegant long-needle syringes used to probe and explore said Pain. The rows of narrow ampoules and capped vials of bitter and sugary-sweet *sirops* and dubious medicines. So many elegant instruments of torture. The Victorians had such style! Such precision.

The visit has given me a hint about where Sel might go too, in search of her own family roots. In my notebook, I've drawn crude sketches of the display of old glass and metal nursing bottles that were once placed on a baby's chest. A medallion with silk ties that once served to identify orphans at the Hôtel-Dieu.

Is Sel an orphan? One born at hospital Hôtel-Dieu? Hmmm.

⌐⌐⌐

The museum has a nice collection of natural poisons and medicines too. White, amber, rust, and blue-green rocks and powders in old-fashioned looking tins labeled *Arsenic* and *Hysterica* and *Sarsaparilla*. Had De Quincey lived longer, he might now be helping me to determine their efficacy per gram weight, the method of preparation of the different tinctures, and—most important to Sel, I imagine—their effect on the body and mind, as well as other Changes, as De Quincey described his drug-induced metamorphoses. Without any help, it's up to me now to ferret out the Dreams and Pains of the arsenic user, the ingester of *hysterica*. Or, more practically, if any of these ancient herb-based remedies might help treat spontaneous sepsis, a condition that has put Johnny back into the hospital, his insides revolting; his kidneys cleansing too little.

Come to think of it, maybe opium is just what Johnny needs. He certainly needs something for his Pains, and to help him sleep, never mind dream.

~

Before moving on, it's important to mention something I just learned this week over the telephone. My father, Raymond, was an intern at the Hôtel-Dieu, a rite of passage for most medical students at the Sorbonne in the 1940s. Again, history knocks at my door.

Surely I won't be able to avoid the temptation to make them meet in my story—Sel and my father—the coincidence is too great. How, when, where . . . none of this matters yet. Just the idea of it gives me pleasure. Even if it becomes an idea for the mental drawer where I'm stuffing many of these fantasy tangent thoughts. I've titled it *Flights of Fancy with Little Clear Purpose to Your Narrative.*

Indeed.

~ 49

I've been a bit lazy the past days, rooted to a spot on Belle's couch. I like the view, the rooftop city with the river just beyond. Sel hasn't moved much either. She's taken up temporary residence in an empty barge that resembles a house-boat I saw in a museum exhibit of Yokohama here. A photo show that made me think of Aldyn, now evanesced, his ashes awaiting further spiritual transport to Japan.

At other times I glimpse Sel making her way to a makeshift laboratory in an abandoned quarry or in a closed part of the underground—down in one of the tunnels, leading to the secret branch of the Seine that still runs under the city. I envision her concocting things, testing things on herself, using the equipment stolen from the city's museums and hospitals. Most often though, I see her walking, talking to herself, loud enough for others to step away a bit. She's addressing her conversation to the men of the state, letting them know just what she thinks of their leadership, their endless restoration of the Marais. *Tout à la rue!*

Belle sticks her head in the room. *Was I saying something?*

No, not to her.

Just to my ghosts, a party in my head.

Steadily, my notebooks are filling up. Sel's own war story to be developed.

~

Later, I'm alone. Belle's out seeing a friend. We'll meet up with the deaf boys later for a drink. I've had a nap, some food, some wine. I think about calling my father to tell him about my visit to Hôtel-Dieu. But he'll be with patients; I'll wait till later. I'm due for a catch-up call with Jersey, who is calling me on her lunch hour. We're staying in touch and I miss her. I'll be home in a few days. When we talk she complains about her job, about how Saint Mark's Place is gentrifying; she hates it. She regales me with stories of small misadventures, nights out with pals, a party she was invited to.

There's a subject we avoid: a girl from work, a crush, someone she sees every day. I'm not sure what it's really all about and right now, I don't want to know. I'm with Belle, hardly in a position to point fingers regarding fidelity. Jersey and I are officially girlfriends now, but we've left the corners of our relationship box open, undefined apart from a commitment to communicate. No lies, is the rule. But I've been lied to before. A lot. I feel a knot of tension at the thought.

You choose your demons, Anne, I remind myself. *No one is forcing you to be anywhere you don't want to be. Focus on what's good. Choose happy.*

⌒

After our call I open my trip journal, review notes and sketches I made earlier. I'm starting to trace what I think of as Sel's fallen family tree, conjured up by my crude drawings of the objects in glass cases that were hidden from sunlight under the gray coverlets in a corner of the Museum of Public Assistance: the fading-blue, silk necklace with a half-broken medallion. Lying next to it a yellowing letter, a plea with instructions from a mother who's abandoned the child, asking the directors of the Hôtel-Dieu orphanage to please deliver her child to whoever appears bearing the other half of the medallion. A letter such as the one Sel's mother might have written.

I study the sketches of the giant jars of dusty powders and silver-plated pharmacy bowls with copper handles into which blood flowed from women giving difficult birth. I look at my drawings of leeches, before and after being placed on a bleeding patient. The fattened leeches look like brown turds. I'm not the artist I wish I was, but I feel inspired. All of which leaves me, as De Quincey felt in his opium daze, with *the creative state of the eye increased.*

VII

New York

~ 50

AUGUST 1994

Almost Indian summer in New York. I'm finally slowing down after a whirl-wind period. The book tour is a success so far, at least to me. Lots of media and great reviews. But not that critical one, that sink-or-swim one. I've had what my writer friends call a reality check: the same day I got a wonderful, full-page *Washington Post* review, I got a snitty little blurb from the small-god critic of the *New York Times*. A reviewer culled from the paper's Haiti desk who was pretty conservative, I was told. The assignment editor thought it would be a great matchup, but the reviewer clearly hated the politics of my Haiti novel. So that's disappointing. I've learned some fast, hard lessons about book publishing. And right now, I'm licking my wounds a little.

I was hoping to take a break, escape the heat, get up-country. Instead I've taken up temporary residence in a small artist's studio run by a friend. He's a rather amazing painter of dreamy frescoes. The studio is a few doors down from my Avenue C apartment, but it feels like a getaway—sort of. I feel the need for stripped-down summer living and an escape from my usual routines. Like a stoic: a bed, a few books, a few cassette tapes.

It's funny: all these years I thought I lived on a pretty nice, quiet block of the East Village. And I did—I do, partly because I live on the top floor at the very end of the street, well above the fray. But down here, with the big store-front window at street level, it's a whole different view and scene. For starters, the local traffic rarely stops; it's a twenty-four-hour shuffle of hipsters and the drunk looking for take-out coffee after midnight to sober up, or traipsing past the studio en route to some party or to find their drug of choice. I'm learning to distinguish between the serious junkies and the tourist ones.

Summertime lures them outside, to loll on the stoops, which is where I'm found, sitting in the open doorway of the studio, trying to direct a little breeze into the room. Directly across from the studio is a squatters' tenement the cops have raided twice. Next to it is an abandoned, gutted synagogue that makes me wonder who used to live on this street. It's entertaining, though not exactly peaceful. The heat is the biggest problem. I only have two small fans. Even with one inches from my body, I'm sweating.

My friend's paintings are like dense Chagalls: moody, imagistic, surreal, with rich pigments—ochres, forest greens, mustards—and fluid dogs that look like Biblical animals. They remind me of the world I daydream about: Sel's world, medieval Paris, old Europe. The pages of history I've been mining for two years as a backdrop to the present.

⁓

This past week I'm reading many things at once, as I tend to do, trying to fill in holes in my knowledge, picking up little details of European life in the World War II period. I'm enjoying Martha Gellhorn's war correspondence from the 1950s up to the Vietnam War, and a book of interviews with Sartre and a friend. I also reread bits of an old standby, *Janet Flanner's World*, a fabulous collection of *New Yorker* essays Flanner wrote as Genêt. There are some gems, including "Paris, Germany," headlined December 7, 1940. She, like me, favors words like *malodorous*. I'm always inspired by her writing.

What else? Oh, a few foreign papers—the Rome-based daily *Il Messaggero*, the *Independent* (for their arts coverage), and *Libération*. I want to follow what the Europeans are saying about the exploding Balkan crisis and the siege of Sarajevo, and the role of Western powers in helping to broker peace. Their newspapers are more like opinion columns; there's less pretense of impartiality. They're also full of historical context. I learn so much.

It's still easy to get distracted from my story research, though. Outside the window, in back, is an open airshaft connected to the studio, and this morning I saw a large rat crawling around. It disappeared into some crack in the building and ever since I've felt jumpy. Is there a more appropriate fear? A rat crawling up to sniff my toes. Like all the old rats of Eastern Europe: the ones foraging among the stinking gravesites of Bosnia and those forced indoors like Sarajevo's residents, seeking shelter in the basements of shell-shocked buildings.

What to do then? If I leave the back door open to let in some breeze, then the rat might get in. I hardly feel stoic about that. If I leave the front door open, the rest of the world may feel invited to peek in, and I'm only ever half-dressed in this heat. So: I can't sleep, I can't get cool, and I'm having a little rat panic. I'm beginning to stink under my arms and between my legs. The sun's rising in the west. I've got my fingers in my ears, wishing I could quiet my mind, get that madman, Slobodan Milošević out of my head, and that damn rat too. It's friggin' hot, I'm telling you.

~ 51

I finally got away. I've come upstate to a friend's cabin, to listen to the birds and feel my chest fill up with . . . what? Some cooler air, for starters. And a mix of emotions: relief, anxiety, and sadness too. The news from Sarajevo is so disturbing. Relief at being away from the city for a spell; away from routine and a busy work schedule. Anxiety because I have a decision to consider, about my relationship with Jersey, and I feel like moving toward it ever so slowly. And sadness, real sadness about Assotto. *Another pox mort.*

Assotto from Haiti. I didn't know him well, but we shared an immediate, deep bond based on a shared Haitian-American gay sense of identity. A kinship. Both of us were writers who became AIDS activists. Whenever I saw him—at an event or, unexpectedly, at a writer's conference—I would feel a connection that comes from being seen in one's complex identity, from a shared cultural experience of what Haiti represented for us. There would be these moments of recognition, a light in Assotto's eyes, and his smile that said, *Yes yes yes, I know exactly what you mean; I felt the same way!* Whenever we bumped into each other, he would say, *Hello, sister.* And I would reply, in my rusty Kreyol, *Ti gason.* Little boy. *Sak pase?* What's up? *Koman ou ye?* How you doin'? *Kenbe fem?* Hanging in there?

We were both outsider-insiders. Native, but exiled, in Assotto's case. I was a *blan*—a de facto member of Haiti's social and economic elite due to my white skin and extended family connections. But we knew that social acceptance might end if my sexual identity was revealed. Homophobia was—is—a deep and often violent chord in Haitian culture, and with AIDS, even more so. I had kept my private life largely to myself in Haiti, without denying anything if anyone inquired. I felt visible already, being from a wealthy *blan* family; being American; being a journalist and a public critic of successive Haitian regimes. We both felt a sense of responsibility about fighting for the rights of Haitian gays and lesbians, of those living with HIV. But we were both careful.

Assotto had left Haiti. He was a member of the diaspora. He felt accepted by his Haitian family as a black gay man with a white American lover in New York, but that acceptance didn't yield enough safety to live an openly gay life back home. He could come and go from Haiti as he pleased. If any threats became real, he could escape.

For months, he had been sick, and that's when I got to know him better. Every so often, he would call me up at the magazine and we would talk about his health and about treatments, what advice I could give him, what I felt most optimistic about. I could hear his fear. I had thought about calling him several times in recent weeks, checking in, but I hadn't. Now it was too late.

⌒

Assotto's memorial service was beautiful. I attended it as a friend, but I was a
stranger to his closest loved ones. I watched them closely, wanting to learn
more about him; listened to their stories. He was a great man—this I already
knew. A Haitian pioneer. A poet and actor and AIDS activist. And he had a
beautiful face and beautiful eyes. When I looked at a flyer they had made up for
the event, I remembered his voice, his flamboyant spirit, his generous warmth,
and the special moments that acted as glue to firm up my own sense of myself
within the Haitian diaspora. My gay *frè*, Assotto, a brother. Gone back to
Guinée, ancestral Africa, where Haitian spirits seek their final resting place.

Let me remember his words, his fierceness:

> Gay boys stricken again then again & again
> Black men broken again then again & again
> Best friends taken again then again & again
>
> *Assotto Saint, "Evidence"*

~ 52

This year the heat is more crushing than I ever remember it. Worse than Paris.
Brutal. I've hit my limit. You can't go out before dusk. The newspapers keep
reporting the deaths of the very young and elderly from heatstroke. It's unbelievable. Everyone blames global warming.

⌒

Week two of the heat wave. The city I inhabit is boiling; the culture of this
country is emitting gaseous ideas and, in Bosnia and Rwanda, it's the putre-
factive odor and heat of death: large-scale, out-in-the-open mass graves; the release of ancient—even forgotten—hatreds; all of it making the air too nauseous
to breathe. It's been a never-ending parade of horror on the radio. I can't even
bear listening to the news anymore.

The Rwandan genocide. A million people—ethnic Tutsis slaughtered by hand,
by machetes, by their Hutu neighbors. An efficient mass slaughter organized
by an ultranationalist group, the Hutu Power. The newspapers are full of it, in
horrible, horrible detail: stories and eyewitness atrocities that keep spilling out.
The human rights groups keep changing the number of dead, but the story is
all there: something unimaginable, worse even than the national bloodletting
of Serb versus Croat versus Muslim versus Albanian in the Balkans.

Just today I read that Macedonia and Montenegro may be the next to blow up in hatred. In Srebrenica—*I can't pronounce that city*—a lot of men and boys are missing, assumed buried by the Serbs. Maybe thousands. *Thousands!* How to capture the scope, the intensity of these large-scale spasms of human hatred, of depravity, of old-fashioned barbarism that we think have no more place in our modern lives? So many rapes littering the landscape. Rape camps in Bosnia. Rape camps in Rwanda. It's unbearable. *Is that why my parents and their generation turned their backs on Vichy, on Hitler? Forgot that justice remained incomplete?*

Fifty years after Hitler, here we are again. *Genocide. Again.* In two places, arguably. Watching the survivors pick through the smoldering ruins of their houses, searching for relatives. Srebrenica, Vukovar, now Kigali. It's unbelievable. So is the response of world leaders, which seems not that different from 1940: words, denunciations, calls to action, a repetition of the lesson, *Never Again.* But not enough actual action, not a real commitment of troops or money to stop the killers from hunting Tutsi with machetes, from snipers training their telescopic lens on the residents of Sarajevo. It's too little, too late, again and again. We refuse to learn from history.

This time, I have to confess, I'm glad I'm not there—in Vukovar or in Kigali. Waiting for the first light of dawn to arrive, to go out and see where the bodies were dumped last night, a reporter's drill in a war zone. What I had to do in Haiti during the elections. I heard that Susan Sontag and her son, David Rieff, are again organizing PEN writers' events, rallying the literary community around the newest atrocity. Sontag has truly stepped up in the Balkan conflict, I have to say. *Been a voice. Been a force.* Put her body on the line all those months in Sarajevo, directing *Waiting for Godot* among the snipers, to prove that art remains a tangible force against tyranny. *Does it?*

Yes, yet the killing goes on. And it's distracting me in this instant. I'm finding it hard to think about writing, about Sel and her story. Art may trump atrocity, but for the moment, I'm overhorrified.

⁓

Later, I read more reports, trolling, as always, for the little details. The Balkan names and places sound so old-world to me. *Radovan Karadžić.* The general with blood on his hands in Srebrenica: *Ratko Mladić.* I roll their names around on my tongue like an awkward language student. *Why must they run their consonants together like that?* Before I finally sleep, I think about the questions that remain in my head: What will we tell ourselves about this chapter of Balkan history in another fifty years? And Rwanda? If the Balkans represent our Spanish Civil War, as Sontag argues, then what of Rwanda? Our African Shoah?

~ 53

Today I was reading about the *hibakusha*: explosion-affected people. A term given to the survivors of the Hiroshima and Nagasaki bombings. I'm living in New York, far away from Japan and Europe and 1945. Far away, too, from Rwanda and Lake Kivu, where the water stinks from so many bodies still washing ashore. I want to consider how this moment compares to those earlier ones, how progressive people before us responded to the sharp political shift toward ethnic hatred and repression, to what Primo Levi called *the unspeakable*.

I'm thirty-seven years old now. I'll be forty-two when the new millennium arrives. I feel the intensity of everything around me and how it is all cyclical, a spiral of forces. I feel like a hibakusha. AIDS, genocide, ethnic cleansing in the Balkans, the rise of new fascists in France . . . the explosions are happening all around me, around us. I'm witnessing it, and I'm fully alive, my eyes and body wide open. Sleepless in the blazing summer. *Hibakusha days*.

~ 54

For the past—what is it?—four, five years, I've refined the idea that my body could actually be sick. Partly, it's due to my increased awareness of microbes and new technologies to detect them, and everything I've learned from my poxed friends with terminal prognoses. When they talk about what's wrong with them, or when I research what might be plaguing me, I begin to feel the detached horror I know my mother felt about her cancer. *The enemy within*.

I've had amoebas mostly, from my trips to Africa and Haiti and, most recently, Mexico and Latin America. But I usually recover quickly. My current travel companion is called Blastocystis, a tenacious creature that likes to delve into the walls of the gut and hold on for dear life. *Blasto*, a friend I've encountered before. It's given me nausea and a vicious headache and the runs, all at the same time. It's made me sicker this time than I ever remember being and the damn bug may not be gone for good. Like me, this blasto is hanging on. And I may have some other pox too, says my doctor, Joe Sonnabend, based on my symptoms. The blood tests haven't proven anything decisive yet. What's clear is that I'm sick. No question about that. On top of the blasto-gastro issues, I have bad joint pain that I've never had. It's all a tropical mystery, says Joe. He's an HIV doc, but we've become colleagues over the years I've been covering AIDS. I profiled him in the inaugural issue of *Out*; he's the man who helped invent the concept of safer sex. He's also from Zimbabwe—formerly Rhodesia— and knows his esoteric tropical bugs.

I've had what I think of now as a state of chronic malady for several weeks. Something I might have picked up from a trip to Belize a while back. Every day I get crippling headaches. One day in April it was so bad I held my head and actually prayed—to whom or what, I'm not sure, my mother I think—I felt that afraid and in *that* much pain. Nothing was working to stop the pain, the come-and-go nausea. That's when I called Joe for help.

I took what he prescribed—his best guess: nearly two months' worth of broad-spectrum antibiotics that my friends with HIV take for pneumonia and parasites. And I have to confess, I've been feeling better. Plus, I'm allowed a twice-daily pick-me-up of my favorite legal drug of choice, Sudafed. It makes me a bit speedy, but in a good way. Extra alert and productive. I've been able to read and write, and still sleep.

I'm sharing these details of illness to explain why I worry about my health in the big picture. Worry that the years of travel and exposure to tropical bugs in Haiti and Latin America may have taken their toll, reduced my natural resistance to the point where I won't regain my good health. I told you how my mother looked on her cancer with detached horror. Now, when I eat something that makes my stomach a little queasy, I get the same feeling: *There is something terribly wrong.*

I know: I'm turning very French; developing some real hypochondria. I'll probably be fine in another few months. But it's been scary, to get really sick and not know the cause. Unlike Sel, I haven't been able to enjoy getting to know my mystery pox. A pity I don't go for opium, à la De Quincey, either. Sudafed is hardly a substitute.

~ 55

FALL 1995

Where does time go? I can't keep track of my days. Tonight, I'm waiting for Jersey to come back from a trip, one of several she's made without me these last months. That's because we're taking a break—a trial separation. We've been together, girlfriends, for a while now. But for nearly a year, on and off—more on lately—she's been carrying on a tortured love affair with another woman; she's been distracted and conflicted and upset. She says she loves me, loves our relationship, but she can't ignore this passion. Our own romance has become rocky as a result: we fight, we try to support each other, then we both feel tired and shut down. It's a familiar pattern—too familiar from my life with the Aerialist.

When I first found out about Jersey's crush, as she calls her other lover, I felt really upset. I couldn't believe it was happening so soon after the start of our own romance. We had recently been to Europe, to Paris and Greece. To Corsica, a great adventure. I was in love. I didn't write about that. I suppose I was having too much fun. It had been amazing fun. We had become good friends as well as lovers—the best kind of romance. I wasn't at all ready for infidelity, not so quickly. I've hardly had time to call her my girlfriend. It tears me up, because I like her so much. We have a lot together.

It's been so difficult for me. I hate being cast as the shrill, suspicious, cuckolded lover, and that's how I feel. And how I'm acting too, I suppose. Unhappy, frustrated, jealous. *Stuck.* I feel stuck again, after what I went through with the Aerialist. *Why is this happening? Is it really true that I'm drawn to unavailable people? Crap! Maybe time for a 12-step Al Anon-style meeting. Codependent No More. I need to break out of this dynamic. It's making me miserable.* Now she's in the doghouse, a familiar place.

A while ago I proposed that we just try being nonmonogamous; I'd date other people too. Go back to having fun. Try to be poly, to use the modern term, openly polyamorous; no cheating. So we had a trial period, but when I began an affair, a light affair, she freaked out. Suddenly, she wanted to be monogamous again. She was too jealous. Yet clearly that won't work. She's too caught up in her crush, in her pattern of triangles. Bottom line: she needs attention. I saw the red flags and chose to ignore them. At my peril, I suppose.

I know I should just go—end this. I've been around this ambivalent block before, for way too long with the Aerialist. Jersey just needs to grow up, confront her intimacy issues, but it won't happen overnight. Can take years and some people never do. Her drama is sucking up my emotional energy. *Monogamy, nonmonogamy, fidelity, ambivalence. Should we break up? Should I go out with boys? Men?* It's the modern lesbian bad drama merry-go-round. I start to question everything again. But, really, I know what I want. To go deep in a relationship with someone I can trust. It's not about monogamy per se; it's about honesty. The lying undoes me. *Is that a word?* Or maybe I just feel too alone in our relationship today. That's the worst.

What else? My close friends are struggling so much. Johnny is going blind, slowly but steadily. It's a terrible thing. The eye drugs don't work; not even the new experimental ones. The CMV has scarred his retina past the point of some recovery, that's what we're told. He's seeing spots in the corners of his eyes. He can't even watch his favorite shows now, unless he gets right next to the TV.

The world is getting dimmer, he says. It's very painful to witness. I do what I can, but it doesn't feel like enough. And my own mood doesn't help. I want it to lift, all this blueness. I want to feel good again, to drink a cup of joy. Life is too short, I remind myself. *Maman told you that so many times. So did Papou. Choose happy.*

~ 56

I've become incredibly busy, following my own advice: have fun. Since Sel's story is still nascent, I wanted to get back into more creative writing. Last May, for some crazy reason, I launched a gayish arts and literary journal, *x-x-x fruit*. It's really an excuse to have a party—or three. Two pals from Gran Fury, Vincent Gagliostro and Avram Finkelstein, are working on it with me; so is Marisa Cardinale, my friend with the Mapplethorpe Foundation. I always rope her into my crazy, overwhelming projects but we do manage to keep ourselves entertained. I'm the editor, Idea Girl; she's Top Girl, the one we hope will help us sell ads and hit up her wealthy art friends for support. Vince and Avram and George Whitman are the art directors, and I roped in a pal from *Out*, Will Guillaums, who's our Best Boy.

For our first issue, I wanted to do a literary exquisite corpse using a text from the O.J. Simpson trial and have the whole magazine be a big corpse. The trial is one of the events that everyone continues to be obsessed about. So we've all been spending a lot of time at Vince's studio, close to Johnny's, in the meat-packing district. We've invited a lot of writers and artists who we admire to contribute to the magazine. Our new issue is titled "Witness: An Exquisite Corpse." I like the tag line: *Wake Up, Darling.* Sort of sums up how I feel about the political climate in general.

It's all taking way, way too much time and we have zero money for anything, as usual. But has that ever mattered? Not enough to stop us. We're going to have a lot of fun doing this magazine. For me, it's been a new opportunity to write and to let myself loose a little. Good times.

⌒

I keep dreaming of a quick trip to Paris, but I can't manage it. I want some of the latest French books written about Le Pen and the National Front. Out of the blue, Philippe calls to announce that he and Marina are coming to New York en route to the south—New Orleans or somewhere. I quickly make up a short reading list. I want copies of *Ras l'Front*, the antifascist paper that's doing a decent job tracking Le Pen. I want a book about that gross man René Bousquet, the famous friend of President Mitterrand, whose case has reopened files on the friends of Vichy now helping Le Pen in Marseille. He's dead now, but his case interests me. Bousquet served as secretary general to the Vichy regime police from 1942 to 1943, working under Pierre Laval, another bad guy. He helped lead the infamous Marseille Roundup in which thirty thousand citizens were rounded up and expelled from the Old Port. He also helped send some two thousand Jews to the camps, including children under two, a category of infants he pushed to include. Another Goebbels.

Bousquet was the last Frenchman tried by the postwar Haute Cour—the High Court—in 1949, but he was acquitted. Then later, when he cozied up to Mitterrand, he found himself a renewed target of French justice. He helped fund Mitterrand's political election in 1965. He would drop by Élysée to talk shop, to talk politics. Only when others began to protest too loudly, when the stench of the past was coming too close to the national palace, did Mitterrand begin to distance himself from his former patron.

I hope you've followed the timeline. I admit: I'm interested in Bousquet because of the Marseille connection. Papou was seeking permits from the Marseille housing authorities to develop the Old Port area, to resettle the re-turning pieds noirs, at the moment the Butcher of Marseille had the president's ear. *Did they know each other?* Bousquet remained a high-profile guy in Marseille up until just yesterday nearly. It sort of boggles my mind. Should we even call his crimes the past? I think we should see where they're extending into the future. He's probably fundraised for Monsieur Le Pen and the Front. The wolves have continued their party in Marseille.

~ 57

I've been reading back in my journals, looking at my own patterns. My life seems to be full of painful events but that's what I tend to record. You should know I have my fun. And even when we date cheaters, there can be some black humor in it. If we can't laugh at ourselves, then we're really doomed. So here's a funny story for my grandchildren, should I ever have them. The story of how I learned that Jersey was cheating on me for real. I was just recalling it. Such a good story, really. A time when I understood the universe is a trickster and I, the fool. A good fool, though. Like in the tarot.

It was at the start of this year. ACT UP organized a protest called Target Rudy against Mayor Giuliani who was hell-bent on cutting the city's Division of AIDS Services for reasons only his shrink may understand. (*We're at ground zero in this epidemic and this is his response? Fer chrissakes*). Anyway, Jersey and I decided to do CD—civil disobedience. Housing Works and Stand Up Harlem and Mother's Voices were co-organizers and Jersey's work pals from Housing Works were there. I can't remember how many of us got arrested, but there were a lot. The Lesbian Avengers too. We sat down to protest, an arrestable infraction.

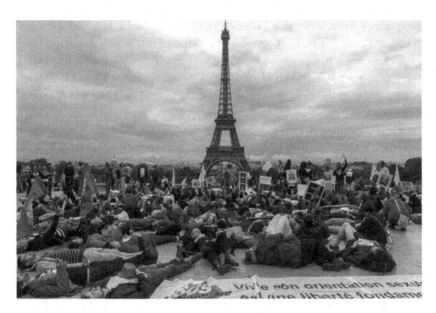

"Silence = Mort!" ACT UP Die In protest, September 2013. (tomcraig@directphoto.org)

I was probably sitting with Jersey but lost track of her when we got arrested. Instead, to my shock and dismay, the cops quickly handcuffed me and put me in a holding cell with Jersey's new crush at the time. It was so bad that it was comic. *Oh my god!* There was just no way for us to avoid one another any longer. At some point, if memory serves me right, Jersey got out earlier and came looking for her crush, calling her name. I'll never forget the look of horror and panic on her face when she spied me too. Her girlfriend and her secret lover, handcuffed, locked up together.

Worse for her, the crush and I had bonded a bit by then, which horrified Jersey. She felt guilty and paranoid at the same time. I felt like less of a victim, too; recognized the crush was a smart, interesting girl who had fallen for Jersey's cuteness but was also vulnerable, hated being the villain as much as I hated feeling a victim. Is a crush a crime? I blamed Jersey more. She was a huge flirt; it was on her, as my girlfriend, to protect our relationship. Who knows what she had told the crush about our relationship?

I didn't forgive either of them, but I understood. I haven't always been a saint. Jersey's never pretended to be one. So the crush wasn't one either. They had been busted, for real. But somehow we were laughing about it. *Dyke drama!*

Why would I stay? My friends ask me that. It's the oldest question. Because the heart loves, without intelligence perhaps, but for its reasons. My reasons are the qualities about Jersey that I cherish and her good brain. I like her spirit the most: she's bold. We really do get along so well. She can be so fun and we share a lot. She's not a bad penny, but emotionally, she's narcy—narcissistic—and immature. She's the wild child who hasn't grown up enough yet. Maybe she won't. I've loved the good and the sexy-hot part; hated the lying and cheating, the betrayal.

The funny thing is, she says she adores me. Capital *A*, adore. Somewhere I know that's true, I really do. We've become best friends, apart from lovers. That's still true. She just needs to be adored by others, too; her ego needs it. But the lies make it emotionally unsafe for me. So I'm in triage mode, seeing if I can salvage the healthy parts and jettison the crap. *Good luck*, my friends say. *Is she worth it?*

Short answer? *Yes, to me.* I don't give up easily on people. *Bend, don't break,* remember?

~ 58

One advantage of being a journalist is that you realize how easy it is to get what seems like privileged information from people. It's just a question of having your sources. I contact a French journalist-friend, Françoise, who sometimes writes for the *Village Voice* and is now in Paris. She agrees to purchase some books for me if I wire the money in advance. Philippe will carry them over to me when he comes. Françoise is following Le Pen closely and recently filed a story for the *Voice* about how powerful the National Front has gotten—powerful beyond anyone's expectations. Philippe revises my list and suggests others.

Two weeks later, he calls from a midtown hotel. He's too busy to see me but left the books Françoise picked out with the concierge. As promised, Françoise found the best ones.

The concierge is all business: *For you, sir.*

Thank you, but actually I've got breasts.

I'm sorry, madame.

I feel good about this little exchange at the hotel, but I'm left irritated afterward. Why is it that hotel clerks and waiters and women my age, modern women with short hair themselves, display confusion, then panic, about my gender? Especially in the women's bathroom? What is the problem, ladies? Gentlemen? What if a man accidentally used the women's bathroom? Could ya live with it? Huh? *Enfin!*

I carry my little bag with the books daintily, saucily, back out into the street. *Merci, Françoise!*

Riding the subway home, I'm a child at Christmas. *Treats. Presents. Goodies. Infor-mation at last.* . . . The books are all paperbacks but appear dense and heavy and slightly unreadable, with teeny-tiny fonts, the way Europeans seem to like their books. Why, I have no idea. They have no sense of making it easier for the reader. I look for pictures but there aren't many. It's an understatement that the French can be serious, especially French publishers. No illustrations, no breaks in the text, and lots and lots of footnotes.

Les Enfants de L'Épuration, by Pierre Rigoulot. *What's that word: épuration? The Children of the Purification? Sort of.* And the book I've been wanting: *René Bousquet*, by Pascale Froment. With a nice postscript by Primo Levi: *Those who are most dangerous are the ordinary men.* I quickly scan it. There's a picture of François Mitterrand sitting at a table with his hands folded, as in prayer. I think in every picture I've seen of Mitterrand he's looked that way. Very French. Very much like my Papou—similar style and gestures. I note the day—June 8, 1993—that Bousquet was assassinated. *What was I doing that very day?*

I know: I was back from Tim's funeral, and readying for Jon's.

It's a hefty book. *Am I really going to read it? I'm becoming such a nerd.* The next one has a weird title. *Les filières noires*, by Guy Konopnicki. The black links. A Polish Frenchman? The book offers a comprehensive survey of the National Front now, what they stand for, and who their supporters are. I scan the back cover: *Saddam Hussein to Vladimir Zhirinovski.* That rings a bell. Zhirinovski. I remember: skinny, scary-looking Polish leader with the sunglasses. I study the covers of the remaining books. How will I have time to read them all?

Fascisme français, passé et présent, by Pierre Milza. Cool. This is the book that links the ideas of the Vichy royalists and colonialist pied-noir generation to Le Pen, now. *Oh, but the writing is so miniscule! What's wrong with these publishers, don't they think their readers deserve to read without glasses? Why do they make us suffer?* Ah, now the Monzat book. *Enquêtes sur la droite extrême.* An investigation of the extreme right. Bigger print; looks comprehensive. Monzat, only thirty-three years old when this was published in 1992. *Another overachiever.*

I'm exhausted by the time I get home. I have a headache. It's too much. All this information, all these footnotes. If only they were all translated. *It's going to take me forever!* I wanted all these books, I remind myself; I really did. But now that I have them, I'm so overwhelmed. I immediately want to forget Jean-Marie Le Pen and his daughters, including blonde Marine-who-would-be-Saint-Joan, and the butcher Bousquet, and the contemporary historical amnesia of the French.

Well, correct that: I want to ingest the information like an IV, without having to chew and swallow to digest. It takes me a long time to read in French, and it becomes work, not the massive pleasure of reading in English. I barely studied French, just spoke it from birth. And these books are so ultraserious, even for me. *Zut alors!*

I feel a stab of frustration. I want to be writing a different book. Something more modern, something fun. Something properly gay, if it's going to be labeled that way. Coming-out stories, lesbian sex, funny, violent, gothic stories—those are the things people want to read today, right? Light things, stories that enter-tain, that make people laugh, gossip. What's my problem? Why do I have to be so damn serious? Ugggh! People don't even read anymore. Who's going to care about this wild-ass road-trip-through-history story about a sexually fluid writer living in New York's Lower East Side who hangs out with her buddies—lesbians, fags with AIDS, Haitian expatriates, anarchists, ex-war journalists—and drinks too much, and never gets to the gym anymore, and fusses and gossips about her complex dyke dramarama relationships, and thinks about high crimes and who got away and asks the drunks sharing her bench in Tompkins Square Park: *What's it all about?*

Then I remind myself: *I would.* A wild ass roadtrip—it sounds juicy on paper. And Sel, I remind myself, is very entertaining—to me. Maybe that's all I get, as a writer-creator. *This rabbit hole: all mine.*

For now I'm stuck with myself and these very dense, very intimidating books that will double as a doorstop when I'm done with them.

Welcome to my wonderland.

⌒

There's a message from Philippe later on the answering machine. *Did you get the books? Did you see my note?*

What note?

Ah, here it is.

Dear Anne-christine, I think it's all here. Whatever is missing I can get for you later. Also, don't forget I have a good friend who's been a chief investigator of the Far Right since the 1960s; you can meet him when you come next. Good luck, Philippe.

Great, I think, staring at my future doorstop. *Just when I was tempted to throw in the towel. Oh well. Maybe my grammar will improve from reading all these books. But, God, someone has to tell the French to use bigger print. It's trop cruel.*

⌒

A postscript for the year 1995: I keep getting calls from Kiki, who's had an extraterrible time of it lately. His pox has gotten even more out of control. He's having trouble walking and he feels murderous. That's what he keeps saying, and it's no longer any kind of joke. *I feel murderous. I want to live by any means necessary.* That's become his mantra, his calling card: *by any means necessary.*

When I stopped by his house the other day, he was in a particularly foul mood, hating the *heteros,* and my own kind, *the HIV negatives.* He's moved out of the first stage of grief—denial—and is now in the full-on *anger* stage. Or maybe the anger that's so long sustained him has gone viral like his pox. He's laced it with humor and dark wit for so long but now it's a bitter anger and it's the only energy that's left. If he had completely lost hope, he wouldn't be angry. But he hasn't. He's still a fury-machine, hurling his words at anything that moves, using his *POZ* column to denounce, to rail, to curse: that's how it feels. Raging with his every breath.

It's worked, though. In November, due in good measure to his tireless rants, the FDA gave accelerated approval to Doxil—now the new Holy Grail drug for KS patients. *Now let's wait and see how much they're going to jack up the price,* he says to me. But there's a measure of pride in his sarcasm. His bitchy queen army has won at least one decisive battle. *Looks like I'll make it to the New Year,* he said as we hugged good-bye last week. *More hell to raise ahead.* He tossed me one of his favorite screen-queen quotes: *I told 'em: Don't fuck with me, fellas. This ain't my first time at the rodeo.*

~ 59

The deepest moments can feel like a single current of emotion, like a poem. Or, in Johnny's case, a song—one long mixtape of songs from the eighties, from Manchester, England, a mix of Roxy Music and Pet Shop Boys and Culture Club and his favorite, R.E.M. Johnny turned me on to R.E.M. early in our friendship. We've bonded over it, over sugary pop music that was so danceable. We danced constantly before he started to lose his eyesight, often in his loft on Hudson Street, above the parade of sex workers patiently trolling truck drivers coming in from New Jersey. We listened to Michael Stipe ad nauseam.

As Johnny fell ill, he started looking more like Stipe, with his shaved head and slightly pale, sickly demeanor. Stipe has a gorgeous, haunting voice. Johnny has a good voice too; theater-trained, but he's shy in public. Alone in the loft, he'll let himself go, sings loudly all day long. He has more records, more tapes than anyone I've ever seen. A great, very private, very beloved collection that reflects his life, his journey as a young man who struggled to come out and relied on music to make him feel better when the boys would leave. Or when he would leave them. Because Johnny, before he fell really ill, had a lot of hookups. It was true love that's remained elusive.

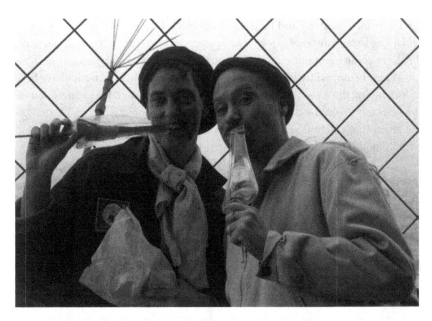

Author and John Cook in Paris, 1993. (Kelly McKaig)

I used to shake my head in wonder, trying to imagine my life as a gay man in the New York of the eighties before AIDS. Even now. The casual daily fucks with friends one sees later at the gym. I don't know how they keep track. It's so easy for them to have sex, with the bars and the culture. It's what the boys do, want, seek. Nothing more; just the sex. Except that isn't true, has never been true, at least for Johnny and Boy Kelly. They're deep-down romantics, like all of us. They want to be loved; they want someone to cook them eggs in the morning.

But sex is like grabbing for cookies in a jar when you're leaving the house for the gym: so tempting. There are so many men, always so many possibilities. It works against love, against commitment. Everyone's eternally on the prowl. And it leaves them feeling alone, feeling emotionally isolated, no matter how many boys they hook up with. The boys don't love them, don't even wait ten minutes for them to get dressed before they're gone sometimes, on to another bar or boy. Random, anonymous, sometimes superhot fucking, but nothing enduring.

I've heard all about it. *I should've been a lesbian,* Johnny complains. He ribs me, makes light of my problems: *All of you dykes have more than one girlfriend. It's not fair.*

What does he want then? Hot sex, then eggs in bed, and then going out and flirting together with boys, and then going home together to have hot sex again.

And being allowed to feel crazy happy about your cute boyfriend, to use the *L* word even. *Love.* That's the recipe that excites him, and evades him. The elusive boyfriend that haunts gay men. On top of that there's HIV. It's always been a struggle for Johnny: when to reveal his status. The boys may bolt. Most don't, but some do. He has to assume they may be positive too; we're in New York, it's the nineties. But it's never easy. He enjoys his hookups. But a steady boyfriend is the goal.

I write all this to stress that Johnny hasn't only suffered with HIV and now AIDS; he's had a big dose of fun too, including a lot of sex, clubbing, great parties, great clothes, and great music. And deep friendships. Boy Kelly, he, and I have traveled together. He's friends with various exes and bar shags. He's got a small but devoted posse. So he's found love, just not a boyfriend.

⁓

When Johnny went slowly blind, I saw a white Ray Charles emerge; a young Stevie Wonder, wearing permanent sunglasses. The way Johnny would turn his head, following my voice or a sound in the street like someone sniffing perfume, searching the air for it. Or sing, to himself, privately, listening to a song on his ever-present Walkman, lost in the music. Still singing to himself, still dancing, but more quietly. Not wanting to draw attention to himself. Hoping to pass—the outcast's eternal hope. I didn't realize, until the moment blindness became Johnny's new life—a new era of darkness—how much music would remain his savior, his lifeline, the only thing keeping him from total despair. Keeping him connected to his soul. Music, more than television, even for a child raised by the boob tube like Johnny.

Blind Johnny. A fate none of us predicted. When we began to see it happening, it made us feel impotent to help him, to spare him. For the first time, I felt I had little to say that was hopeful. The cytomegalovirus had quickly damaged his optic nerve, scarred his retina. It rendered his line of vision slightly spotty on one side, then increasingly hazy at the edges. I imagined a camera narrowing its focus on an object in the center, leaving everything else a slight blur. It was the spots that bothered him the most, an eternal desire to clear his vision. While a new eye drug had reduced the infection in his eyes, there was no coming back from the dimness, the spottiness. Instead, more darkness was predicted, especially if his HIV advanced again. Johnny's world was reduced. *Severely.*

It isn't easy to go blind, virtually overnight, and to live in a third-floor, walkup loft in Manhattan with very steep stairs. Everything that had been so familiar was now a challenge, a threat. Johnny would panic constantly, searching for his medicine and fingering the pill bottles to try and determine what he had taken, and when, to make sure he did it right. He had adopted complicated, tedious routines to make sure he could remain independent. It exhausted him. He would get short with me and his other friends. He didn't want to be more of a leper. And he felt so alone now. He couldn't see himself—that was the most terrifying moment. *What do I look like?* he would ask me. *Am I okay? Is my face okay? Are my clothes okay?* He had lost himself.

He was inside the blindness, and it wasn't a friendly place. Only music helped. And touch. I would give him back massages, and Boy Kelly too would come over and keep him company for hours and even days. Hold him sometimes. A touch that wasn't sexual but was the love he had so long desired from Boy Kelly: a real love, lasting. A kind of boyfriend.

Boy Kelly, in my eyes, was the other hero, aside from Johnny, who refused to stop living in the world. A true, true friend who had done a hard thing: opened his heart, not closed it, when Johnny admitted his deep fantasy crush. What they shared is its own song, its own love story of profound friendship. Johnny had other friends who showed up to walk beside him in the streets as lookouts, when he began inching his walking stick down the sidewalk, navigating a new world. Learning to find his box of Entenmann's at the corner deli because nothing, not even total blindness, would deny him the chocolate donuts he so loved.

Johnny's willingness to venture out alone was also the clearest sign that he hadn't given up hope. He planned to remain among us, living and not being erased, not merely suffering awfully and dying, for as long as possible. He would show up at our loft parties looking dapper, wearing a beret bought in France that made him look like a film director, with his fashionable shades, holding his walking stick more confidently, like a pointer. He eventually switched to a cane, favoring it for small sorties in the neighborhood.

A final year of gradually diminishing vision. Until the day came when he confessed to me, tearfully, that he really couldn't see much of anything at all. He couldn't figure out what was what in his sock drawer. The time had come for a visiting nurse, an idea that he abhorred but would adjust to.

It's hard for me now, in retrospect, to remember the fine details of those last days, months, and moments. I remember the *tick-tick-tick* of Johnny's walking stick. I remember him sniffing the air—he developed an appreciation for changes in the weather. His inner musician blossomed. He gave himself over to it; let music mother him.

In the hospital, he would listen to his Walkman music and we would sit by him. I would read aloud to him too. Sitting in pre-Shiva. It was almost peaceful, until I had realized the day was coming when I wouldn't see him again. Then I would feel the stab of grief, advance grief. And he would sense it too. He couldn't see but he knew I was crying silent tears.

I barely remember the week of his death. I didn't record it in my diary because I must have been too far in it, my emotions elsewhere, locked up with Johnny's heart, his about-to-leave soul. But it happened and, in the end, I felt not only grief but a tidal wave of tenderness for Johnny—and for his battered body. That last part surprised me.

In the hospital, Boy Kelly and I took turns at his bedside, along with his family from Baltimore: Johnny's brother, his sister-in-law, his beloved mother. They would come up often in the last year, to show Johnny the unconditional love that families can sometimes offer. It hadn't always been there for Johnny— or he hadn't always felt it—but it was now. He was beloved and he was dying. He looked so handsome, still, with his pale face, his blinded, beautifully searching eyes. His mother would murmur that, running her hand over his face, the remaining thinned hair that was growing out into tufts at the nape. It was hard to see him in pain, which is what dying can bring: more pain before we're allowed to go, to be in peace in some other place. What Johnny wanted, then, even then, was his music.

After he died, they took his body away quickly, to be washed, cleaned, and prepared for the funeral. I was left alone in the hospital room. In the end, it had happened too quickly. I still wasn't ready to say a final good-bye. I didn't want him to be alone as they prodded him again, so, I confess: I went to find his body in the morgue. It was in a waiting area. Hospital limbo.

There was Johnny as he died: poxed, diabetic, gay, hair thin from chemo drugs, muscles shrunken from disuse, poked daily by needles as the dying are; the body prodded to give up its secrets until it takes control in the end, stills the heartbeat. A body with velvety-soft skin, smooth and quickly hardening into marble but still soft enough to caress. His naked body, his privates covered with a sheet as I let them be. He was always modest about his body, never wanting us to get too close. He retained his dignity and we respected that.

But that body, that dead body. *It was so beautiful.* Even in death. It was Johnny, my good friend. *The body poxed yet majestic.* With strong, capable arms and legs; with a whole world that had been lived and contained in it. With his hands and delicate fingers that had given up piano too early but learned to touch and feel again in his blindness. And his face: a good-looking boy who had never felt handsome enough because of his desire for other men. A body once caked in childhood fat, a protective armor. There was little trace of it here, just the softness of his chest, above the heart. And his stomach. I stood, looking at his body, caressing his fingers, his face. A human Caravaggio, paler than ever, a whitening body in final repose. Finally allowed to stop fighting.

Before leaving, I couldn't help it. I snagged his toe tag; a final indignity, I thought. Besides, there was a medical chart still hanging from the gurney, identifying him. *I'm going to let you sing again, don't worry, John. I'm taking you inside me now—your spirit, your dreams, the unfinished business of your life; our gayish world. I'll do what I can to honor you in it. You fought so well and bravely, my friend. I was there. I saw it all. I'm your witness. Good-bye, Johnny,* I told him. *Au revoir, mon ami.*

$\mathcal{VIII}$

$\mathcal{N}ew \; \mathcal{Y}ork, \; Still$

~ 60

1996

Weeks become months. I remain in a too-familiar place where my relationships seem to head: *sorrowland*. Johnny's gone, and my relationship with Jersey is a failing romance. She keeps cheating. She's having yet another affair. She's admitted it this time at least. But that doesn't make it easier.

We've had amazing times. We get along so well. She's a soul mate of sorts. We've traveled. She came to visit me in Europe, to Belize. We've had bliss. I still find her sexy, and we laugh so much together. I love her, I do. I truly love her. But she frustrates me. She's so immature. Amid our good times, we keep hitting the shoals. I'm so over the cheating.

I review the conversation, my internal conversation, my 24/7, nonstop, *detach-with-love* therapy lecture. There's only one healthy answer for me here: *let go*. So I have. But I'm still not willing to completely lose our closeness, the deep friendship that roots this romance. I'm looking for a new box that fits what we still mean to each other. I want her to become family.

All my friends say that's impossible—a true exercise in masochism. Codependency, the other therapy buzzword. But I disagree. I've seen too much loss. Life is too short to reject people we love because they can't give us everything we want or need. Like my father always says: bend, don't break. There's a lot of love here; let's transform it. It's something I want to try and Jersey is game. The question remains: at what cost? I won't let myself over-suffer either. I have new mantras. *Trust yourself. Build your ship and sail it. Build your house and live in it. Let love trump loss.*

In the meantime, the novel—Sel, AIDS, Le Pen, fascism, Henri, the Balkan and Rwandan genocides . . . everything I've written or researched to date—lies in a drawer, too complicated, too untamed, to simply pick up and move forward with. I want to avoid my inner world. Since Belize, where I wrote every day for two months, where Sel rose with me before everyone else, I'm back in my fitful

189

sleep state. Not quite insomnia, but not proper rest. I wake, stare down at the street, at fellow night crawlers avoiding the inevitability of tomorrow. Talk to Johnny in my head.

⁓

The end of love is such a familiar spiral to me by now, and I hate it, hate feeling powerless to avoid the pain, the dissolution of the dream. It's been lonely even with Jersey close by. It's the loss of the conversation, the openness, that hurts in breakups. *But I chose, didn't I? I did.* Change takes time. I know I'm in mourning. It's bigger than Jersey and bigger than Johnny or Aldyn. Each loss reveals another. Last year we lost David Feinberg, Joe Franco, and Robert Massa, all friends of mine in ACT UP. David was so angry at all of us; he held nothing back. He raged the way I wish my mother had. She was bitter but she never let herself explode. We should all explode and rage at untimely death.

If I were in Paris tonight, I would walk, let the Seine soothe me as only that river can, past my little ball of self-sorrow. Instead, I keep choosing other routes of escape. I've been hanging out with friends in Tompkins Square Park; enjoying a nightcap whiskey and other stimulants; had a little hookup of my own. I've had some small hangovers, but nothing worse. It feels good to open myself to affection too. It was time.

⁓ 61

Another week gone by. Every day I've tried to write, but the words swirl around my brain with my head still on the pillow. Fragments of thought that I know I should write down because I'll lose them. I've carted my research material— my notebooks, those damn doorstop French books—from here to there, to the beach with me and back even, just to sort through pages, to read and reconnect, like a patient probing herself after an operation, to feel if the body is ready to take up its living.

Then, one day, without any effort, I wake up and Sel is there, waiting on the edge of the windowsill where I've set my cup of coffee. On the second floor of the Avenue B loft, where I now share my life with Jersey, my ex and friend, and two other roommates. Where Boy Kelly and Jersey moved in first. Where Johnny used to dance, spinning a bit blindly in the end, to my favorite Morrissey song: *Everyday is like Sunday, everyday is cloudy and grey* . . . A song about England and the war and lost boys that inexplicably cheers me up.

Hello, Fish Girl.

That's her new nickname for me, the girl with the buggy blue-green eyes. *Ready for that fishing trip? We've been waiting.*

A fishing trip? Let's go.

And who is we? Some new friends I'm about to meet? I'm ready, I think. But first, you know, I need more coffee.

It's warm in Jersey's bedroom. It has a cozy chair and a kitty-corner view of Tompkins Square Park and the Korean deli below that has good coffee. I like to sit by the window and write late at night. New York can be so lovely this time of year. I love the late afternoons especially. I only recently learned about the park's history. It's a site of historic protest, many strikes. It was redesigned by Robert Moses in 1936 in an effort to curb the strikes, but that hasn't stopped anyone, has it? The protests go on.

Just a few years ago, the park became a giant camp. It's been full of old-timer Bowery winos and newer homeless people evicted from shelters that are being transformed into fancy student housing as NYU encroaches on more of the East Village. I have to admit, the park got so dirty and out of control and there were a lot of rats and a lot of drugs. But the city acted with force, illegally, to evict the tent squatters without a proper plan to resettle them, despite our best protests. It viewed them as vermin, tore down the makeshift tents without warning sometimes, threw out furniture and lives like so much garbage. Soon the dogs will have a nice place to run around and shit, and the kids will be able to frolic in the playground without stepping on a dirty needle. Those are two key arguments supporters of the cleanup made. The park should be for every-one, they say. Our kids can't play here. But who's everyone? The NYU students? Everything's changing fast here.

And those homeless people: where did they go? Where are they sleeping? That's what no one talks about, now that the news cameras have left. *Where did they send the undesirables? To jail? To New Jersey? To Queens?* It's a question I should know the answer to; I'm a citizen of this city, after all. I do care, and I'm upset we're losing the gentrification war.

Of course I'm a gentrifier too. I know my privilege. But I support afford-able housing for the poor and I'll keep protesting for it. I'm not happy to see the Ukrainian stores with their pretty painted eggs disappear. I want to be able to go to Delancey Street and get a cheap egg cream and a late-night blintz at Ratner's or a cheap beer at the Lansky Lounge. Kill the culture, you kill the city. They're killing the soul of the East Village and we can't stop it.

Downstairs, I see a flow of people stop in the deli, headed for the park. A group of musicians, instruments in hand. A group of young gay men in bright dresses, chatting with excitement. There's a Wigstock event happening at the other end of the park, near Avenue A. Lady Bunny is in charge. Wigstock has been happening here for years and has always been the best party. Then it got too big and they shut it down. Now Bunny is hosting mini-concerts to raise funds. It's certain to be good.

I should go. I wanna go. Maybe later.

I settle into the cozy chair, tune out Wigstock. Open the window a crack, put on Sade. "Smooth Operator." I close my eyes. I've been invited to another party. Let me tune in.

Fish Girl, I hear a moment later. *You're here. Pay attention. They're coming.*

~ 62

I see Sel ahead. She's by the square, the Place de l'Hôtel de Ville. People are setting up for a party. They've decorated a large barge that's tethered close to the bridge. Is this the festival of Saint Joan of Arc? A band is warming up on a stage. I see well-dressed couples, some of them young, getting out of parked cars with tinted windows. Young fascists or undercover cops? Not far from the barge, lurking near one the pillars of the bridge, I spy a group of young men, including Henri, and his friend, whose name comes to me instantly: Maoud, a young man from the Saint-Ouen flea market. A burly, handsome fellow dressed in soccer shorts, a T-shirt, and Adidas flip-flops, the uniform of the urban soccer fan. He's hand-rolling his tobacco, laughing. He has a nice gap between his front teeth.

Oh, and here's Torn Stockings, a newcomer to the scene. A once-pretty junkie from Marseille who looks like Marianne Faithfull. Who's slowly walking the perimeter of the square, keeping an eye out for any unattached handsome men. And there—the child I would recognize anywhere: Piglet; my future Judas. He's holding a red-and-white kite with a blue tail. So, the gang's all here, it seems. Now where's Sel? There she is, by the crowd gathering around the bandstand. I can only see her shadow, but I know it's her.

Then I see the car, driving slowly up a side street toward us, escorted by two policemen on motorcycles, like a funeral cortege. *Did somebody important die?* There are young women in the back of the car, an old man between them. *The Le Pen clan, all dressed in white.* Then other cars. The passengers inside waving to the crowd. Known faces. Famous people. Who are they?

Behind Sel, I see a large-scale replica of Saint Joan on her horse. This is a National Front recruitment event. Le Pen and his daughters are speakers, guests of honor. Two handsome young men, National Front youth leaders, are handing tourists and passersby a little pamphlet. *Le Front National: Premier Parti de la France.* Already the crowd is growing in size. The celebration will be marked by fireworks over the Seine.

Over there, Sel barks. *Do you recognize him?*

A group of men are laughing together, greeting officials who've emerged from the crowd. It's Jacques Vergès, lawyer to the Vichy Nazis, with Sauveur Vaisse, lawyer to the new divorcé Jean-Claude Duvalier. Vergès ushering Le Pen through the crowd, shaking hands.

That's right, Fish Girl. They always bring their lawyers. It's Laval's old cronies. They must have driven up from the south. I think the party's about to start. I'm sure we'll see a lot of the old wolves today. I hope you're paying attention. . . .

⁓

I sit in my New York window, pad in hand. I close my eyes, let the scenes come. I'm so tempted to go over to the Tompkins Square concert, wonder if any drag kings I know will perform. Several of the younger Lesbian Avengers are exploring boi drag, a new trend. They're talented. Maybe if I work for a few hours I can go after. Wigstock parties always get best at the end of the night. For the moment, I'm content here.

My research box is at my feet, the French books tagged with Post-its. I pull one of them out. Look for a face I just recognized in that crowd of men. René Bousquet, the Butcher of Marseille. Posing for a picture with the French police, looking handsome and happy in a fur-trimmed coat like my mother bequeathed to me. Stylish, smoking a cigarette. Happily in charge. Is that before or after he oversaw the thirty-six-hour lockdown of Marseille, the house-to-house sweep by twelve thousand police, who then blew up the Old Port area and put two thousand Jews on trains headed for Fréjus, then the camp at Royallieu, then Drancy, a point of no return? The caption doesn't say.

I put the book aside, pull out some recent Xerox pages from the French newspapers. The newer wolves, my contemporaries. *The women.* Catherine Mégret, the Front's newest It Girl, recently married to Bruno Mégret; he, a rising star who's just fallen, charged with corruption. Catherine may run for office in Vitrolles, a suburb of Marseille where unemployment is close to 20 percent and immigrants from North Africa are taking all the jobs. That's the message the Mégrets are peddling to their core base, the children and grandchildren of the pied-noir generation who voted for Bruno.

Catherine Mégret is attractive, slim, intelligent looking, with bright-brown eyes, a good haircut. She's wearing a good suit. These fascists are always so much younger then I expect. Catherine is my age, also a Pisces, born eighteen days after me—on March 16. Two days after my father's birthday. She looks younger than I do though, like a university student. Easy on the eyes. She's also a calculating opportunist, like her husband. She's jumping in where he got booted out. *Financial irregularities*, the papers call it. Dipping into the municipal coffers to fund a white supremacy program, and make sure he got well paid too. The press has dubbed him Le Pen's Goebbels. So Catherine is now Madame Goebbels.

The women of the National Front do seem to have taken a page from Hitler's chief of propaganda. They clearly understand the value of presentation. They're media telegenic, like our kind—ACT UP, the Avengers. They're a fashionable bunch of fascists.

I think Philippe may be wrong about Le Pen and the Front. He's definitely right about the economy and the unemployment trigger, but I think he underestimates the draw of beauty and couture to a French person. Some good lipstick, some killer heels, and Madame Goebbels may wow them. They'll underestimate her because they always underestimate women. She'll court the housewives who are tired of seeing their men striking for months against falling wages. The falling white middle class. I need to keep my eye on these young conservative women, there and here too. All these would-be Joans of Arcs.

~ 63

What day is it? What week? What month? It's all a blur, lately. The mad rush of New York life. I've had so little time outside of magazine work, of reporting, to keep up with my journal, to spend with Sel and this book. And I realize I skipped over a very important event—one that's also related to why writing has had to take a back seat to real life lately. It's Kiki. He's left us now too.

Even in his final moments, he staged a last party, his swan song. It was time, he announced. He removed all the medical supports: the chemo, the albumen drips, the morphine, the lung drains. *Time to meet Mr. Buddha.*

There was Kiki in his bed, surrounded by his Barbie doll collection and his pictures of Saint Lazarus, looking every inch the picture of his diva-muse, Joan Crawford, a woman who had given him some of his best one-liners. His legs were huge, released at last from their confines, his bald head wrapped in a towel, like a debutante stepping out of the shower, hair washed, readying herself for the ball. Holding court, in other words, as he always did. In charge of his own party, up to the last minute.

It's such a sad thing to think about, and it was sadder even to witness, to run into a parade of old faces and friends en route from Kiki's house for the final good-bye. He knew so many people and his magazine columns had reached so many more. I stayed for the after-party, a small gathering of close friends. One by one, we leaned in for a final good-bye, to kiss the brow, to give a final, deep hug.

In the end, then, he hadn't killed anyone and he hadn't killed himself, either. He had cried and mourned as much as he had screamed, with his best friends, and endured as long as he could. Even with AIDS, even as a proud champion of Lesion Liberation, he had remained the life of the party. Now he's gone. Another loss that I feel like a sharp inhalation, not an exhalation.

Looking back, Kiki won a big fight—faster access to Doxil. A fairer price. It didn't save him, but it helped him live longer. And it's going to save a lot of others still in desperate need of lesion liberation. He didn't leave us his southern belle memoir. But he's left us his furious words, his diva rage:

> I am someone with AIDS and I want to live by any means necessary. . . . I am being sold down the river by people within this community who claim to be helping people with AIDS. Hang your heads in shame while I point my finger at you.

~ 64

It's easy to lose your way. In life, in love, in work, in your thoughts. Another truism. A few days ago I met with Ann Rower, a close writer friend who's been struggling with her new novel for as long as I began keeping this journal. Months ago, after I came back from Belize, we exchanged material, determined to spur each other on. Now she keeps getting ideas for how I might structure the journey, as I call it; how to integrate my research, my real life, and Sel's narrative—and how not to. She leaves random musings on my answering machine without any introduction:

Hi, it's me. I was just thinking that Sel could keep her own diary. Don't you think you might? blah, blah, blah . . .

I like her ideas, but I have to be careful. I can be influenced so easily. Still, her entry into my inner world has been so helpful, and it's so gratifying to share the creative process. It makes Sel all the more real. Ann loves Sel—*her dirtiness,* as she calls it.

I've tried to do the same: to give Ann pep talks, to urge her to dream even larger, take more creative risks, ignore the internal voices of doubt that keep blocking her because so much time has already gone by and the book still isn't ready. She's writing about the art world, about Lee Krasner Pollock and Elaine de Kooning, and their circle, including Lee's more-famous husband, Jackson, who sounds like a genius asshole artist, and the great gay poet Frank O'Hara, who my friend Brad Gooch adores, and Stuart Davis. Her book is a pseudo-biography. She's bringing Lee and Elaine back as lesbians, imagining what the girls would have done without Jackson and his alcoholic rages. But it's tricky.

She's had to get permission from the artists' estates to see certain works, to reference certain correspondences. She keeps seeing detractors in her mind, the gallery owners and critics she knows, and anticipating their dislike of the book.

They just might hate it, she says. *Hate me. And then I won't be invited to any more of their great Hamptons parties.*

We like to joke, but the worry is real. People get so prickly about their dead loved ones; about how history will remember them.

You think people will want to read this book? she asks for the umpteenth time. *Who, besides the people who aren't going to like what I have to say?*

Think of Virginia Woolf. Think of Djuna Barnes, I remind her. All the great women experimentalists. Look how they were rejected, right and left. They would have huge problems getting published today. But so what? They wrote the books they were meant to write. And thank God they didn't hold back. Or maybe they did. Who knows how much farther they might have gone with more support from fellow writers or editors? But, the point is, this is yours. So run with it. *Get out of your own way,* I say, a jewel I picked up from a self-help book at the airport years ago. This is what you have to offer, I argue. So do it. But at least take the journey yourself first and try to enjoy it. Everything else is gravy: getting published, read, reviewed, appreciated, making some rent money. *Also,* I remind her, *hate sells. If those art critics hate it, that means they've had to buy the book and read it. Think about that.*

That makes her laugh.

Plus, I add, *you're making Lee and Elaine lezzies? How fun is that!*

The problem is that we're not writing enough. Me, due to the drama of an unfaithful lover; due to heartsickness over losing yet another close friend to AIDS. For Ann, it's the opposite problem. She's seriously falling in love. She's having an unexpected intense affair with Heather Lewis, a woman who's a good fifteen years younger than Ann, and a talented writer—a lesbian lit-star, if such a category exists yet. It sort of does, now. So, Ann's disappeared into the world of lust and discovery.

When we run into each other, there's a guilty apology: *I haven't written much. You?* Our books trail behind us at the end of every day. Like shadows; afterthoughts that follow a last shot of tequila at a corner bar on a weekday night. *Get anything good done today?* A cock of the head, a quick shake, *No. Well, a little. A few pages.* Then we both smile, knowing it's all right, that it can't be any other way. I'm slightly miserable and she's suddenly extremely happy. Neither is conducive to a calm mind. *Oh well. Let's have a short drink then, shall we?*

I'm not stuck on my book, I tell Ann later, I'm stuck about my life, my choices, love, a partner. I'm back to square one—or, nearly, it feels. I'm almost forty, you know. The idea shocks me. How could it be? I feel thirty; no older. I'm young in my head. I haven't settled. I want to—and I don't want to. I feel out of sync with people my own age; that's what I complain about to Ann. It's not an age thing or a body thing—not the number of years, but the energy; the spirit. At the same time, my younger lovers make me feel, well, older.

Ann has it even worse. Friends her age, nearing sixty, make her far older than she ever wants to be. *They remind me of my mother,* she jokes. *It's terrible.*

She's another one who's not ready to stop living for the moment, in the moment; who's watching her body fall apart a bit, but so what. *Give me a beer, give me a bit of that cocaine. Who's young? We are. It's everybody else who's old.* We're like the two drunks in *Waiting for Godot,* waiting for our books to happen while life confronts us: the sum of what we're hoping to do, to shape, to like and possibly love—people and ideas and ideals, especially, but also our failures—all of it, up for discussion and review until it's closing time, and we've done it again, out-lasted everyone, and we crawl home to our respective small apartments, to our beds, to our incomplete books and dreams.

~ 65

It's high time I got back to Europe. I'll go soon. First, to London for a few weeks, then to Paris, to my original source of inspiration. But before then I want to get a lot of writing done: to arrive at the end of the book, not even a midpoint. Europe. It gives me a deadline, a frame for pushing myself a bit.

Have I been writing? A bit. But I've been surviving. Thank God I haven't been too self-destructive, though my liver might be damaged from drinking too much Bushmills. I've failed to put myself on the wagon, though I keep vowing to, as a precaution; to prove that I've got some willpower left. For now, the goal is harm reduction: wine, not whiskey, and more naps. It's helping.

I'm also having sex with a younger woman—Jessie. She's too young for me, I sometimes think, but don't care enough to stop. I know it's an affair and I want to enjoy it. It feels good to have sex again, to be loved, physically, to be desired. For so many months now, with Jersey emotionally distracted, with our romance failing, I've felt like I was in still waters, without even a ripple of desire for anyone, or like a computer that's offline, ready to be turned on, but charging its battery. I've been still and quiet, like the packed earth under my feet as I walked barefoot up-country, desiring nothing, trying not to think too much, feel too much.

Now I'm coming back—my energy; I feel emotionally lighter. And with this shift of emotions comes an opening through which Sel crawls, invading my daily thoughts. Just last night, when I was kissing Jessie, Sel appeared. It was her tongue, her desire, taking me over. A rush of thoughts, about what her sexual story is, who her lovers have been; are? I feel oddly comforted by this reappearance; grateful she survived my depression.

Old tart, I think, *welcome back.*

IX

London

~ 66

Europe again. En route to London, writing on the plane. It feels like it's taken me too long to get back. I have some new research I'm doing, maybe for an *Out* piece, but also for the book. Sel's story. I'm ready to see friends, meet new people, see art. London: *tea and toast and the Tate*.

I'm spending ten days in England, then on to Paris. Traveling with Jersey and her best friend, Jeane, from college, a lesbian farmer from Vermont who wants to become a public radio reporter. She picks my brain, listens to my stories of working at WBAI Pacifica Radio in the early eighties with Laura Flanders. Days of cold, damp weather, tall glasses of beer, and tense moments navigating the highway to Wales, driving on the left side of the road. Jersey and I are fighting, nervous, as always, with each other's driving, even though we're both excellent at it. I'm enjoying the trip but feel the undercurrent of our relationship's long tension; the emotional tide that will inevitably ride back in, reminding me of what's still not resolved. I'll be glad when they leave and I have a few days alone.

I've made a short mental list of things to do here and in Paris, wanting mostly to soak up the atmosphere again, to capture on film the images that speak to me, that will inspire me when I'm back in New York, sitting again at my desk, far away from the damp, salty spray of the Seine.

⌒

London. Lousy weather, gray and rainy; very cold, but nice buses and taxis. Tea: good in the morning but better in the afternoon. The English budget hotel is a good place to set a movie about a pornographer or a serial killer: thin walls, pretty wallpaper, chilly, soft mattresses, lousy breakfasts. *Did I say chilly? I can't get warm.*

I have a few people to see; questions to pursue. Not much time to get my interviews done. I'll go alone; leave Jersey and the farmer to their fun. I need to make some money while I'm here, if I can, and I'm interested in the new pox. *Bovine spongiform encephalopathy*—BSE—also known as mad cow disease. There's been a major outbreak in cattle here—for years apparently—and many thousands of cows have been rendered (read: killed), their carcasses burned instead of ground into food. So says my friend, Oxford, who wonders if we've been told the whole story, or whether, as has been rumored, the rendered bone got exported overseas to America and fed to other livestock. Oxford is studying at the university and has offered to introduce me to some scientists who are following the story.

I've been boning up on prions, pronounced pree-on. A still-mysterious protein that acts as an infectious agent but isn't a virus or a bacteria. It has no DNA or RNA, the two things we've always been told are the essential building blocks for life. Right? Wrong! Apparently, a prion is a whole new creature, and practically an indestructible one. Oxford says she's been told you can't even nuke a prion to death, it's such a tough little protein. You can bury it deep underground, but it won't die. So, it will never disappear and, so far, it can't be treated—and it's fatal. *So scary.*

Prions attack tissue and cells in the brain, causing infected cows to walk loopy, like drunks, before completely collapsing and dying. Hence the name: Mad Cow. Its human equivalent is Creutzfeldt-Jakob disease. The million-dollar question everyone is asking is, how contagious is it, cows-to-people? *Can you get it from eating a mad burger?*

The British authorities have been slammed for initially denying the epidemic, though I'm not sure that's fair. What's clear is that the meat industry has been hit, very hard. The UK meat lobby is apparently launching a major PR campaign to try to stop the panic. But everyone is freaking out, says Oxford. Everyone's going veggie.

~~~~~~~~

It's a train ride up to see Oxford. I call to set up a visit, but she's out, so I leave a message. I still have time to kill before meeting Jersey and her friend Jeane later. I put in a call to Simon Watney, a writer, columnist, and one of the leading UK AIDS activists; a man I've always wanted to meet. He's with ACT UP–London and helped found OutRage!, a gay rights group, a few years back. He's home, working on a book manuscript. *Are you free for a beer?* I ask. *When?* he asks. *Um, well, uh . . . right now?* He laughs. *You Americans are spontaneous, aren't you?*

⌐◡

I'm seeking an update on AIDS activism in London now. Simon's been in charge of one of the major foundations funding HIV programs in the UK, the Terrence Higgins Trust. When we finally meet, over a pint, he's friendly, though dismissive of gay leaders I plan to interview. *Don't bother*, he warns. *They're all buggers.* But there are some younger activists who are, he puts it, very promising. There's a major generational split, he explains. There's the old, tired crowd, the ones who are afraid to really call out the government on its failing AIDS policies, and the younger ones who don't give a toss.

I like Simon. He reminds me of Kiki with his wicked wit, suffer-no-fools attitude, and his passion for AIDS and the survival of his clan: gay men. I also like his accent. I mean, who doesn't love an English accent, really? Look at Madonna.

Later, when I'm back with Jersey and her friend at yet another dim bar, nursing yet another strong lager, I recount my day. We play darts. I'm terrible. I hear myself happily throwing around the words I've picked up. *Bugger that. I don't give a toss!*

X

Paris, avant tout

~ 67

November 1996

Paris, again, at last, at last. My friend La Folie, as I jokingly call her, one of the Crazy Girls, owes me for a giant phone bill from when she lived with me in New York last year. She's a student again and I know I have no prospects of getting the money back anytime soon. I figure I have years of credit in exchange, so I'm going to cash in my chips for a bit of it by staying with her. Her flat on the Quai de la Seine is a small, crowded room with a junky balcony overlooking the city's largest artificial lake, the Bassin de la Villette. It's a beautiful, industrial corner of the city, the nineteenth arrondissement.

In the morning I wake late, and the sky is inevitably gray with the promise of rain. I stand looking at the river, which is riding high, threatening to overflow the banks if another big storm comes along. I'm delighted by the idea: the Seine exerting her dominion over Paris again.

The air along the canal is freezing. Men huddle in small groups, watching each other play boules. I have my Super 8 camera out; I film them discreetly. They're a living postcard. But, then, everything looks like that to me. I'm so glad to be in Paris again. It's so beautiful, as always. Even gray and so cold my hands hurt.

In the subway, I see an older Arab woman begging for money, then, down another passageway, a blind man with glasses and a Muslim skullcap. Down the escalator at the Gare du Nord a young man hops onto the train and plays a large, red accordion. I'm happy; I love the accordion. He plays the standards, including "La vie en rose."

I study his fingers. Everyone avoids his eyes; they don't want to feel they've entered into an implicit contract to pay him. I don't care, though. He clearly loves his instrument and he duly notes my pleasure. He directs his musical flourishes my way. He's a burly, unattractive young man, with stained teeth. His accordion has lost a black key as well, one in the upper register.

202

In another life, I'll be a musician. I'll play the saxophone and the accordion —
play shtetl music; working-class, dance-hall music, saucy tangoes, zydeco. I'll
be a chanteuse, accompany myself on the accordion, lift my skirt after a song, à
la Dietrich, and slip the money I'm given into my garter belt.

I've invited Oxford to come to Paris for a few days. She's easy, fun company:
perky, smart, and mellow enough to accept my *don't-feel-like-talking* mood without
taking it personally. She's packed her briefcase with documents comparing the
penal systems of the United States and the United Kingdom, determined, as I
am, to get some work done.

Oxford is tall and androgynous; like me, she constantly gets mistaken for a
gay boy. A cute one. We hooked up at the Vancouver AIDS conference. I had a
great time there. The news from the conference was a breakthrough: protease
inhibitors, a new class of drugs that work in combination with the old standbys,
AZT, 3TC, ddI, even d4T, though it's starting to get phased out. Toxicities.
The PI drugs are gonna be tough too, but the trial results look really good. It's not
the cure but it's a line in the sand; a brake slowing the runaway train of AIDS.

ACT UP was celebrating hard in Vancouver. I really let loose; even joined
a friend, JD, on a stage at a gay bar after-party hosting a wet T-shirt competition.
The prize was $100 and only gay boys were competing; we couldn't let that be.
No way. And we won, unbelievably. JD had Manic Panic, long, green hair; it
ran all over my wet T-shirt. I remember how freezing that damn stage shower
was, such a shock. The next day I had an interview with one of the scientists
about the new PI drugs. *Congratulations*, he had smiled. *I saw you on stage.* I remember being a bit mortified. *Holy Jeezus! What kind of professional am I?*

The kind that drinks and dirty dances, obviously. Luckily, a lot of these
scientists do too. In Amsterdam, I had felt like an innocent, seeing so many of
the best brains in AIDS smoking a legal spliff as they relaxed outdoors in between
sessions. *No, I thought, you can't get high! No, wait. We need your best thinking in here.
C'mon. Straighten up!*

Anyway, Oxford was part of my Vancouver good times. It was nothing
planned. She had needed a bed to share. *Sure, of course.* She was part of my
summer of casual sex; my need to push myself out of the Jersey doldrums. Part
of that *I-should-have-sex-with-someone-already* action one takes to feel better after a
breakup. An escape, nothing too serious. My season of sex with younger women
and the third wheel with monogamous couples. Funny times. And good fun.
My threesome rule: wine me, dine me, no drama.

Oxford says my eyes are bright here in Paris; she's never seen me so enthusiastic. I can't stop filming: long, still takes of the river framed by construction

cranes, of partly demolished buildings, of ordinary window displays I find beautiful. I take her to all the neighborhoods I like: the African market at Belleville, the gay area around the Bastille where all the street sex happens. It's the Paris I love.

~ 68

Along the Rue des Rosiers in the Marais, I pause every few feet, capturing the garish neon displays of kosher foods, rows of Middle Eastern delicacies. The colors and textures excite me. I tell Oxford about the summer of 1982, when this Jewish quarter was bombed; when I discovered the underlying strains of anti-Semitism and anti-Arabism in the French press. That was the summer I partied with a new journalist friend, Peter Brooks, from London, and his friend, Haoui Montaug, a flamboyant gay party promoter from the East Village. Haoui became famous as the doorman-to-befriend at the happening clubs: Hurrah, Danceteria, Studio 54, the Palladium, the Garage. He also hosted an East Village cabaret night, *No Entiendes* (You Don't Understand, or as he put it, You Dunno); it was a good time.

Haoui developed AIDS and staged one of the first suicide parties. At the time, it was very hush-hush. No one admitted to being at the party, afraid they would be blamed, somehow, for not stopping him. Or maybe afraid of the legal implications, because it was a bit of a mess and things didn't go as planned. Haoui took a bunch of Seconals and went to sleep while everyone waited for him to die. Instead he woke up again the next morning, furious to be alive. He had to swallow more pills. Can you imagine?! That's beyond drama. Madonna couldn't come, but she called in. I heard about all of it thirdhand, so don't hold me to the details. I wondered if Peter was there. We had lost touch long before.

Haoui died in June 1991, another Jewish fegallah who, like Kiki the Lesion Liberator, refused to go gently into that good night. I've made note of the date: two months after Bousquet was indicted; three months before Klaus Barbie died of cancer of the blood, spine, and prostrate. Cancer in the balls, just like Kiki. Maybe Haoui will show up at one of Sel's planned parties. *The emcee.*

On the subject of parties, Pete brought me to a great party here in Paris in 1982 with Fela Kuti, the Nigerian pop star. That's where I met Haoui. I've heard rumors that Fela has the pox too—HIV—but it's not something I've confirmed. I've just heard the gossip. If it's true, it's especially sad because he's known to be a polygamist and has something like a dozen wives. Which means they're probably at risk of exposure. Has anyone written about that? It's such a very touchy subject.

I didn't know much about Fela back then, but everyone there seemed very excited by his presence along with a group of superhip Africans, all dancing in the middle of the living room. There were a lot of white French hipster kids too. After a while, I noticed everyone kept disappearing into the bathroom for what I learned was cocaine. It was impossible to get into the bathroom to pee, so I had to leave the party to find a toilet.

When I came back, it was a serious bash, like the East Village parties I later attended, and I remember feeling like I had stumbled into the heart of some important cultural moment. It wasn't just that Fela was there but the excitement of the French kids about the new Afrobeat music. I also remember passing on the coke, which I had never tried at that stage, because I was afraid of it, and because I didn't know Pete well. I thought he might judge me; think I was not a serious journalist. Of course, I later found out that Pete was a first-class party animal who probably jumped into the loo for a snort when I slipped away to pee elsewhere. I do remember thinking, *Damn, I'll probably never get another chance. Ha!*

All this was back when I was trying to get my first real journalism job at a French news agency, Agence France-Presse (AFP). I was fresh out of Columbia journalism grad school and I had scored a paid summer internship at AFP's English desk. It was a weird, intense time. I lived in one half of a dentist's office that belonged to a friend of my father's. I woke up to sickly sweet smells like chloroform. I was lonely and conflicted; still closeted at work. I wore skirts and sensible shoes and felt like more of a drag queen than ever. I'm not surprised they didn't hire me permanently, just on the basis of my bad fashion. The point is, I wanted to fit in, but I felt on the outside of the chummy Paris reporter's club.

That was also the summer that I first began to confuse the names of two groups that were engaged in some intense rival massacres: the Hutu and the Tutsi, of Rwanda. At the English desk, we had to quickly translate and edit updates of hot stories coming across the wire. The job often consisted of adding one or two lines to existing copy. I was quite confused by the Hutu and Tutsi conflict. I kept stumbling over the words: *Hutsi? Tutu?* It's like the Balkan crisis, same problem for me. I've had trouble figuring out who's who, who's done what, when, and, most importantly, who's the bad guy now, and who is the West backing? Looking back, I realize now that we were receiving the early field reports of the genocide to come, a decade later.

I remember how my colleagues and I would quickly scan the copy to see what the numbers were like: if the initial death toll had climbed a lot, or if one side had issued a denial for the massacres, which would almost certainly warrant an immediate wire update. I remember the story feeling very far away; a part of Africa I didn't know much about, and the AFP bosses didn't seem to care to know more either. It was a bad African bush war; all sides bore guilt.

In the Marais, I film with intent, capturing the things I cherish: a Michelin sign, Arab graffiti, the juxtaposition of new and medieval. I tell Oxford about the Rue des Rosiers bombings in Paris that occurred years back, how this whole quarter has become gentrified since then, a posh gay district. How it's depressing too, because whatever is new has surely displaced the poor, the elderly, or the immigrant. In fifty years, the parts of Paris I love the most will be gone.

Walking back to the apartment in the evening, I share bits and pieces of history that I've learned about the local neighborhood with Oxford, who's a history buff too: morbid details of executions and scandals, about this canal, where the victims of past epidemics were piled onto ships and taken to be buried in unmarked cemeteries beyond Montmartre. About Sel and my archival rabbit holes.

She talks about her own PhD research, about the connection between AIDS and the prison system that is spreading the pox to American black men faster than even we activists realize. About how a lot more people everywhere are dying of AIDS than we think. Once again, it's all a case of too little, too late.

~ 69

Before coming to Paris this time, I wrote a short note to Belle, asking her to call me if she wanted. I doubt she will, but I'm hopeful. I feel her distance. Walking around now, I'm full of her, the memory of our past times, of that magical soul connection. It makes me sad, then a bit grim. *She withdrew; it wasn't just my fault. I told her I wanted a closer relationship and she didn't respond. She never showed up. If she's mad that I got involved with Jersey, then I do feel bad, but I did tell her I needed to move on. I gave her plenty of chances to choose. Inaction is still a choice.*

I'm tempted to just call her, to make sure she's actually living at her old address, but I haven't yet. I don't want to hassle her. Instead, I fantasize about running into her at the movies, at a bar. In my fantasies, she's with some man, or some friends from work. She's uncomfortable, but polite and distant with me, making small talk before leaving. I'm the same, but less uncomfortable. It feels crazy to have her out of my life. But I have to accept if she's just moved on forever. I wonder if she heard about me and Jersey, our breakup. If she knows I've now moved into Jersey's loft and we're becoming friends.

Two, four, six, eight; if she calls it will be great.

⌒

Quick Notes. A summary of this week's highlights:

- Reading up on the *sans papiers* movement. Very exciting to see movement on this immigration front. My friends in the Haitian community are getting involved but are wary of being pawns in the French political scene. Theodore asked me about the status of his lawsuit; wonders if they'll ever see any money from it. His ear still bothers him.
- Antifascist demo being organized for this week near the Bastille. I plan to go. Hoping to interview the organizers. Have put in calls to Ras l'Front, left messages in a few places.
- Belle, Belle, Belle. No call. She has the number. Frustrating. What did I expect?
- Sebastien is arriving in Paris for a few days. We plan to shop around Barbès. I want some henna and some presents for friends. He wants to introduce me to a cute Moroccan guy he met last time he was here.
- Need to write more about the boys, the last days: Kiki, other friends.
- Met with my step-grandmother. Love her! Sweet lady; always so kind to me. Only relative who always seems to really care about my sister and ask about her. She finally told me the real story of how and why my mother was lined up to be shot by the Nazis. A few new details, but the basics were all there. Amazing that they weren't shot. A miracle of timing. A few minutes more and there would be no Anne-christine, or any of this life of mine.
- There's a strike going on by French truckers over unemployment and shitty government policies. *L'opération escargot.* The snail strike. They may block the rail line back to England. What to do? Solidarity with the snails, 'natch.

⌒

Postscript: Belle called today, on my last afternoon, just as I was packing. I'll see her in an hour. Expectation and disappointment go hand in hand. *Why did she wait?* She says she misunderstood how long I was staying. My heart is beating a bit, with feelings of familiar sadness and a small glint of hope: maybe we'll be friends again. Maybe she'll tell me what happened, finally.

XI

New York

~ 70

December 1996

A new era has begun. I'm home again, still in Alphabet City, but on Avenue B, not C. In Jersey's loft. Jersey, my friend, my roommate . . . but not necessarily my lover. Everyone still thinks we're crazy. But we are making it work.

It's early December, and cold out. I just woke up from a deep sleep. It's 3:30 a.m. and I'm up at my computer. Rereading my trip notes. Glad I'm back but wishing I was there too. Wishing I could have done more and stayed longer. Still, I have a lot to work with.

When I was in England, I picked up a book by Bernard-Henri Lévy, one of France's contemporary philosopher-politicians and Renaissance men. He's the same Lévy who's made an excellent documentary about Sarajevo, *Bosna!* It's about the abandonment of Sarajevo and the embodiment of democracy it represented before the Balkan war. This book is a collection of edited interviews, fleshed out from a film project he did about the political attitudes of French intellectuals from 1890 to today. Lévy is interested in the fact that intellectuals could—can—be found on both political extremes, right and left, and wondered what he would find as he dug more deeply into the positions they held and the creative work they produced. He points out something that resonates with me, something that I suppose has shaped me strongly, since at least two of the writers he looks at, Jean-Paul Sartre and Simone de Beauvoir, influenced me as a young woman.

It's this: in the past century, being an intellectual meant that you had or could have a certain role to play in the culture, one that was publicly recognized. People read more and writers enjoyed the privilege of feeling they had a purpose, which was to engage themselves in the pursuit of a greater social good. In other words, a writer or an artist wasn't living solely for herself but for others. Even though the creative imagination was the terrain, the object was social justice, or something close to that. As Lévy stresses repeatedly, it was commonly accepted

208

that at times writing or painting would not be enough; that the pen, words, images, would not suffice.

That's when they took off to the Spanish Front to take on Franco, or, like Sartre and the Beaver, trucked to Moscow to interview Lenin and Marx before belatedly rejecting Stalinism. They *had* to put their bodies on the line. That kind of thinking is what drove Susan Sontag to go to Sarajevo and also to stage her production of *Waiting for Godot*. She sees art as an essential in times of atrocity, a creative action that calls us to remember our humanity, our connection. To elevate us above barbarity.

AIDS has drawn a line in the sand of my life. I find it difficult, in a time of such suffering, watching so many friends die or go blind like Johnny without a cure in sight, to step away from reporting on this disease, or the next protest; to take the time and internal space I really need to develop my creative writing. I feel too pulled. We need to witness and we need to act, says Lévy. I agree. But Sontag's right, too: art amid atrocity is an act of witness and its own call to action. So I have to find the way to do both.

~ 71

Sel's story is in the news again today. That's how I feel, anyway, reading the *New York Times*: so many current events seep into her story, into the issues I'm researching, both directly and covertly. There's a page-one story about the Balkans, with a picture of Serbian university students waving victoriously from on top of a tank. There's an update on the unwinding Gulf War syndrome story and the Pentagon's admission—too late; so sorry—that officials there withheld information from scientists reviewing the complaints of veterans of the Persian Gulf War who have since fallen ill.

Do you remember the Gulf War? It wasn't long ago. It made Peter Arnett of CNN an international television star and changed the way we watch wars. Now, we're really up close and personal, right out on the balcony of the hotel, being attacked with an uncensored view. We can hear the bombs exploding, see the balcony shake. Though we still don't feel the actual heat of the battle or suffer its bombs. It's all the more exciting for that reason, I suppose. Like the greatest digital war game yet.

My long-ago ex Laura Flanders has been interviewing Gulf War vets for years now, looking into the impact of low-dose exposure to toxins like sarin gas in U.S. troops. Five years ago or so, thousands of these vets were apparently exposed to a cloud of sarin gas that was released during the destruction of an Iraqi chemical-munitions dump in Khamisiyah. This was in March 1991. (That's the same month the butcher Bousquet was indicted and right before

Haoui killed himself—just to show you how events and people stay linked in my brain.) Now, so many of these vets have a host of mysterious illnesses, including terrible headaches and loss of fine motor skills, which suggests their brains and nerve cells were affected.

A year ago, Laura told me she had all the material to write a big exposé book on Gulf War syndrome, then didn't. Too bad, because it would have been a good book, and timely—she had the story when most journalists couldn't care less. Now everyone is jumping on board, but the denials are still coming from all sides.

Anyway, what caught my attention this morning and made me think of Sel is the theory of how low-dose sarin impacts the brain. I had a narrative brain fart: perhaps Sel chooses a biological agent—maybe a rhabdovirus, a fish pox—that can impact the brain or nerve cells. Some kind of viral weapon to go after the old Nazis who continue to evade justice. She could put it into a skin cream, one that also darkens the flesh. That would really trouble an old racist like Le Pen too. Anyway, the sarin story has me thinking. Rabbit holes, but creative fun.

Am I done with the *Times* for today? Almost. There's also a story that's more directly relevant to my—okay—Sel's obsession with the resurgence of fascism in Western Europe. It's an article about whether the formerly Communist countries of Eastern Europe will join NATO. Five or ten years from now, all of Europe might not only share a European common market but a unified border, manned by a pan-European police force and military. That could really keep new immigrants out. Let's not forget: it's not only the Eastern bankers and citizens who might benefit but the Far Right nationalist parties too. Chew on that little German deutsche mark for a while.

~ 72

The phone call I've long feared comes unexpectedly. There are three calls, actually, but I've missed the first two. The first is from Sebastien, who's left a message: *Call me, it's really important.* The second is from Jersey, a simple *call me* that doesn't convey any particular sense of urgency. I missed both calls because I was out, spending the night with Jessie—my younger what? *newish affair?* paramour? something more than casual and less than a girlfriend?—who lives in outer Brooklyn. She's the call I take first, make plans to meet her for a date, maybe go dancing.

When I finally reach Sebastien the news isn't great. But it's also not clear how bad it may be. It seems that somehow, after years of being more chaste and sexually careful than any sane gay man, Sebastien has the pox. *What* pox is the million-dollar question. It all began as a skin infection that the doctor thinks is shingles, the latter an infection that affects men over sixty-five but rarely someone in their thirties, unless it's related to HIV. The doctor isn't 100 percent sure, but he's warned Sebastien of the risk.

No one mentions the pox by name, or the threat—AIDS, or death—the subject clearly on our minds. But it doesn't matter. The possibility spells disaster for Sebastien and his family, an explosion that's hit like an implosion.

But it's not the worst news in the world to me. Because death is no longer a given with HIV; it may never lead to AIDS or even illness. We now have protease inhibitors. Taken early enough, they can slow the virus and, the hope is, maybe even eradicate it inside dormant cells. The prognosis is longer life, not death. The worst, I explain, would be Sebastien not getting access to the newest HIV drugs immediately, especially if he's seroconverting, is in the earliest stages postexposure.

I project another reel of the future for Sebastien. The best outcome: survival, restored health, a long life. But not death. If Sebastien was exposed to HIV, I stress, he'll be among the lucky ones. He's landed on the right side of the history in this epidemic. *You'll be all right,* I tell him. *If you have it. You have to trust me.*

None of this lessens the impact on his acute fear and anxiety. It's all too new to him, and terrifying.

Tell me what to do, he asks again. *You've studied this disease. You know the science. If you were me, what would you do?*

Sleep on it, I suggest. *Seriously. Get some rest. You're exhausting yourself. You still don't have a test result. But if you have it, you're going to be fine,* I stress, meaning it. *Trust me.*

Really?

Really. You're not going to die. Not anytime soon. I mean, maybe from eating mayonnaise or drinking, yes, maybe you could die earlier.

And, for the first time in the tense hours since the news, I can sense him relax, at least a little.

We talk about what I've learned: what's behind the media message of hope, the clinical trial results I know about that haven't yet been reported much outside HIV journals, how the new protease drugs actually work, the synergy with older drugs like AZT. He takes it all in like a drug itself—a dose of hope, of life—directly into his veins, into his heart. Until at last he says, *I'm really tired. I'm going to go. I think I can sleep now.*

⌒

As Sebastien sleeps, far away, in another city, I stay awake, late. While he tries to rest, I become a machine, energy in motion, wasting no action. I know time is of the essence, if he's actually been exposed to HIV and seroconverting.

There's a small window to act, quickly, to try to slow the virus at the gate, to reset its pace. He'll need a test for the actual virus, not just an antibody test. It's past midnight; I've placed calls to colleagues around the world, to experts carrying out clinical trials with protease drugs. I want their opinions: what are the options; what's the best first combination?

All of this is familiar to me, the rush to unearth hope. I've done it for Johnny, for Kiki, for other friends, always with the same urgency. All of us have, the activists and journalists, armed with information that could help. What's different now, what's been missing from the past decade, is my internal feeling of certainty. This time, we have something that works. Sebastien's going to make it, *if* he's got HIV.

The big factor is time. As always. If he's newly exposed, the virus is multiplying millions of copies of itself hour by hour. The sooner he starts treatment, the greater his chance of resetting the clock on the disease. Or, so goes the theory. I'm not completely convinced by all the details of the emerging science of early treatment, one involving a protease plus two non-nukes (non-nucleoside inhibitors, a different drug class from AZT, a nuke), but I think it would be the smartest of his choices on the table. But the new protease drugs also cause serious side effects, because they are potent like chemo. That could immediately and seriously limit Sebastien's quality of life. If he starts, he'll have to take drugs from now on, every day, on a set schedule. Forever, or until we know more, or have a cure or other drugs to work better. That is a very bitter pill to swallow, especially overnight.

Still, he's being offered a chance, a rare lucky one compared to millions of people who can't get these new drugs. He can try to blunt the impact of the virus by starting treatment early, or do nothing and wait. He won't get sick— it takes years to develop AIDS, at least a decade usually. By then our understanding of HIV and AIDS will be so much greater, and we'll likely have new drugs. Waiting is a real option. I would probably wait. But by then, his immune system would also be weaker too, his ability to stay healthy compromised by years of living with a quiescent or slowly reproducing viral infection.

Sebastien has made it clear to me he's too anxious, too terrified by the very idea of AIDS, to do nothing, to simply wait and see. If he's got it, he wants action. He wants the weapon now. Of course, it'll be his decision, not mine. His life, his body. I'm a laymen's expert. But I'm not the one who will have to swallow that bitter pill for life. I'm going to suggest he see a counselor as well as his doctor. Living with HIV is a journey unto itself. It's not one to enter lightly.

By morning, I have the information I need for him: the very latest results from all the recent and ongoing trials. I've reviewed them with some of the best

minds I know. It's not me, so I can't say what I'd do for myself. But knowing
how he feels, what he wants, I would probably suggest he start now. *The sooner
the better.* Knowing his life as he's known it will change forever. Knowing it will
change the second he gets that positive test result.

   Get a confirmatory test, I tell him. *As soon as you can. Then talk to your doctor. You'll
need one who knows about these new drugs.* I tell him everything I know. There are no
guarantees. *We're talking about therapy for life. You have to be ready. And you don't have to
do this now; you could wait and see.*

   These drugs are still very new and hard on the body, like cancer drugs. But
they work. They do. So he'll have to decide. *First, let's get that test done.* Then I
can talk to him again. Still, bottom line, he's gonna be okay.

   After we hang up, much later, I begin to say my prayers for Sebastien, for
the test, and, pending its result, for the possible long road ahead.

~ 73

My life intersects with fate and with my creative instincts. In my search for Sel's
story, I've researched the history of syphilis. Now, it turns out that Sebastien
has Columbus's pox—not shingles, which are an indicator for HIV in younger
men. Syphilis is a less scary infection, and one that leaves open a possibility that
HIV isn't involved in his skin infection at all. But he's not out of the HIV woods
yet. He still needs that other test result.

   On the phone again, I ask him a set of routine questions like the doctor I
will never be. Do you have the bumps on your palms? *Yes.* On the soles of your
feet? *No.* Are they hard? *Yes.*

   From this I deduce he was exposed recently, maybe ten to twelve weeks
ago. He had sex with a man and the condom broke. It was his only risky contact
in years.

   Life is a spin of the wheel, a game of chance and sometimes misfortune.
Sebastien is starting to spin out in his anxiety. He needs help. *I'll come down and
see you soon,* I say. *I need a break anyway.* Keeping it light, as if I'm just wanting a
weekend vacation. I'll be a good friend. I can feel his relief over the phone. He
wants someone else to handle his life right now. His own is too scary.

~ 74

Sebastien picks me up in his new car, chewing his lip, clearly worried, but
relieved that I've come to help him. The news, in the end, is what we feared.
He's been exposed to HIV. By now, the initial shock has worn off, days have
gone by, and he's more able to deal with the information. He's made an initial

appointment to see his doctor, and I'm riding shotgun, staying for a few more days to help him weigh the hard decisions.

Before we've left the airport curb, he's peppered me with questions, the most important one being: *What should I do now if I want to start? Enroll in a clinical trial?* I answer his questions one by one, trying to relax him, fiddling with the radio. *No, no clinical trials. Just focus on staying healthy, on reducing your stress. That's number one.*

From this moment on, the rhythm of our days is fixed. Questions, plans, explanations. By the time we meet his doctor, Sebastien is on his way toward mastering his fear. Knowledge is a God in the age of information, as ACT UP knows well. I can feel it lifting him, new terms and questions filling in the expanding hole created by HIV and the uncertainty of life. His skin looks bad, but not as bad as he described. And by the end of day one, he's making awful jokes at his own expense, happy to have someone with him to appreciate them.

I test the waters with my own joke. *You're lucky you didn't get crabs too, you know. Lie with dogs, get fleas. Where'd you pick up your sailor boy, anyway?*

He doesn't quite laugh but rolls his eyes. I see he can take the joke. Gallows humor will be the way he manages this disease. It's what's helping everybody else, including me.

⁓

There's the time of dreaming and the time of writing, and the time between the two, when I wake from a nap, remains my favorite time. Slow, sensuous, fluid. I've been cat-napping all day on Sebastien's bed, in between phone calls to doctors, dropping into a heavy sleep that leaves a drool mark on the pillow and long creases down my left cheek. It's the exhaustion of an emotion that I don't feel during the day, of a current that pulls me under so quickly that I have to struggle to get up again. But I do. The phone rings, Sebastien hands it to me, and I'm all business, precise and urgent, racing ahead of my tired mouth and eyes and brain to ask the critical questions, to assess this one's opinion.

What would you do? This is not my body, seroconverting, but I have to imagine it could be. *What would I do? What's the very best step forward?*

⁓

Sebastien is utterly concentrated, learning the science as fast as he can. I'm already trying to slow him down, to balance his new singular focus on AIDS and survival with downtime, wishing he would stop reading and rereading HIV literature that's out of date, or reports that don't contain messages of hope. But I'm not overinterfering. He has his own journey to make; he has to live with this new reality, not me. I can help him now, but I can't be him. It's a critical distinction.

There's no subject that's taboo, including his acute fear of dying and getting sick. He knows rationally that it's not in the cards, at least not death and not AIDS. But he needs to talk about it, about what feels like a small death anyway. The fear he now has of telling his family, his friends. His need to hide it at work. His awareness of the stigma and discrimination. More than anything, his loss: the loss of his life before this time, when he didn't have to think about any of this, to be afraid, to worry about exposing others. How is he going to live? It's a new world. He hasn't been part of the AIDS movement like I have, doesn't know any activists in his area, has never been to an ACT UP meeting. He's not even ready to join a support group for newly infected individuals, something his doctor suggested. He just wants to do what he's doing: reading a lot, asking for explanations. He's soothed by the knowledge, and the balm of my confidence. He's been able to sleep, finally.

Right now, he's also very healthy aside from his skin thing, and he's dealing well, I remind him. He's doing more than fine, all things considered.

Throughout all this, I feel the edge of sadness for this unwanted event, this tough new chapter. But I give my sadness little room. That will be for later, when I'm back in New York by myself. Right now Sebastien needs my best, my brightest, my most optimistic self.

⁓

A month has gone by. Time for a quick update: six weeks since Sebastien got the news and he's now undetectable for HIV after two weeks on his protease drug cocktail. He's coping well; he's adjusted to his new uncertain sense of life. He's on his way to living with HIV and getting healthier too.

~ 75

FEBRUARY 6, 1997

I'm marking this date because it's like the first day of Smokenders, the day when good intentions crystallize into action, into that small but determined step to willfully change. Lately I've worked quickly, focused intensively, produced a lot. Sel's stories and my own are taking shape. Her own tale, separate from mine in wonderland.

The second priority has been my relationship with Jersey. In the past months, we've cleaned and repainted the loft and worked to incorporate our separated lives and relationships more fluidly. That means we fight less and that the issue of having other lovers has become a more acceptable reality. We're looking at what we have together as something akin to family. Occasionally I still miss having sex. It feels like a void, small and muted, but the hurt is still there, a pang that reminds me of the joy we first knew, that coming together. I miss the soul-sharing union we had and wonder what will replace it. If anything will. But I certainly don't miss the conflicts and the pain. I'm happy to be out of that cycle at last. It's good—very good—to finally hit this place. I'm testing myself.

Number three? Well, that's a big one; a really new source of happiness. In the midst of the tough news about Sebastien, I recently met someone new, and I'm so excited about her, about us. Bridget. An artist and someone with whom I really feel a deep connection. A sensitive soul. A tender button.

~ 76

Bridget. What can I say about her? She's a bit saucy, sweet, and vulnerable, and I like what I've seen of her art. She lives in San Francisco but was visiting New York when we met. She's applied to go to graduate school here, which is exciting. Right now, she's back in San Francisco but we plan to meet soon. Before I was seeing Jessie—sweet younger Jessie—but that's now moving into a friendship because, well, because it needs to. We're just not well matched—the age difference, for one thing. But also, Bridget. I'm smitten.

All of this is also taking place without any lying or covert activity, and with a great deal of conversation and clarity. I even made out with a boy recently and it was fine. Not that exciting, but fine. And not weird. Now that I'm technically single, I can have my little fun. But the truth is, I'm falling for Bridget. I feel it. I want to be with her. And I think she feels the same way.

I feel like I'm in a *Cosmo* magazine moment: *if it feels good, do it,* as long as you're careful, as long as you take responsibility for yourself, as long as you honor your commitments and aren't self-destructive or harmful to others. Personal freedom is finally a concept that feels a bit more real to me, that has some muscle, that I can wrestle with—it's not such an abstract notion. I've never felt freer from the judgments of others. And love. What an amazing feeling. That great, exuberant joy of connecting with someone else. It just feels so good.

I turn thirty-nine in two weeks—a little frightening, since I'm vain about aging and want my life to last a long time. But I am trying to live by Papou's philosophy: I am having fun, amid the many wars.

I'd be remiss if I neglected to write down here what's happened with Jersey's health. She's been diagnosed with precancer of the cervix and had three biopsies taken this week. I saw her cervix before and after the operation. Before, it was a pinkish-white oval, egg-shaped. After, it looked like a cigar has been stubbed into it: ashy spots, almost gangrenous due to a coating of something liquid that was nitrous or ferrous—had nitrogen or iron in it—that was put on her cervix to stop the bleeding. This information went right into my brain and into Sel's. I know I'll use it.

What does it mean for me? I've had a new Pap smear done and I'm waiting for the results. But even before she heard about her own condition, I was in the process of researching breast cancer, deciding it's high time I faced the demon of my own fatalism about inheriting my mother's disease. I'm going to pursue a path of prevention. I'm going to enter a clinical trial; somehow get myself tested for the mutated BRCA1 gene and, if I have it, figure out what I should be doing.

Life is serendipity, I keep telling everyone I know; everything is coming together. I've spent more than ten years reporting about AIDS so that now I can help Sebastien. I'll spend the next weeks and months doing the same with cancer and it will help—if not me or Jersey, then someone who needs it. There's a popular modern term for this feeling: *flow.* I am flow. I am the awareness of flow. I am being borne along, creating the next moment. I'm feeling some De Quincey-high flow. This is the essence of life.

~ 77

Here we are, a month later, and so much has happened, even in the past week. I feel like I'm living extra-intensely. The biggest news first, then: I'm happy. Really happy and excited. I've also learned from the last years. I want to slow down time with Bridget, to let it match the feeling of deep expansion that comes with new love. I'm not lost in love this time, though I'm enjoying as much romantic fever as I can. I'm not so wide-eyed I don't see that this woman, like me, is just a woman—human, flawed, not an apparition.

Yet she's amazing in a way I can appreciate. I'm truly excited and interested in who she is, in her raw edges, in what's not always so nice. She's complex and very smart and creative and it's a relief, a profound relief at times, to have met her. I've been waiting for someone like her, for someone who I can talk to in a way I can with her, someone who isn't afraid to open up and isn't afraid to want more, to ask if more is available. She's really intense, but then, all my lovers have been intense. Because I'm intense too, though I'd like to think I'm easy-breezy. In a very short time, we've gone very deep.

I'm also pleased by what's happening in my relationship with Jersey—the transition to friendship that we're attempting. Ours is a bond that's been tested by the betrayals. But we're on the other side now and I'm building something with her that I have with M: a real feeling of family. It's not a lover's bond anymore, but it's still really big and close. I'm happy we've made it this far.

I'm loved, then; I'm loving as many people as I can in many different kinds of relationships. That applies to myself too. I've put self-care and self-love higher on my to-do list. *Gotta keep my own soul shining.*

XII

New York

~ 78

Long Island. There's an edge of heat to the dawn. Somehow, another summer has arrived. Time is elastic, bending itself out of shape. I've been attending to personal relationships, doing medical research, launching and writing an HIV supplement for *Out*, traveling to Haiti, taking a cross-country trip through the southern United States . . . in short, life. A busy life that competes with writing but complements it.

Meanwhile, the political landscape in France is radically transforming. The postmodern fascists are moving more quickly than I have. I can no longer attempt to be a Cassandra or use my book to warn about their arrival. They are here; their movement is more popular than ever. They have outpaced me as a writer. But the day is not yet done.

What's been happening in France, then? With one of my subjects, the modern wolves? Here's a quick summary: since I started this writing in 1992, Chirac graduated from being mayor of Paris to becoming prime minister and the strong head of a conservative coalition government. Beyond the infected blood scandal, he's also been embroiled in personal scandals after members of his government were found to be living in fancy apartments and paying extra-cheap rents—the benefits of patronage.

Meanwhile, ex-president Mitterrand, friend to ex-Vichyites, also continues to enjoy his share of *scandale*. He died not long ago—in January 1996—and has been posthumously exposed as a polygamist of sorts. Turns out he was a married man with a longtime mistress and an illegitimate daughter, and divided his time between the two families. He lived with one during the week; the other on weekends. That trumps the worst of my lesbian drama and complex family making, *définitivement*.

Mitterrand also managed to dupe the country about his health, hiding the fact that he had been living with prostate cancer for fifteen years before it finally killed him. He chose the same final course of action that Kiki did—to stop his cancer drugs—and quickly died. But the questions about Mitterrand's early life and long friendships with the men of Vichy like René Bousquet continue to invite public scrutiny and condemnation. In hindsight, he looks less and less an innocent man. *Au contraire.*

What I find interesting is how it was so easy for Mitterrand to escape public scrutiny for so long. Enough people in high places certainly knew about *l'affaire Mazarine*—his illegitimate daughter, Mazarine Pingeot—and that her mother wasn't a mere mistress but more of a second wife. But they preferred to look away, to allow their leader this privacy. Even the media. A separation of the man and his political office. It's a cultural thing, goes the argument. *Really?* Is it the same cultural habit of looking away that impacts the unsolved Greenpeace boat bombing affair?

Let's go back to Bousquet, rich friend of Mitterand and ally of Le Pen. What about the unresolved accusations of the murder of dozens—maybe up to two hundred—Algerians by Papon when he was head of the police in Paris? Why hasn't anyone faced a courtroom? What about the nighttime raids that continue on new immigrants with legitimate papers but no lawyers they can call on the spot, no ability to make their case to an antiterrorist policeman who sees a link to a Muslim terrorist? It's not scandalous, this lack of interest; it's criminal. Two hundred Algerians, swept into the Seine in 1964. Doesn't that qualify as a mass murder? *Où est la justice?* Not here, not present.

Economically, France remains in major crisis. The wave of labor strikes that started two years ago have shaken the public confidence in Chirac's leadership. This culminated in the *opération escargot*, or snail strike, that took place while I was last in Paris, in which convoys of trucks laden with products moved at a snail's pace through the main arteries of France. A protest against Chirac's economic policies and against unemployment. An unhappiness that deepened as the country more fiercely debated the benefits of membership in a greater European union at a time when the French franc is weak.

All of this may read as faraway politics if you're a reader outside Europe, but these are political flashpoints in France, and for Europe, where the recent combination of a weak conservative government and high unemployment has set the stage for further advances by the Far Right and the National Front. This past spring, underestimating the nation's dissatisfaction with his leadership, Chirac called an early election, convinced of his party's victory. Instead, Prime Minister Jospin's coalition of Socialists, Communists, and Greens did surprisingly well in the initial round. I've heard all about Jospin and his potential failings from Philippe, who's happy Chirac is out but worried Jospin will disappoint too.

Interestingly (*well, disturbingly*), Le Pen is given credit for this surprise turn of events. Last year, his National Front split from the moderate-conservatives and left the Right splintered and internally feuding. The National Front has won over 15 percent of the seats in one hundred smaller departmental assemblies. A bit better than last year. They are gaining ground. Where did the new votes come from? From eastern France, from the colder Alsace and Lorraine regions close to Germany. Yes, I'm inferring a connection—that these areas may be riper for Le Pen's message than other areas because of their geographic history. As for Paris, the cosmopolitan heart of France, it remains less vulnerable to the xenophobic tide than I feared. The Front didn't score big there.

Clearly, Le Pen's proving to be more shrewd and daring than other politicians, an attractive and dangerous combination. A clever man with a sense of history. He would rather lose now and lure more conservatives to his extremist brand of nativist populism than dilute his politics. He's in this for the long haul. His daughters, notably Marine, continue to be groomed to rise in the party ranks and one day inherit the mantle.

I would be remiss if I failed to report that Le Pen's new popularity has finally scared French progressives into panicky action. They recently held a few huge antifascist demonstrations, mostly in Paris. But now, with the Socialist victory, I wonder if the scared citizens will feel lulled again into complacency? Possibly. Probably. Which is unfortunate, because Le Pen's party is more powerful now than before. The conservatives are hurting and need Le Pen's supporters, so they'll be ready to compromise. So may the Socialists, who owe Le Pen their victory. It's scary to think that the fragmented Socialist party, which did little to stop Le Pen until now, is charged with leading the antifascist fight.

~ 79

Though it is somewhat tangential to my story here, I'm keeping my eye on the continuing Nazi Swiss money scandal. In these past months, the Swiss government has begun to return to families millions of dollars stolen from German Jews and hidden for fifty years in Swiss banks. It's reopened old wounds left by the war. A bit of history that has bitten the Swiss in their polite neutral butts and sent officials there muttering in shame and public embarrassment. An admission, after initial denials, of grand theft; of major complicity. And now we see the Swiss Far Right fighting back, questioning the whole affair. They're led by a nationalistic businessman who thinks the Swiss are being bullied by a Jewish cabal. Another man who's gained instant popularity for saying the unthinkable, for defying the government. Another strongman to watch out for.

This is a bare outline, one that leaves out the important events unfolding in Eastern Europe, particularly in Bosnia, where the perpetrators of genocide are

on the run but still popular among their supporters. As I write, Radovan
Karadžić is hiding out in a bunker while NATO finally acts to arrest him and
deliver him to the international war crimes tribunal at The Hague. I feel deep
satisfaction reading that Karadžić's face is being plastered on wanted posters
all over the shattered villages of former Yugoslavia. A little bit of collective action;
un petit brin de justice. A crumb.

⌒

A few days ago, my father called to tell me that he's worried about my older
brother's second child, still unborn, whose head seems to be too big, so my father
reports; a grandson he fears could be mentally impacted. A child with bad
genes is the implication. A baby whom I'm now praying for, in a secular sense,
meaning I'm sending him good psychic vibes. A being I feel for because it is
extravulnerable and may die.

   During our conversation, Papa tells me that he was similarly worried about
my sister because she was a blue baby for seven minutes and, look, she developed
schizophrenia as a young adult. I remind him that all my life he said this about
me — *that I was the blue baby!* It even became part of my personal mythology,
something I referenced as the possible source of later poor short-term memory
(*not enough oxygen, maybe?*). But Papa insists I'm mistaken: *You were not a blue baby;
you were the one I thought was mongoloid because your eyes stuck out like a little frog,* my
father clarifies. *It's true you didn't breathe right away, but you didn't turn blue. You had
other . . . problems.*

   Oh?

   *You were hyperactive. You rocked yourself back and forth. You always wanted your
mother to hold you and she didn't; I think that's contributed to — you know . . .*

   To what? My sapphic side?

   It's amazing how far my father continues to search for someone or something to blame for what he regards as my skewed gender identity, for my early
preference for *pantalons* and not *robes.*

   When I report all this to Bridget, she's sympathetic about my future nephew
but warns me that mongoloid is considered a racist term. Sigh. Should I bother
to inform Papa? Once, I was a blue baby, not quite ready to breathe. Now, I
look back and discover yet another crack in my personal history. Not exotic
bleu, just a little froggy tomboy, with jutting eyes that prompted other children
to taunt me, endlessly. *Frog face!*

   For now, I'll pray for this water-on-the-brain boy, this little nephew of
mine, send him my strength and life force, my belief in universal energies, in
hope, enough to counter my father's negative projections.

   Meantime, I just got a clue about Henri. Born a blue baby? *Très possible.*

~ 80

JULY 27

Mattituck, Long Island. It's early in the morning on the North Fork, a lovely spot. Since June, I've been sharing a summer house with friends, including Jersey. A bunch of close friends who all party too much, like me. We're going to try to be more healthy here, though that's going to be hard. There are some great dive bars around, hard to resist with this bunch. At least I'll swim in the ocean twice a day.

This is the place where I hope to finish a draft of Sel's story. Everyone else is working on their creative projects so that helps. I've started writing her story, finally, but mostly I have a lot of scenes. The central narrative—her mission— is still evolving. She's going to go after the wolves, yes. But many details remain— what would De Quincey say?—in a state of creative distillation. I've just had too much magazine work; too few stolen weekends. And now it's almost August. Still, I've started writing again and I wake before everyone else, already typing in my head, hearing a stream of conversation before I'm even out of bed.

I'm going to share a little about my posse. They're outside on the porch now, drinking and talking shop. They're such a talented group—as individuals but also as collaborators. We've had a rotation of friends out here on the weekends and I've enjoyed hearing them talk about their projects. They're all even more obsessed than I am, I think; it's just 24/7 immersion in the worlds they're creating, their scripts mostly. Rose Troche is working on a new film; she made *Go Fish*, which is a cult lezzie comedy movie now for young lesbians. She made it with Guin Turner, who isn't here now but probably will be; she and Rose used to be lovers.

My good friend Alison Kelly, who's a DP—she sets up the camera on big film shoots—is here too, taking photos and talking shop with Rose. Then we have Kim Peirce, who's writing a fiction film based on Brandon Teena, a transgender guy who was murdered. She's working on the script with Laurie Weeks, who is about the funniest, edgiest writer and wild girl I know. She makes my partying look very tame by comparison. I'm not saying it's healthy but she's really an amazing person, just hilarious.

Then there's Lisa Cholodenko, who's also a director who's writing a feature film, and her girlfriend, Cheryl Perry, who's a great chef. So we're eating well and drinking and partying like fish. I almost forgot: there's also Robin Vachal, who's an independent film programmer. Then there's me and Jersey, and also my good friend Marisa, from Mapplethorpe. She's been putting together some great shows of his work for the foundation. Lastly, my pal Sarah

Pettit, who is my erstwhile boss at *Out*, who was supposed to come with Amy Steiner, who also is the photo editor at *Out* and very talented too. Sarah's hoping to get some writing done; she's a good poet, though she hardly shows it to anyone. So that's our crowd. I may have forgotten others who were here before I got here.

I'm writing about us—my crowd—because I had that same feeling again earlier this afternoon that I had at the Fela party in 1982, and that I get at Wigstock, or when I'm at the protests. A feeling of being in a moment that is making history, not living outside it. I've felt that with several political groups I've worked with, and certainly felt it as someone reporting on AIDS in the early eighties, at the *New York Native*. It's not that I or my friends are so special, but we're living in a unique cultural, social, and political moment. We're part of a particular generation of LGBT culture makers and feminist activists and the way we're living and trying to love, and make family, and play, and make work is all part of that feeling I get, that we're in a moment, a specific zeitgeist queer cultural moment.

I was just watching everyone outside, playing badminton and drinking gin and tonics, and flirting and listening to Rose and Lisa and Kim argue about how to direct straight actors in a gay sex scene (which everyone has a lot of opinions about), and I just felt: *Hey, look at this; this is my life, these are my friends. Let me freeze this moment and not forget it. We're part of a changing gay world. And we're part of what's helping to change it too. Us and a million queers and women. A nineties generation. We're living in a special time. This is a special moment, right here, with my friends. Let me not forget it.*

I'm going to spare you the sordid, juicy details of who is sleeping (or not) with whom; and how many of us can play the six-degrees-of-separation Kevin Bacon game of who slept with whom and how are you connected to them? But I'm noting that here too because it's also part of our subculture and I think it matters. It's a reflection of how we—meaning us lesbians—are trying to live our modern values of both sexual freedom and sisterhood, of being ethical sluts, as we joke. When I look around at my friends and I, and our friend's friends, and their friend's friends, I see the waves of six degrees rippling out. We're all very connected, us lesbians in America, and in the larger gay world in the nineties. We're the fruit of a lot of people who fought for the rights and lives we're living now. So I'm writing it down here, as I feel it tonight.

~ 81

The other night, instead of drinking cocktails or renting a video, our little group caught a cable program on the Nazi Swiss gold scandal. I felt myself getting all worked up again—excited and a little desperate—the way I get when I feel something is important and I want to be a part of it. I immediately fantasized about quitting my day job at the magazine to volunteer as an investigative reporter with one of the three teams searching for the Swiss Nazi-era assets. It took me back to the Duvalier fortune-hunting days.

As I watched the old newsreels of the Nazis and the Nuremberg trial, I also felt a little panic, as if (this is a familiar feeling) I was missing the more important life I could or should lead: working as a court reporter at The Hague, or tracking down the Serbian killers. On this issue, I was watching the important drama on television, a historical couch potato.

Of course, it's partly about my ego, how I'm often drawn to events and work that feel larger than life, that give my life some greater sense of purpose. I have to admit that's in there, somewhere. There's also a current of historical guilt, surely a small-*c* Catholic imprint, some of it stemming from other obvious sources, like my family background—my inherited mix of former European aristo-cum-Haitian *blans*, ex-colonials with stripes of color in their blood and a dubious family notion of noblesse oblige. Even if I was raised in America, I picked this up from my parents: a sense of social duty; to be of service to others. That doesn't fully explain my personal passion for seeing justice done with a capital *J*; for historical redress in cases of genocide. I'm just offering a few ideas.

Anyway, as I watched the Swiss gold program and listened to details of how the Germans melted dental fillings from murdered Jews into gold bars then sent them over the border to Switzerland, I kept thinking about my mother's mother, Grand-mère la Comtesse, who revered the pope.

Here's the recap: After she remarried her rich count husband, they settled in Menaggio, a village bordering alpine Lake Como in northern Italy, one of the most beautiful places in the world. Rome and Il Papa were nearby; so was Switzerland, land of stability and safety for the money of the Euro-rich. I spent many end-of-summers in Menaggio as a young girl. It was gorgeous. In the summer, huge lightning storms would come rolling quickly across the *lago*, spectacular and scary.

My grandmother taught me to watch the sky carefully for the first signs of a storm. But she read the sky for a different reason, like a reader of tea leaves. She was very superstitious and considered a coming storm an apt metaphor for Italy's unstable political climate. When she heard the first rumblings, even if the sky was clear on our side of the *lago*, she'd check the radio for news. More than once, after the storms had died down, she would quickly dress and force her husband, Count Dedy, as we called him, to navigate the narrow cobbled roads in their tiny Mini Cooper *vite, vite!* to withdraw her valuables from a safe-deposit box. Then, in a matter of hours, they would be driving through the long, dark tunnels toward Geneva or Lausanne—savings passbook, cash, and important jewels tucked under the seat—to redeposit their money into a safer Swiss account.

When I accompanied her a few times, she would tell me what the pope had said that day. Her real papa. She organized her day around his schedule. Every day, she woke at five to listen to the Mass from Rome, then again after her lunchtime nap. The pope reassured her. Like the Swiss. They weren't crazy, like the Italians who couldn't rule themselves. The Swiss currency was stable, just as they were, not impulsive and superstitious like she was, passionate like an Italian yet a bit mistrusting like a stereotypical French aristo. A complex creature, my grandmother. Anyone like the pope, who could make her sleep well at night, deserved her devotion.

She's dead now, a year after I saw her for the last time, shrunken and nearly bald and very much two feet in the grave, breathing only with difficulty in her bed in a nursing home in France—a splendid nursing home; one that provided her with doting attendants. She was already a bit senile and looked miserable as ever and even more fearful; alone, it seemed, with her demons and the pope. She did recognize me for an instant, though, and I saw the gleam of her old sharp spirit and a smile that reminded me of her face—flush with a gambler's instinct for victory—as she surveyed the passing storm over Lake Como and predicted Italy's political future and her own.

What would she think now, if she were alive, seeing how very unneutral the Swiss were and remain—how very complicit? Would she click her tongue in disapproval like my mother also did when something vexed or excited her, or give a quick, dismissive French *enfin* shake of her shoulders? What would she think of her beloved pope and the Vatican, if she knew that more evidence has emerged about the Italian church's role in sending Jews away? Or how much Italian money flew into Swiss banks then. It's an ongoing investigation, but I won't be surprised by future discoveries.

Here's what I would say to her, my pope-loving Grand-mère la Comtesse: your famous Swiss banks were the financial *engines* of Nazi Germany. An amazing, but not overstated, charge, it seems, based on the documentary I just saw. Avarice, greed—*not neutrality*—were the motivating factors behind their actions. And anti-Semitism. Let's not forget that. There's been nothing neutral about the decision of Swiss leaders to help the Nazis before and after the war, nor about their longtime effort to conceal this sordid past and hold onto the loot, and, most recently, to shred the documents that prove all this. It's all taken a consistent and organized effort. And your beloved pope, well . . . the Vatican's deeply implicated. *What do you think, Grand-mère? Hein?* Your popes and the Vatican have a lot of Italian and French Jewish blood on their hands. What do you think about all that?

~ 82

JULY 28

Another week gone by. Since my moral spasm of excitement over the Nazi gold, I've sobered up. I can't track stolen Swiss gold, do my daytime job to track AIDS treatment, and look more deeply into what Monsieur Le Pen and his fascist friends are up to this week in France. Never mind follow what's still unfolding in Rwanda and the Balkans, our modern genocides. I don't know how I'll resolve this problem, morally speaking. I'd like to do it all of course. I'm putting this new temptation on hold until the end of the summer. There will be enough to do if I ever get to The Hague, that's certain.

Now I've actually written an outline of narrative action for Sel and her good friends, as she calls her crew. The key scenes and a possible ending. The whole thing sketched out within minutes, longhand, in a Chinese elementary school writing tablet with a pretty, yellow cover. And I've assigned myself a small but critical role in the whole affair: as a scribe, naturally. *La journaliste.* Why didn't I see that immediately? It was so obvious, no?

~ 83

AUGUST 15

Ever since I got back from Haiti in March, I've been sick. Again. Suffering from what I assume are parasites. An old pox, new, mutated? Always so many possibilities. Main symptoms: gastrointestinal problems, transient headaches, brief night fevers, and, now, more consistently, mild arthritis in my fingers and a stiff neck that, like my headaches, begin mid- or late afternoon and make it hard to turn my neck in the morning. These symptoms last for a day or two, then go away, although I've had lousy bowels the entire time.

Since Jersey and a friend of ours traveled to Haiti with me not long ago, we've been comparing notes. They got sick in Haiti too—a version of turista—and Jersey is still feeling lousy, with a poor appetite and minor digestive problems. But no intense joint pains or headaches. I keep wondering if I have an entirely new pox, or a reactivated chronic infection of the blasto bug, since Jersey's test came up positive for that. Or whatever creature invaded my system post-Belize last year—a mystery pox no doctor was ever able to diagnosis, only treat by throwing various antibiotics at the symptoms, hoping one would stick.

There's a crazy little story to recount about Belize and why I got sick. Why I'm still sick, and it's a sort of come-and-go malady. My go-to doc pal Joe Sonnabend is pretty sure, based on some matching protein bands, that I was exposed to some viral cousin of dengue, some tropical creature not yet seen here in the United States, or not often enough. That's why we don't have a specific diagnostic test that will pick it up. He thought maybe I had breathed it in from the dust of rat bats in the eaves of an old house we rented in Hopkins, a Garifuna seaside village. The house had been empty for years. They were happy to rent it to my friend Pascale Willi, who had found the place for us. It was cheap and had a lot of rooms and a hole in the ceiling of the bedroom where I set up my writing desk.

I had never heard of rat bats, but they are native to Belize and rather scary as hell. They aren't that small, for starters, and they're vampire creatures. Mostly they attack cattle, but any hot-blooded mammal will do just fine. As I sat, calmly having my morning coffee in Belize, imagining scenes of battle for Sel and her clan, the rat bats of Hopkins were probably keeping their eye on me, readying their attack too. I would hear rustling in the walls but thought it was just mice. Island mice; no big deal. Luckily, we discovered the rat bats one day when two little girls from the village were visiting me, and they shrieked, pointing to a tail hanging from the ceiling where I had put a piece of cloth over a hole. I saw the bat spread its wings like in a B horror movie, and the rest is a total blur of their screaming and my yelling and us running and the whole village soon rushing to the house to help.

In short order, we smoked the bats out. The village was familiar with them, eventually teased us, a bunch of foreign white women from New York with short hair who were so afraid of some bats. We hired some local young men to stand on ladders by holes they made in the upper outside wall of the house and watched as the rat bats slowly emerged, driven out by the smoke. They efficiently chopped off the rat bats' heads with machetes in a glorious, disgusting, medieval scene of battle so bloody I couldn't quite believe it. It trumped whatever battle I was creating in my head for Sel. A slaughter.

All this happened; it's a real, bloody, wild, gory story. Those village boys killed dozens of vampire rat bats emerging from holes in the house where we had been living for a month, and it was amazing. Blew our minds. But neither I nor Jersey saw the whole thing because we ran away, horrified and disgusted and freaked out that the rat bats had been watching me for weeks like their next victim. I think Suzanne Wright, one of our posse, did stay. She still reminds me about it: *Remember those rat bats? Remember how crazy Belize was?*

How can I forget? It left me with a mysterious illness. What I've learned since then is that bat shit is a glorious world for a pox. Viruses, bacteria, molds . . . they thrive in it. I've researched it; the theory is possible. *Dengue, Joe? Really? Jeez.* I gradually got better, but maybe that was my body just healing itself.

That's Joe's theory. That's what poxes can do too, he says. The body fights
them and eventually, it's like détente.

⌁

I keep freaking out, now, secretly and for hours, despite my faith in medical
science. I hope it's not the return of my mystery pox. Part of the problem is that
I don't know a good specialist in tropical medicine. I've approached this new
crisis like an AIDS activist, with a surfeit of knowledge about parasites, but a
lousy HMO insurance policy. This time Joe has quickly ruled out the most
common bugs and any sexually transmitted diseases. He's advised me to take
Flagyl for a possible parasite anyway, since Jersey had that in Haiti, and the
drug is such a poison, so toxic, it kills almost anything that may lurk in the gut.
Not dengue, but a lot of the nastier bugs.

   I really like Joe. He's been very good to me and hardly charges me any
money for his advice and blood tests. He has a great reputation as an HIV
clinician with unorthodox approaches to treating unusual problems, which
pretty much defines the seemingly endless range of problems caused by HIV.
He learned his craft treating patients in rural southern Africa. He even makes
house calls, which is almost unheard of in this day and age. He's just that kind
of nice guy, plus he has a social side and enjoys a glass of wine to decompress at
the end of his day. I know I'm a minor case of mystery disease compared to his
daily caseload of dying gay men. You go into his office and it's like stepping
back into 1985: so many young guys.

   Joe's been very responsive as always, calling me back soon after I've phoned
and going out of his way to follow up. Besides, I rarely ask for help: only every
few years and then usually I have weird things wrong with me that give him a
break from HIV. I don't want him to think I'm a hypochondriac either. So I
agreed to the Flagyl, a drug I hate to take.

   Ouch! On day ten, I had all but two of the possible side effects to Flagyl,
including swollen, itchy eyes; a metal taste in my tongue; nausea; a migraine;
and a case of vertigo so bad I had trouble walking from my office door to the
bathroom at work. I'm so damn sensitive to drugs, it's a problem. By doing some
detective work, Joe managed to lower my dose and maintain the drug's power.
I finished the course of treatment. But instead of the joint pain getting better,
now it's gotten worse. And it's taken another week to stop feeling nauseous and
having vertigo.

   I don't think the Flagyl did much for this bug. My colon and gut haven't
quite recovered and are now producing similar symptoms to an actual infection.
Joe gave this turn of events a fancy term I've forgotten. It has something to do
with my having become toxic and now needing to detox from the treatment. I

dunno. My other big thought is that I might have Lyme disease. It's all over the newspapers these days, and I visited the east end of Long Island not that long ago. They have deer and deer ticks that carry Lyme.

Joe remains skeptical.

Joe: *Did you get a tick bite?*

Me: *No.*

Joe: *Then why go looking for something like Lyme disease?*

Me: *Because my joints hurt—a lot.*

Joe: *Well, how old are you? Thirty-nine. Maybe you're getting a little arthritis. Do you exercise?*

Wrong, wrong, wrong! I wanted to shout to Joe.

Instead, I've accepted his lack of conviction as wisdom. But I feel neglected and a bit scared. Joe's worried about me too, I know. He likes to solve his medical mysteries.

He thinks the mystery bug from Belize is making a return appearance. *Re-colonization.* Bottom line is he has no solid idea what it could be and no suggestion about where to turn now. Maybe it will go away by itself, he's proposed. It did last time.

Eventually, I remind him. *But I suffered for months!*

Then roll up your sleeve and let's take that blood sample. It can't hurt to do the Lyme test, I suppose. And lupus, he throws out. *Just to rule out the obvious. There's MS too, of course. So many women are getting MS.*

That's the downside of seeing an expert like Joe. He doesn't hold back on his theories either.

I don't have MS, I say tartly.

He smiles. *No, but you are going to be forty. Now relax your arm or I'm going to hurt you.*

~ 84

Surprise, surprise. My Lyme test came up positive this time on the ELISA antibody test—although, it's a not-so-sensitive ELISA test that does yield a lot of false-positives. The lab forgot to do the lupus test. While Jersey and others began panicking about my Lyme results—*is it contagious?*—I did more research and went back to the lab a week later to get a confirmatory Western blot test and the lupus test.

Now it's the end of August. The lupus test was negative and the two confirmatory Western blots came out as *indeterminate* and *negative.* Joe says I had one protein band that was responsive to the Western blot Lyme test. The Centers for Disease Control calls that *negative* so I need to repeat the test in two to four weeks.

I'm back to square one, then. And the afternoon migraines plus stiff neck and joint pain in my fingers are back every day, arriving in the afternoon like the daily monsoon rains in India. What to do? When I recount my saga to my father, the pediatrician, seeking some paternal support, I get the opposite. He's a Western medicine man; his advice is simple: *take some antibiotics.* If it's Lyme disease, I need to treat it before it gets worse.

He adds a familiar barb: *What can I say, Anne? It's your lifestyle.*

What do you mean? I ask. *What does Lyme have to do with my lifestyle?*

Of course, I know exactly what he means, and he knows that I know he's talking about my sexuality, using this as a pretext to once again punish and blame me for my deviation from the conventional social path he wants for me. I play dumb.

Your lifestyle, he repeats, knowing that I'm on to him. *The way you live; your bohemian life.* He tries to skirt it. *You sleep here and there; you stay in poor motels instead of good places. You slept in houses with bats in the roof in Belize. What do you expect?*

I'm impressed by his ability to stay the course, to actually attempt this association. It's quite a stretch.

Papa, I remind him, *you slept in a cheap motel in Belize when you visited me. I don't see the connection. In fact, there really isn't one.*

What I don't say is, *Why must you always attack me when I'm vulnerable, when I'm seeking your help, when I need you to be the parent who will tell me everything is fine, who will let me be a child? Why is this always your response to feeling scared, to feeling unable to help me? Why can't you open your heart? Why can't you just be nice? I feel like shit and I'm scared. I just need you to tell me it's going to be okay, the patient will make it.*

No such luck. *Get some good antibiotics,* he repeats. *Call me in a week.*

———

There is someone who does make me feel there's a reason for all this suffering. I don't have to research in any archive to know how it feels like to have shooting pains in my head or joints, the kind of Pains that the Victorians treated with opium. I can acknowledge the power of an organism that is slowly seeding its way inside me. I do feel the need to surrender to this migraine right now. It's killing me. I know, in other words, just how my muse Sel feels.

My body is sending me a message. It's breaking down, even further, the boundaries that divide internal and external, imagination and reality, health and disease, fiction and memoir, author and character, Sel and myself. I'm feeling so poxed today, and internal Sel, not any real person, is the one who best consoles me. The circle feels complete.

I also have a name for this hybrid literary journey I'm taking. *Biological fiction. A biological historification. A poxed memoir.*

XIII

New York, Round 27

~ 85

OCTOBER 1997

I haven't written enough about Bridget since she arrived last July. When I'm happy, it seems, I don't write in my journal as much. I've told you how the relationship was instantaneous: an immediate, powerful connection. On a creative level, Bridget is the companion I've been waiting for. She's a wonderful artist, one whose vision and expression I truly appreciate. She makes me envious sometimes: I love everything she does. We share an aesthetic sensibility. She seems to enjoy my writing as much as I enjoy her art and that is a rare, wonderful thing. I feel very lucky to have found someone like her after so many years of wanting a creative romantic partner.

On the relationship front, though, things have proven more challenging than I expected. We're in love—there's no question of that in either of our minds: we really adore and appreciate each other. But different needs are fast cropping up and keep knocking us around to the point where we don't know what to do. We did well long distance but, up close, we're clashing a bit.

Here's what I can tell you: the issue is one of timing, I think, more than temperament or personality. So she presents it to me. When Bridget got here in July, she had left behind a tight circle of friends, a home, a satisfying job—in short, security. She felt a sense of family. Here, in New York, she feels uprooted, isolated. She has her best friend living here—they moved here together—but there's a real gap created by this transition to life in New York. She's missing her old friends, her social circle. I'm her girlfriend but can't fill that shoe, even though I'm trying.

On top of that, she's not happy that I share a home with Jersey, even though she's been my ex for almost two years. It's the intimacy that threatens Bridget. Jersey and I really are very close and we have a lot of fun together. There are unexpected challenges. And, in reality, things got complicated too fast with Bridget; things I couldn't predict and certainly couldn't control. For starters, as Bridget and I were moving her here from San Francisco last July, Jersey suddenly started a relationship with Jessie, my previous, still-lingering dalliance. A classic power move. More triangulation, as her therapist calls it. *Super bad boundaries*, says Bridget, and I agree. It's almost embarrassing and I'm very annoyed at Jersey. I hate finding myself in a lesbian soap opera but somehow I have. I swear Jersey is addicted to triangles. And me. I'm in one so what does that say about me? I'm not avoiding them.

The bad tension between Jersey, Jessie, and me has affected Bridget negatively. It's encroached on the private space she hoped for and needed to have with me. Even though I've been up front with her about my relationships, and about being in transition, it's all been a bit too much, too soon. I can't and don't blame Bridget. I wish it were all different: my feelings, her feelings, Jersey's feelings, Jessie's feelings. You make a plan; it doesn't work out. We spend a lot of time at her place, and in truth, we're avoiding my loft a little. I don't like that either.

Bridget supports what she views as my unconventional approach to relationships, my European bohemianism, as she jokes. But she feels like she's gotten the short end of the stick, emotionally. I'm living with an ex who's involved with another ex. It's messy. On top of that I'm uneasy about changing my living situation, and about living with her so soon. I told Bridget I need to move more slowly, to make sure it's good. And that I need this transition time with Jersey. *You don't just leave your family because there are problems; you work them out. I think I can work this out. We're all adults here, aren't we?*

Sure; adults who act like juveniles in Jersey's case. I'm mad at her but also annoyed at myself. Why did I think this could work? Why won't Jersey cooperate and grow up already? Or is it me? Am I really in denial? *Why can't everyone just get along?*

One reason is because Bridget wants to make plans for the future. She's a planner. And why shouldn't she? She wants a full-time partner and the picket fence: sleeping together every night, the prospect of marriage, children—all things that represent personal security and happiness to her. Many couples want that and have it and say it's great. I worry that too few of them keep having sex after a few years and often cheat on each other—things I don't want to do. Especially lesbians. We nest and our sexual lives die. I've seen the corpses on the battlefield of sapphic love. I don't want that. I want a passion that endures. I'm not sure living together too soon is smart.

I've also had my share of being on the wrong end of cheating. I want honesty, commitment, and a relationship in which we follow through with whatever terms we agree to. At least, that's my goal.

Bridget's astro sign is Cancer. It's in her nature to nest, she says; she can't help it. She lost her father when she was young and still feels this loss acutely. She wants a family—her own family—and she wants a future as an artist and a mother. She also wants to be pregnant now or very soon and she would like me to be her partner on this journey, something that makes me feel honored and awed and a little despairing that I can't just say yes immediately—a big fat yes to the whole package, today.

But I can't, not without worrying that I'm selling myself and my own needs short. I want so much to give her the dream, to share it, but I'm also in a different space. Slower. I need time and internal space to heal, to process what feels like a pattern of bad past choices and bad relationship dynamics. I'm not feeling that confident that I can go forward quickly without repeating the same mistakes. I do want a future with Bridget, but I want a happy today even more—or, at least, one that's more peaceful than what I've had in the past. I want to experience a healthy, committed, loving relationship that doesn't sour quickly or become codependent in all the wrong ways. I want one that leaves me feeling like an individual within a couple, something I stopped feeling in my prior relationships. I'm damaged, I tell Bridget; you're not the only one.

Shell-shocked is another word. Clearer too. With the clarity of the cuckold. I won't make these mistakes again, I dearly hope. I won't tolerate a serial cheater. I know what I don't want and won't relive. I do learn lessons the hard way. At forty, I want to build solidly but I don't want to lose myself along the way. If I'm rushed, I might. I hope I don't lose Bridget because I need to move slowly, but I am a slowly moving turtle right now, not the madly race-ahead hare.

~ 86

Sebastien has been calling more lately. Quick, clipped greetings that always begin and end the same way. *Hey what's up? This is me calling. Call me back.* Brief communications I try to decipher for their emotional content. It's in the lilt of his voice: whether he stretches out the *call me back* and leaves it on a happy high note. If he doesn't, if it's very short, I know he's upset. And these days, he's upset, deep down.

Sebastien is the kind of reserved, outwardly cynical man who's secretly a young boy you want to tickle so hard he screams. He's a bit type A; a buttoned-down, by-the-books Gap boy and admitted control queen. Or, king, really; he's not girly. He sometimes tries to control his friends as well, but gently. With sarcastic humor. Like me, he's hardest on himself.

We talked on the phone last night. He was in a good mood, but grim, giving me an update on his health. He's got a sharp, dry wit. He's a boy who sniggers and giggles, putting his hand up before his face to guffaw. As if, when he does laugh, it threatens to reveal too much of himself, a core of mirth that feels explosive, something to control. Like his feelings. These tend to be expressed indirectly, passed through a sieve of light sarcasm. But I'm never fooled.

So far, he's been doing well on his HIV cocktail with one exception: his hair is falling out—well, thinning. Not just on his head but on his legs. It's falling out in clumps, leaving his calves patchy. *My friends tell me I should shave*, he jokes, but tonight there's no chuckle. He feels exposed, vulnerable, and a bit afraid, uncertain if this is a side effect important enough to warrant a doctor's attention.

Of course it is, I reassure him. You're not being a hypochondriac. Losing your hair isn't okay, not just because we're all vain. I'm sure I would feel the same way. It's scary. It's a sign that something's wrong and it makes you feel like you're not in control. I understand. Plus, I can see it's affecting how you feel about yourself, making you depressed and scared. That qualifies as a quality-of-life issue. Health is about feeling good, remember? Just because you have HIV doesn't mean you have to look sick, especially since you're healthy. *Don't forget, you're in charge, even if you don't feel that way. If you're having serious side effects, you can change your regimen. You have options, remember?*

My little speech lifts him up. I promise to swing into action, call my contacts, get on the Internet, find out everything that's published on unusual hair loss and anti-HIV drugs. A week later, I'm nearly empty-handed. I've found two citations. Hair loss is not listed as a commonly reported side effect of the protease drug he's taking. The top researchers I talk to are doubtful about his story. Perhaps it's stress, one suggests. I call Paul Bellman. Perhaps baldness runs in his family?

Listening to these experts, I admit I hear echoes of the lousy advice I've gotten all year from the specialists about my mystery Belize bug (except Joe, who's at least open to the improbable). I start to get angry on Sebastien's behalf in a way I haven't gotten angry about my own health problems. Did you hear that, reader-therapist? A classic example of feminine conditioning and transference; I'll own it.

I avoid calling Sebastien until I have some definitive information, but he's getting more anxious every day. His messages stack up on my answering machine. *Any news? It's not getting better.*

When I finally call, I share with Sebastien the frustration of not being able to get a proper diagnosis for my recurring joint pain, the lingering low-level headaches, the vague skin itches, the lousy bowels. I ask him to keep close track of his alopecia, the fancy term for losing your hair, and to give me more time. I tell him I'll talk to his doctor myself if he wants. And the whole time, inside, I'm feeling a renewal of the old grief. For him, for me, for all of us. At the reminder that he may still suffer, even if he doesn't get sick from his pox, and so may I, with my own obscure prognosis.

Two weeks later, the reports I've digested are skimpy and hard to compare. The researchers continue to annoy me with their calm, assured skepticism of Sebastien's story. They think his hair loss is likely to be a transient problem, one that may resolve itself naturally but isn't life-threatening. I agree to disagree, politely. It may not be serious, but it shouldn't be ignored. I give Sebastien my studied personal opinion.

Bugger the data; I think the protease drug is the villain. Switch that drug, I suggest, *and you may get an answer. Or stay on the drug combo and accept your temporary baldness.*

Sebastien is torn. Under his microscopic scrutiny, his hair appears to be growing back, but maybe he's imagining it? He's afraid of switching to a regimen that doesn't work, afraid of doing something his doctor won't approve of. What if that backfires? Searching himself, he admits he's becoming more depressed. It's freaking him out. He doesn't want to go the gym, reveal his hairless legs. He's stopped wearing shorts.

It's disgusting, he says suddenly, angrily, finally speaking his own truth. *I feel like a freak,* he whispers, near tears. *Maybe I should wait, to see if it gets worse?* he suggests, rising doubt in his voice.

How much worse? I ask him gently. *How bad does it need to get? You're not sleeping. You're very depressed. You can't ignore how this is making you feel. Your biggest obstacle right now is the fear of change, fear of the unknown. You may have to take a risk—a calculated risk. You can switch back later, but at least you'll know.*

But he can't. Like my mysteriously inflamed hands, his hairless legs have shaken his confidence. All is not right in the world and all may not be right again.

I'm becoming a Buddhist. *Surrender.* I say this to myself a dozen times a day. *Surrender to that which you do not control.* Turn it over, accept the mystery, consider the lessons, and do what you can to overcome your fear. Act to change what ails you, but, in this moment, *surrender.*

I keep this advice to myself, giving Sebastien a more positive version: *Relax. You're doing fine. Life is always throwing you curveballs—this is one. Stop analyzing and follow your heart. If your heart tells you it's not okay, listen to it. You'll feel some relief when you do.*

Two weeks later, he calls again. *It hasn't gotten better,* he reports, *so I've made a decision.* He pauses dramatically. *I'm going to kill myself. Just kidding.* He sniggers, his old self again. *I'm going to switch the meds.*

~ 87

DECEMBER 1997

A four-month rumble-tumble of work, love problems, research, late nights, and too much processing. I should dissect it all for you but don't think it's worth the trouble. Too many details; too many tangents. But a big problem looms. Bridget calls it my ambivalence, my refusal to fully engage with her, to set more boundaries and have more distance from Jersey. Even though she understands it's not a sexual thing with Jersey anymore. That's it, though: the emotional intimacy. She doesn't trust it. Doesn't trust me. She sees emotional infidelity and bad boundaries where I see a genuine effort to develop family and embrace different, flexible kinds of relationships. To be committed to a lover but evolve with my friends too.

The bottom line is that Bridget wants me to move out of the loft, away from Jersey. She feels threatened and dissatisfied with the whole setup, feels that I'm unconsciously controlling our relationship by holding back, by having these other intense friendships. Emotional polyamory, the therapists call it. Hmmm. *Am I?*

I blame Jersey, but I blame myself too. Maybe I'm being too idealistic, for thinking Jersey could act like a grown-up because she wants our family bond too. Because now she's acting out too, expressing jealousy and insecurity about Bridget in her own way.

I haven't reacted that well, either to her dating my ex-fling, or to her being a jerk, or to Bridget's equally fierce reaction to all this. I want out of the dyke drama, and right now, I mostly wish they would all just *chill the f——k out.* And I wish Bridget could feel more trusting of how deeply I care for her. Because I do. She just doesn't trust it. And that's on her.

Even if I did move out of this loft, I'm not sure it spells living with Bridget. I'm trying to fill the emotional gap she feels from having moved here as much as I can, but Bridget's loneliness is not mine to fix either. She made the choice to move here. She misses her friends a lot. *Does that mean I have to leave my house? No.*

So . . . can you tell I'm having problems? I am, and it's really discouraging me. It also takes me away from writing. I'm a less-than-happy camper today.

XIV

New Orleans

~ 88

DECEMBER 1997

End of the Year. Almost. And tomorrow, New Year's Eve, is the seventeen-year anniversary of the day my mother went into a coma and died a week later. A sad memory, but one that makes me think of her with acute love. I'm in New Orleans today, thinking about how different my adult life is from the one she created.

When I first arrived here four weeks ago, the Mississippi looked, from the plane, like a great muddy moccasin dappled with dark spots where the clouds blocked a strong sun. I've wanted to drive the length of the river and tomorrow night I'll get my chance. Several of my New York friends have joined me here. We're going to go to Gramercy, a district on the fringes of New Orleans, for the traditional French *feu de joie*, a grand bonfire made of rafts and old boats piled high with wood that is lit to show Papa Noël the way to the big city. I've decided Sel could light a *feu de joie* on the first night of an open-street tribunal on the fascists. So you see how ideas keep creeping in. More sparks taking flame, always.

I've come here for the history, the salt in the air, the French-Cajun *argot*—a close linguistic cousin to Haitian Kreyol. For the first nine days here I was alone and I enjoyed it. Spent my days walking in the French Quarter and unfamiliar poor neighborhoods like Bywater. After the second day in a guesthouse I found a house to rent for a month, though we're only staying three weeks. At least, I am—the others will do whatever they want. Jersey is here; so are some close friends from New York. I'm thrilled they decided to join me. I invited Sarah Pettit, but she's mad at me for leaving her with the closing of the magazine. I told her she should come; she can edit and proof from here, but she's being a martyr. *Too bad!*

I'm hoping Bridget will decide to come down. I keep asking her to consider it. She'd love it here. We could take a long drive alone along the *Mithithippi*, as my mother would say in her butchering French accent.

Everything about this city inspires me: the architecture, the fading glory, the pastel and ochre colors, the culture, the sense of time moving more slowly. I've bought a few history books, reading folk tales of Louisiana and academic narratives about the first slave and vodou communities. Being here puts me in touch with my French roots and my southern ones, and Haiti and slavery—all of this is me. Which make me feel closer to Sel and Paris.

I'm remembering what southern racism feels and looks like too, in the comments and attitudes of white people I meet here who warn me that my city sorties are risky, that I shouldn't go to listen to jazz bands in Tremé, a black neighborhood beyond a patchwork of streets across Saint Claude Avenue that sees its share of crime. Or that, if I do go, I should only go by car. I'm not a fool; I listen to the neighborhood veterans, but I also hear racism in some of these neighborly warnings. Mostly I'm struck by how it feels to live in a climate of insecurity here in Nola. People in this neighborhood feel under siege by unpredictable violence. It's worse than the Bronx used to be. It's not gang violence here, just ordinary stickups and break-ins. Poor people driven desperate by drugs to commit crime. So I've come to learn. There's a lot more real poverty here than I appreciated.

Just an hour ago, a lady outside my door told me she was carjacked across the street, at ten thirty this morning, around the same time and place I was out walking to get a cup of coffee. A man—a crackhead, she assumes—pulled out a gun and forced her to turn over her cash and turn on the ignition of her car and he took off. He was going to shoot her, he said, to kill her.

Now Jersey and I are sitting inside our short-term rental feeling worried, feeling like maybe this Bywater neighborhood is too rough for two white girls from New York who aren't fools and who like mixed neighborhoods and a little squalor even. But not to be murdered. We're feeling afraid is what it is. This boho quarter might just be too rough, even for veteran New Yorkers. Too bad we prepaid the rent. Good thing Bridget hasn't decided to come. We might have to move now. This would *not* be her idea of where to have a dream New Year's.

⌒

I'm scheduled to go back to Europe in a few weeks. First to The Hague, to get a close-up look at the international war crimes tribunal and, hopefully, to interview the chief prosecutor, who's a woman. I've fantasized about doing this for the past three years and now I'm finally going to. And, after that, another bit of historic opportunity awaits that justifies my trip since it directly relates to Sel: the Papon trial.

Over the past two months, proceedings have begun against Maurice Papon. For a little while, it looked like he was going to avoid a trial on the grounds that he's too old and frail to withstand the stress. He's in his eighties and has a bad heart. (*But tell me, what old fascist doesn't have a bad heart, eh?*) The court activity has started and I hope that it will be going on when I get there. Witnesses have come out of the closet of history, testifying to the complicity of their *confrères*—their countrymen—to round up and send away Jews. I want to be in the courtroom, to feel how it feels to be in this historic moment. This is only the second time a French citizen has been tried for Vichy-era war crimes. The first was Paul Touvier, who served under Klaus Barbie. All the others were allowed to get away or have died. The trial has reopened old wounds, much as the Swiss Nazi gold hunt has divided Switzerland. My own story has hit a rich, fresh vein.

I want to look around the courtroom at the faces that are there. To speculate, like Sel, on who's who—who's there out of curiosity; who has a shameful hidden story; who's a surviving son or daughter of those sent away? I want to read the French papers, to see how Le Pen and the National Front are reacting to the trial—*if they're reacting*. I want to fully satisfy my own need to witness and testify and defend and judge.

But first, I have to survive these last two weeks in New Orleans. Hope some doped desperado doesn't put a pistol to my head. Hope I can shake this terrible awareness of mortality that pushes me, nevertheless, to venture into uncharted and sometimes unsafe domains, out into the nightclubs of Tremé. The music is just so good. I've discovered Kermit Ruffins, who plays at Vaughan's Lounge, the dive bar almost across the street from our house. I'm in heaven, sitting at Vaughan's listening to him hit that trumpet. I'm living out my Nola fantasy. He's fantastic. It's all fantastic. I love New Orleans, never mind the crack-a-jack stick-me-ups. I don't like the violence but I don't want to be afraid to go out here. Gotta take some risks, as Papou would advise, gotta have fun while we can.

Since I'm in New Orleans, land of vodou, and I'm a grandchild of a vodouist and gambler—my Haitian grandmother—I'll light some incense and candles for good luck and protection and ask the spirit of my mother, *Grand Defender of My Early Soul and Life*, to watch over me. I'm surrendering to that grander force, Life. Protect me, all you who can, from some crackhead knucklehead here in Nawlins. And then I'll go meet Bridget and get back to work. Go check out what Papon has to say to the survivors now that the trial is finally starting. Go witness me some real history.

⌇

A postscript: days later. I'm still in New Orleans and still alive. Happier, because more close New York friends decided to join us for the New Year and afterward. I've got an instant girl gang. With numbers come safety. We've gone exploring, driven on back roads throughout the bayou region, hit almost every thrift store in the state, eaten crawfish. I'm really happy, though in the end, Bridget didn't come. I so wish she had. Neither did Sarah. She missed a serious party.

Truth is, Bridget's furious at me. For ditching her, as she sees it, for choosing to come south to get warm and hang out with Jersey and my friends, versus joining her in the 'burbs in Massachusetts with her family, who, she readily admits, aren't keen on lesbians. Not at all. They're Catholics and they disapprove. They love Bridget though, and she felt she had to go. She couldn't disappoint her mother. So now she's angry because she feels stuck there, and I'm here, having fun with the girls. Fact is, I miss her and really wanted to spend the holidays with her. And I do feel guilty. But I have very little vacation time. Why spend it with people you don't know who are primed to really dislike you because you're gay?

After much debate, Bridget just decided she'll go with me to Paris instead. We'll have our vacay time there. We're going in two weeks. I really hope things will be better when we're alone again.

I also keep trying to reassure her about Jersey, but it's no good: nothing I say or do has that effect. Quite the opposite: she's become explosive on the subject. It's all very difficult and depressing to me. It's also so frustrating, given that I seriously love her. I think she knows that too. But this relationship with me just isn't what she was hoping for, I guess. I realize too that we are different. I really do like having my close friends very nearby, very involved in my life. And I have to appreciate and respect that they're not her friends. If she had her close posse here, her San Francisco gang, I'm sure it would feel different. But she doesn't. So we have a conflict—of timing in large part. I only hope we can get through this. There's so much that's good between us, so much that works. It should outweigh what's not easy. I keep telling myself that anyway.

So we're going to Europe. Just us two. Three weeks, three countries, just like we planned. I'm super excited. I so need to have a good time with her, to feel the connection that drew me to her in the first place. And vice versa. Bad dynamics bring out the worst in a partner, and I know she feels like she's been needy and overbearing, while I've been cast as remote and unforgiving. Whatever has gone wrong here is a mix of many issues, but not, I think, any fault of our hearts trying to love. We are each trying, each a big fan of the other. But we both have emotional baggage and it's getting in our way. I just hope we can lose some of it on the next trip. I'm getting worn out from the conflict.

$\mathcal{XV}$

Amsterdam

~ 89

Europe is gray, wet, and very cold. Amsterdam feels like it has no daylight and, because we're so tired, we sleep past checkout time. We're disoriented and foggy but happy to be away. We've made no schedule beyond seeing art, which is good for me, because I'm exhausted. So is Bridget. But she's happy and so am I. I'm so happy to see her again. I've really missed her.

Art brings us together. It reminds us of our shared passion, of who we are as people and why we were drawn together. We avoid the contemporary museum, head straight for Rembrandt and then earlier artists. The pictures match the weather outside: low, brooding skies, quiet, somber visitations of the Virgin and the Saints, an intense emotion conveyed in a palate of browns and blood reds. The Dutch paintings delight us and we can't say why. But everything has the feel of a swoon to it: the elongated torsos of infants; the strange, long hands; the pinched faces.

Bridget is taking a class on Van Eyck and here they are: huge, busy pastoral scenes teeming with hidden meanings. Her eyes are shining: she loves being in Europe, being here with me. She loves sleeping on a tiny, uncomfortable cot with a lousy view and the red-light district just down the street. That's why we stay where we do; for that pleasure. A pleasure we don't have as women, living in the puritan United States.

At night, we walk along the narrow streets and say hello to the women working in the windows. We half-seriously talk about going inside, but only one woman actually beckons us. We walk on. I imagine Bridget staying here for a few months, painting these women in the windows. Portraits that would look fucked up in some way because that's how Bridget makes art, adding little skewed details that make me laugh, like a bunny rabbit in the window with the hooker, or a messed-up Bambi in the pastoral scene with the Virgin. Portraits

242

that would convey the domestic kitsch of the scenes, and the sexiness of this Dutch housewife working the night shift.

That's what I appreciate about Amsterdam's red-light district: the lack of sordidness, the matter-of-factness of this sex industry. I like to think that the women here have a bit more control over their business, which is what I've been told. Though I doubt such things. It's about money and money invites trouble.

The only thing that's missing here are male prostitutes sitting in the windows for the women of Amsterdam to enjoy. *Would I prefer being with a woman or a man in these windows? Hmmm. A man, maybe, just for the novelty of it. No, because, well, women are sexier. They're almost always sexier. Why is that?* I ask Bridget. *Is it just because they're women?*

I think so, she replies. *Women are just sexy.* On this point at least, we agree.

⁓

Late one afternoon, we visit a requisite coffee shop for a hash joint. Here too the mood is so laid back, no one pays any attention to us, mulling over the various types of weed before selecting our *cocktail*, a blend of three kinds that we plan to smoke some of now and keep some of for later. This is the Amsterdam version of our American craze for fancy coffee. There are dozens of variations of *cigarets*, as the joints are called.

Bridget is tired, so we decide to smoke and take a walk and have a late dinner. Dinner never happens. The hash hits us late, an hour after we've been walking, meandering slowly over the dark canals, looking inside even darker windows. Even though it's a big city and has been drawing tourists for decades, Amsterdam feels small, manageable. We get lost, but never too far. Even though it's quiet, the weed has taken control of our tongues. We get chatty, staying up half the night, giggling. And, again, we can't get up when it's time to check out, so we stay, buried deep down inside a cool room, with our stomachs rumbling for food, rather happy.

⁓

It's so bitterly cold I buy a pair of sexy, very warm, leather, motorcycle pants at the flea market at Waterlooplein and never take them off, except to get in bed. Bridget prances around in new lime-green tights worn under fishnet stockings. She's feeling saucy, inspired by the hookers smiling and knitting in their cubby windows. During the day, we museum hop. More old Dutch art, more Van Eyck. We marvel at how perverse these artists were, how dark and earthy their palettes, the bodies they painted so fleshy and sensuous and morbid. We've sworn off coffeehouses and more space cake and strong hash in favor of long walks, late breakfasts, and even longer naps. It's all very healing.

⌒

One night, we track down the lesbians. There's a regular tea dance at the local gay center. We slip back into our leather pants and slut tights, but the evening is a dud. The women strike us as too conventional: too many bowl haircuts, no freaks. It may be an unfair portrayal, but that's how it feels. After a half hour, we run away, disappointed. *Where are all the wild women of Amsterdam?* Bridget asks. We know they're around somewhere, but clearly not here at the gay center.

I tell Bridget about my past visits to Amsterdam, way back when it was a hot punk scene. Everybody looked a bit more interesting then, the lesbians edgy. Or maybe I was younger. But to us, right now, Amsterdam feels too tame; very pleasant, a bit like a cow, placid and dull and chewing its spliff. Or maybe we're feeling too old for the trendy young rave clubs but too young to be sleeping. Instead, we drink tea and beer late into the night, freezing, but feeling good together again, feeling excited and open and ready for adventure.

The days are flying by. I was planning to go to The Hague to interview the war crimes prosecutor, but now I realize I haven't organized myself well enough in advance. This is Europe, land of bureaucracy and protocol. I needed to have written far ahead to get this meeting. She's traveling and may not be back. For now, we're jumping over to Brussels to see some of my relatives and look at even more dark European artists and then plan to arrive in Paris ahead of schedule. It's freezing there too.

X𝑉𝐼

Paris

~ 90

FEBRUARY 1998

It's good to see one of the Crazy Girls again. French Ann meets us at the Canal de Saint-Martin. Whenever I stay with her, my story with Sel comes immediately alive. I only have to look out at the water to see the scenes.

The apartment is tiny and French Ann has an active pit bull, so it's too cramped for a long visit. She's giving us the apartment for the week and will stay with her ex, Crazy Girl no. 2, aka Diane, who's tall and cerebral and Jewish and likes psychoanalytic theory. Like me, the Crazy Girls are modern sapphists, which means their relationships are a bit complicated. *Did I say messy? Okay, messy. Modern lesbian messy.*

These two *folles* have the same kind of relationship I have with Jersey: ex-lovers turned best friends, family. It's a general trend among a growing number of my peers; something unique to the lesbian subculture I inhabit. We hang on, as women, to the love and the person, and it all slowly transforms, albeit with a lot of processing. We become sisters of another sort. A passionate sisterhood of exes.

~ 91

Bridget has her Paris agenda set up: all art, all the time. None of that Eiffel Tower and Champs-Élysées crap for her. She's taken to Paris like someone who's been dying to speak the language and easily could: she has a feeling for French; she can make faces like they do, gestures; she loves wine and cheese. She's happy to be on her own a lot, practicing French words that make her sigh dramatically because they're so romantic to her, a girl from a small town in Massachusetts, who dreamed of living in France as a child, though why, she doesn't know. *Because it's so romantic,* she says, laughing and doing a little dance on the quai. She's having a great time. New York, New Orleans, our bad times,

245

the possible breakup talk, Jersey . . . it's all back there, across the water; not something to think about today. We're free. It feels great.

While Bridget discovers the Louvre, I reacquaint myself with Paris. I walk and film with the Super 8 again. I feel Sel's story move around, new scenes suggesting themselves, new characters. Most of my time is spent crawling around the neighborhood where the Crazy Girls live. The neighborhood I remember has changed even more. I slip into construction sites, run my fingers along the walls of the buildings that remain standing, along wallpaper and vestiges of paint, the outlines of bedrooms and bathrooms. *All that living. Where are they now?*

I watch a huge crane swing a giant steel arm toward a squat building with fine architectural details, a chain of stone fleurs-de-lis framing the second and third floor. An hour later, when I swing by again, the royalist touches are history. The France I love visually is disappearing. No more French francs. Enter the euro. France is becoming like everywhere else: a glossy, shining thing. A fast-paced, homogenous capital, with a stylish McDonald's on the Champs-Élysées. But no place for the poet, or the romantic, or the dreamer. In my ear, a voice whispers. *That's it, sugar. Leaves you with a bitter cup of coffee, doesn't it?*

Sel. Always at my elbow.

Now that you're back, she adds, *we've got our work to do. You're going to see Monsieur Papon, aren't you? It's about time.*

~ 92

Midweek, I head south, to Bordeaux and the Papon trial. *The Trial of the Century*, the French are calling it. *Is it really? Because it's the only one they really got behind in all these years? Ah, yes, I have my own opinions.* Anyway, I'll write about the trial on another day because there's a lot to say but, for now, this quick bit: before I saw Papon in person, I saw him in my head. I was talking to him, dreaming about him, imagining the trial and my reaction to it. All of this was better than the trial itself is turning out to be, which I somehow knew would be the case. The trial will provide me with fact, but fantasy and fiction is more satisfying, a more accurate reflection of what I'm seeing and feeling.

Arriving at night at the hotel in Bordeaux, I watch the trial on late-night television with Sel. I'm not feeling very good. A touch of some gastrointestinal problem that I fear is the avian flu that made my aunt in Paris gravely ill last week. A new pox, I'll note here.

I awake early and tired for my appointment with Papon the accused. My reporter-friends, including Philippe, have been clipping articles for me, keeping track of the trial in anticipation of my visit. I scan them, but they're not really what I'm interested in, this national breast-beating, the lengthy legal arguments for or against his conviction. I want to see the man's face, to see how I'll react. I want my one-on-one audience with history. This trial feels rare, a last occasion to confront the beast, one of the wolves of this specific period of history, the only war that Europe ever seems to talk about, Hitler's war, before it's lost to us forever. Lost to France, that is—or, at least, that's how the political pundits view it.

Papon is France's last chance. After him, there will be no more Nazi-era trials because there are too few survivors left, too few witnesses. That's why this trial suddenly means so much to them, to this guilt-racked nation. They know they've failed to punish the crime, to act in defense of that thing we all hold sacrosanct (or at least believe we should): our humanity. The Papon trial is less about him than it is about them: his accusers. About France. Everyone knows this, even the journalists who spill their ink over him.

This is my concern, and Sel's too: *indifference*, rather than banal evil. *Passive complicity*. The muted response of France rather than the actions of Papon, a rather arch civil servant who performed his bureaucratic duties without much afterthought; with the precision of a French waiter serving an espresso. Cold, efficient, shrewd, superior, defensive. Papon is making his *confrères* uncomfortable because they easily recognize him, I think. Every one of them has a little Papon side, that French penchant for efficiency and following the rules. Under the same circumstances, they fear they'd do the same. And they probably would.

How many did? This isn't being talked about in the local newspapers, but it's easy enough to see that Papon is a mirror for this troubled nation. And that's why he's going to have a hard time here now: because he's being judged by a jury of his peers. They're not innocent; nor is Papon. But someone has to pay. That's the story being played out here now.

⁓

I definitely have a stomach virus of some kind. I've secured a day pass for the trial and sit inside a big room with other journalists to follow the Papon proceedings on a giant screen. It's too crowded to get inside the courtroom itself. But the bathroom is close by, which is very good. Papon himself may not show up, only his lawyers. But today's testimony is particularly relevant to me and to my research: Michel Bergès, an academic, is scheduled to argue against the validity of the trial itself. He's a historian who was among the first to uncover Papon's name among old archives and bring his case to the attention of investigators. Upon examining the evidence, he decided that Papon can't be properly judged after all. *A turncoat historian?*

Bergès is actually testifying on behalf of the defense now. All this I've gleaned from an American journalist, Adam Gopnik, covering the story for the *New Yorker* who's agreed to meet me for a coffee beforehand to fill me in.

Now we're supposed to meet and I can't find him. I don't know what he looks like and no one looks very American to me. I decide to grab breakfast instead, hoping it will settle my growing nausea. I worry about projectile vomiting inside the hearing room. *Why, of all days, is this the day I fall sick? When I have sought a personal date with history?*

~ 93

A lady in a white lab coat at a corner pharmacy gives me a tablet that fizzes in water; the kind I hate. But I have no choice today. I pray it works. *Are you going to the Papon trial?* she asks me. *Yes,* I say, adding, *Do you think it will be interesting?* She considers her reply for a second. *Everyone knows he's guilty,* she says, looking around for a second, even though I'm the only customer. *But he was hardly the only one, was he? Why now? That's what I ask. Why now?*

A good question. One the journalists I meet will ask over and over again too. *Why now?* Because, they agree unanimously, this trial is not about Papon; it's about politics. They could have gone after Papon earlier. France needs this now; the Socialists need this now. With the rise of the National Front, the regime is worried about the elections. Papon's trial offers them a chance to detach themselves from men like Le Pen, to gain some moral leverage.

I'm a bit surprised at the French journalists, at their independence. Most of them are admitted leftists, like Philippe, or at least liberals. They're quite convinced, like the pharmacist, that Papon is guilty of rather horrific actions. But this trial is like a giant suit being hung on a skinny, old man: it doesn't fit neatly.

One journalist explains it to me: *This trial should be much more narrow; then the charges would stick. But to hang the entire subject of the Vichy regime on Papon is wrong, and it's not fair to the cause, which is justice. Even the survivors aren't happy with the trial for that reason. It's not their trial, and it never was. It's about the future of those in power right now. Which is sad because we really need to try Papon and people like him for their crimes. With this charade, we are being robbed of the opportunity.*

As he puts it, the trial is primarily a showcase public history lesson. A kind of window washing. A chance for the French, who have never wanted to confront their past, to do so now, a little; to look at the past from a safe moral distance. Schoolchildren can attend and many do. Papon is a field trip, a living museum, a warning against the past.

Papon hasn't shown up; probably won't. He's not feeling well either, apparently. (*Surprise, right? I mean, who would, under the circumstances?*) Instead, his defender, Bergès, treats the audience to a long, meandering lecture. He makes a complex argument that I totally disagree with, claiming that we—members of today's society—can't judge past events because we weren't there. We can't possibly have access to all the facts or know the context in which certain actions were taken. And, for this reason, he, the scholar with his years of research, is better suited to interpret the historical record than we are. Bergès concludes that there are serious gaps in the historical record; black holes that will never be filled. The past is lost. Crimes were committed, yes. But it's not right to commit another, to judge a man like Papon, given such omissions.

After he finishes and is cross-examined, it's time for a lunch break. I feel stimulated and perplexed. *What is the role of this man, the historian, in this trial? Is he offering to let France, everyman France, off the moral hook?* I agree with parts of his argument—that most law is a matter of interpretation—but not with his basic conclusion. It *is* our duty to judge, based on the facts as they are presented, as long as we rely on a system of law. A flawed system, to be sure. Omissions aplenty. A system that definitely reflects the values and might of those in power. A system vulnerable to corruption. But law is the instrument nations and societies have created to maintain social order. Crimes should be punished and the punishment should fit the crime.

I say we can judge a man like Maurice Papon, and we must, just as we can judge those in power in France who have shielded him from justice for so long. Both are culpable. I might argue that France is paying for its complicity and long denialism. They now have to contend with Le Pen seducing a new genera-tion of French youth who were never told the truth about what all-too-ordinary local officials like Papon did to help send Jews, and later Algerians, to be mur-dered, all in the name of preserving order, in the name of *liberté*, *égalité*, and *fraternité*.

History is not black and white, I want to say to Professor Bergès. *It's usually gray. Muddled. The gray is what we base our own daily actions on; its shades make up our actions and our lives. And, against the gray, Papon's actions come up a dull red, the color of old blood. There can be no denying the fate of the Jewish children he sent away to be killed, can there? You can't omit that, as much as you might try.*

I'm speaking to the jury now, in my mind, to the assembled audience: *There are some facts that provide a context for judging. To avoid judging is itself a crime. And that seems to be the more interesting issue being played out here in front of millions.*

A few rows behind me in the viewing gallery, the schoolchildren fidget and quietly fight. They are politely bored though excited by the media's presence. Every day, outside visitors queue for a number of allotted tickets to attend the trial. For months, this case has dragged on; it's nearing its end, but not for another month at least.

Hours later, my stomach still roiling, I decide to leave. Papon's a definite no-show. I'm still brooding over the big question: *Can France judge its past? Not well*, I conclude. *Because it really doesn't want to. That past is very ugly. It's a harsh mirror.*

⌒

A footnote: I don't see Papon on the trip, not in person. I only see him later, on the television news. He looks like a thin, fatigued, elderly man, slightly defensive but dispassionate. Resigned, it seems, to the long trial and these endless legal maneuvers. This is his real punishment, I realize, this endless parade of legal experts and revisionists and witnesses and ordinary folk who, like me, have come to make up their own minds about the whole affair. It's unlikely, at his age, that he'll serve much of a sentence even if he's convicted. This is the best there's going to be, and that's how they're making him pay, as it were. By making him an immoral example, day in and day out. *A Sanson for the nineties.*

~ 94

Back in Paris. I spend the evening channel-surfing the news programs on television, catch recaps of the trial in Bordeaux. Up close, Papon looks as he did in the books and newsreels I've looked at. Ordinary. Unexceptional.

I bring my face up close to the TV screen so Papon's face is virtually inches from mine. I'm looking into his eyes. He so reminds me of my grand-père—his sartorial elegance. Papon was rather handsome as a young man. I call my grandfather Papou; here is Papon. Two ordinary Frenchmen. A consonant of difference.

He's the face of evil, I remind myself of Papon. *Banal, ordinary. The careful civil servant. That's who may be drawn to a man like Le Pen now. Those craving order, those raised to feel privileged, to feel they are special. Isn't that all of France?*

⌒

Some of the trial attendees in the news footage are dozing, tired by the slow process of justice. *You're the faces we should really care about*, I pretend-lecture them. *Every one of you who saw then and see now, see a man like Le Pen, but don't care enough to act, who stay too quiet, who see him as someone else's problem. You, your parents and grand-parents. Your family's friends. Then and now. We're all complicit when we refuse to bear witness, when the crime is evident but we step over the corpse. We—you—continue to let them get away. Men like Papon. We shelter them with our indifference. We relegate their actions to the distant past when they are happily living among us. Our all-too-ordinary neighbors. We decide to find them when it's expedient, when it seems to serve the leaders of the nation again. So I view the crime, the failure. We can accuse Papon but what of our indifference? The mirror never lies.*

Gas chambers were a detail of the war, unless we accept that the war is a detail of the gas chambers.

Jean-Marie Le Pen on French television,
April 2015

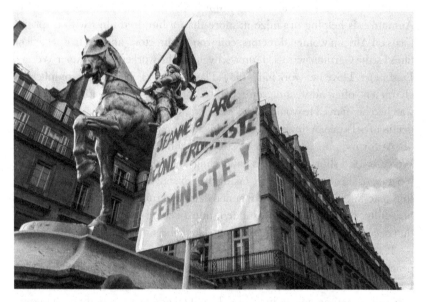

ACT UP–Paris protests against National Front, January 10, 2013. (tomcraig@directphoto.org)

$\mathcal{X}\mathcal{V}II$

$\mathcal{N}ew\ \mathcal{Y}ork$

~ 95

MARCH 1998

I'm back in New York but already planning a return to Paris, to attend the twentieth annual Créteil women's film festival. A friend of mine, Martine Aumaître, is helping organize it: more than a hundred films with a special focus on African women directors, cult women directors, and a retrospective of films by the German actress Hanna Schygulla. She worked with Rainer Werner Fassbinder. I love her work in his films. Playing edgy, sexy, morally complicated characters, often addressing some dubious postwar past. I wonder if Kiki ever watched her films. He would have loved her. I know the trip will add a few more details to Sel's tale. A final seasoning, I think, before the dish is ready to be served.

As for me and Bridget, we're still struggling, but there's some progress. We've started short-term crisis counseling to figure out whether and how to separate or stay together and are taking the next few months to give the relationship space and time to breathe. Planned dates and romance and less processing, hopefully. Bridget also had a sudden, unexpected breakthrough with Jersey that occurred on my fortieth birthday in late February.

It's too complicated to go into here but, somehow, they made some kind of peace with each other; found acceptance. I think Bridget now understands that Jersey really has become my closest friend, even if remnants of our lousy lovers' dynamic sometimes bite us in the ass. That it takes time to work through important relationships. But we're human, and we're trying.

I really wish the transition with Jersey had been smoother. I feel guilty for how hard it's been for Bridget to deal with her. And Jersey too—it hasn't been fun for her. I've done my best and tried to be true to myself in the process—true to my need for space and time, to my desire to respect all my relationships and not sell them short—but I admit it's been a rough ride. The opposite of what I was trying to do, the difference between an ideal and reality. So goes life, I suppose.

~ 96

Today I spent hours in the bookstore below the Writers Room, which serves as my daytime office, just off Astor Place. It's my refuge, with twenty-four-hour access. Many of my writer friends work and often sleep there. This week I've been gabbing with Sapphire and Nancy Milford, a biographer who wrote *Zelda*, a book about F. Scott Fitzgerald's troubled wife. We talked about mental illness and depression, the sources of artistic creativity for some. She's been researching a biography of Edna St. Vincent Millay for so many years she's stopped counting. Twenty?

Whenever I'm frustrated, questioning my sanity, my choice to pursue the writer's life—to spend another sunny day lost in the archives of history, or searching news clips for information about Le Pen and his cronies—I spy Nancy or Sapphire pecking away in their cubicles, equally obsessed. It's comforting. Yes we're crazy, somewhere, but it's our crazy, our choice to creatively torture ourselves, to take these journeys. I always want to hear what they're up to. Writers are a good bunch. The Writers Room does provide a fellowship.

I got sidetracked perusing books on heraldry downstairs—the old science of genealogy. The more I read about our fascination with bloodlines, the more I realize that all of us engage in the kind of thinking about purity that underlies fascism. How can we avoid it? Our fundamental social concepts of being, of self and identity and society and culture, are rooted in essentialist biology, in genes. *Blood=Life=Family=History*. A pure bloodline is a trump card, an ace in the pack for the genealogical historian who relies on the same tools the state uses to distinguish rightful citizens from foreigners and criminals, to identify who is or isn't entitled to a piece of land, a job, health care. Our tools are birth certificates, DNA tests, hospital records, social security cards, passports, school records, the marriage license. Today, the state is as obsessed with keeping the nation's blood clean as it ever was.

All this reading about blood history has also made me think more about what's happening in the Balkans and in Rwanda. Our contemporary genocides. Armenia. Cambodia. How can such events still take place, in this day and age, knowing all we do about the Holocaust? Our love of purity is instilled early on and constantly nurtured. We ask ourselves why people are drawn to a Hitler or a Le Pen or Pol Pot. Because they touch us where we are vulnerable, where we have some longing for order, for control, for purity. Someone to blame for the chaos and insecurity in our lives. The Other.

It makes me think about how much we have in common with our perceived enemies. It's so much easier to hate them, isn't it? To distance ourselves from them on the basis of perceived differences. But it's what I have in common with a Hitler or a Karadžić that I'm compelled to think about—not how I'm different.

Look at Rwanda. A whole nation doesn't just turn evil overnight. They may do what we call evil. But that's because we all can, under the right circumstances. We're all quite capable of being the beast because we're all ordinary humans. Once we—the world—begins to truly understand and accept this inner notion of ourselves, of our *normal*, not abnormal, nature, we might be able to direct attention away from human psychology and refocus it on the external and material conditions that allow people to abandon civility, to allow deeper primal, but quite natural, instincts to take over. Our deeply held fears and prejudices. Our petty egos and insecurities. Our capacity for hate and cruelty— the Janus face of love and tenderness. Our ability to disconnect as easily and quickly as we connect.

There's also the false story we've invented to let ourselves sleep more easily: that those who wrong us can't possibly feel anything positive about their actions. But they do; that's the rub. They absolutely can and do, at least while they're in those emotions. Like love, like hate. Have you not witnessed the exuberance of the victor, whether in a football match or on the battlefield? They're not weeping for the enemy; they're mad with joy for themselves, for their side.

It's the *we* that's so critical here, in my mind. The *we* that replaces the *I*. The group that replaces the individual. That's what we must focus on. The need to belong, the need for safety or power that a group provides. The transcendent feeling of collective *connection*. Of ecstasy, and religious belief. That's the key to these large-scale events, these genocides: the connection, not the disconnection, to one's group. It's no different from soldiers being taught to forget their individual needs, to put the army first, is it?

Look at how easily schoolyard and teenage cliques become cruel, gain cohesion by accepting or rejecting members. The desire to belong, not to be rejected, is normal and deep in us, social creatures that we are. Once we view the *group's needs* as our own, then they have us: the risk exists. We've lessened our ability to act or think outside the group. That's the aspect of the human psyche the psychologists should forcibly dwell on: our need to belong, to be protected. All I'm arguing here is: *forget the monster.* He or she is too different from us. We can't relate. *We need to see ourselves in the mirror.* Let's start telling stories that involve normal men and women and the all-too-human course of human genocide. That's the modern story of genocide. How it's a slippery slope from love-thy-neighbor to kill-thy-neighbor.

I can hear you protest, reader: I'd never do that, be that way, hurt anyone; never kill or torture. So said many good Germans and the French, ordinary folk, who let Hitler's men lead their Jewish friends and neighbors away. So

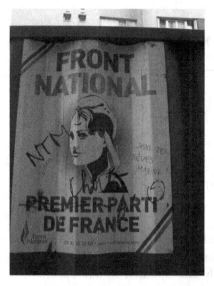

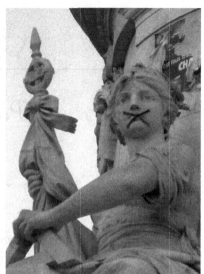

Marine Le Pen poster graffiti. (AC d'Adesky)   Justice silenced. (AC d'Adesky)

felt—so feel—the Hutu in Rwanda, driven by terror, by a sense of being historically persecuted, put down, as a group. That's what the generals understand, when they train their boys and now girl soldiers to think as one. That's
what the ethnofascists understand and count on: how easy we feel slighted, how
much we want to be superior to our neighbors. Our petty, malleable, human
nature.

I know: none of this may make you sleep better at night. But it should. Because once we understand the origin of the problem, we can focus on the suffering of our neighbors. Those who may be vulnerable to the messages of a
Monsieur Le Pen. *Ordinary people, then. Good people. Good neighbors.* A group, I'll
stress again, not so different from the Hutu in Rwanda or the Balkan Serbs or
Croats. All good people. Petty grievances writ large. That's why I say, start
small. Start local. If you want to stop a genocide, if you want to stop Le Pen or
a strongman, talk to your *voisin.* Convince the neighbor, help them.

X$\mathcal{VIII}$

$\mathcal{P}aris$

~ 97

APRIL 1998

April in Paris, yet again. Only two months since I was last here. This time, the weather's changed for the worse. Not only the natural climate, either. When I left New York, the sky was explosively blue and hot, an unusual seasonal warming. But Paris is menacingly gray, rainy, and cold, a turn that mirrors the chill brought on by the recent elections.

I visit with the Crazy Girls again in the nineteenth. They say everyone can't believe Le Pen's party has done so well, especially with youth. No one can believe their neighbors would vote for Le Pen's smooth-talking protégé, Bruno Mégret. It's not the France they recognize. Who are these young people? they wonder, disbelieving. *C'est pas possible. C'est dégueulasse.* Disgusting.

What about the people next door? I suggest. Those moving into the tall, fancy apartment buildings that keep replacing the torn-down ones?

Dégueulasse, French Ann repeats. *On se reconnait plus, en France.* We don't recognize ourselves anymore, in France.

Ah, I think. The critical first step: alienation. *Loss of self to the group.*

⟶

To my surprise, Philippe, my journalist friend, isn't as worried about Le Pen as I expected. Two years ago, he was braying, snorting, fuming. Now he's wearing the posture of the seasoned pundit who saw it all coming and sees how it will go in the future.

Le Pen's strength is misleading, says Philippe. The only reason the National Front has 15 percent of the vote is because they stupidly restructured the electoral system and established proportional representation. Right away, overnight, Le Pen's numbers doubled. It's a quota system, but it doesn't reflect political reality. Anyway, there have always been 15 percent who vote the extreme right; nothing has changed, not really. *It's just cosmetic,* he insists. What matters is what's happening on the Left, which has been forced to mobilize against all this stupidity. Prime Minister Jospin has done well. The Socialists are regaining the confidence of the French people.

Really? I find his confidence hard to understand. What about the people who openly tack up Le Pen flyers in the hallways of apartment buildings? I saw that, I tell him, during my last visit to see Théodore, who's been relocated to a new apartment in a nicer part of town. A pamphlet for a National Front rally, slipped under every apartment doorway, and pinned up on the bulletin board by the telephone. What about the liberal journalists who have taken up their pens to argue among themselves about whether the National Front constitutes a legitimate party? They seem plenty worried.

Non, he says, waving away my doubt. *Non, non, it won't happen like that.* It's a small victory, yes, but that's as far as it will go, he is sure. *You'll see. Well, of course, it depends on whether the Socialists deliver on election promises. We need that. If the Socialists fail, then, yes, we could have a problem. But I'm more worried about Socialists than Le Pen right now. There's been so much fighting, like cats and dogs. We need more unity.*

I wonder if Philippe doesn't suffer from a bit of myopia too: the blindness of denial that comes from ignoring the enemy in order to render it less visible, less powerful? His impassioned attention remains steadily on the Left, on his Socialist colleagues—their thrusts and counterthrusts—now that the Left has a more visible target: the populist Far Right. Is the political Left in France, whatever creature with ten legs it is today, guilty of the same self-aggrandizement as the Right? I suspect so. Politics is a game of ego; why should anyone be spared? I think it may be as inconceivable to Philippe as it is to the Crazy Girls to imagine that a group of fascist leaders could take power in France.

~ 98

The main reason for Philippe's optimism, it turns out, are the street protests that picked up greater numbers across France. Sixty thousand people turned out in Paris on the day of the elections. French Ann told me all about it. She said it was a big party, with all the old faces: grizzled Communists, fiery Maoists, all the unemployed and sans papiers, the ACT UPers and guerilla radio pirates and RAI soccer fans; a whole spectrum of society.

Of course none of them could believe things had come to this point, either. But to Philippe, it was a sign of the strength of the progressive movement, the resurgence of the spirit of '68. *On avance,* he says. *We're advancing.*

We'll see if Philippe's right. I would like to believe it, anyway. I would like to think what's just happened here in France, a step forward by the National Front, is very different from what's just taken place in the East, where the strongmen and women in the Balkans have ousted the democrats. Politically, the situation appears very different.

France is a seemingly solid republic, with a functioning democracy and, most importantly, a strong economy, in spite of its high unemployment. It's not as vulnerable to the passions of nationalist or ethnic hatred. But you can anticipate my argument: is it difference we should be focusing on, or similarity? Such insecurities and fractures exist in every society, and are always vulnerable to exploitation. How deep are these fissures in French society right now? How well will the Far Right exploit the fears and dreams of a disenchanted populace? Will the old wolves in new clothing appear less rabid?

If Philippe is right, France may actually gain something positive from Le Pen's agitations. I'm applying the ideas of France's famous homosexual Michel Foucault to this picture. Foucault explored the role of the Other in society, the thing cast aside, pushed to the margins. How what is made taboo functions as a limit, to frame our desire. We make things or ideas taboo in order to overcome them. When we make something forbidden, we also elevate it in some way; we give it a certain power, allure.

If Le Pen and his racist, xenophobic ideas are being made taboo to most people in France, is that because they also represent some suppressed collective desire? Foucault would say yes. By preaching racism and intolerance, is Le Pen reframing and redefining democracy, forcing the Left and those who support a pluralistic society to reorganize and defend its ideals? Without a frame, a taboo—without a clear enemy in sight—it's harder to advance. What about here in the United States? Is that what the Christian populists are doing? Falwell and the KKK?

I can hear you protesting. As if I were saying France needs a Le Pen; as if dictatorships are useful. They certainly provide a jolt, don't they? I'm merely arguing that men like Le Pen emerge and movements like fascism gain power within a socioeconomic context, and to support what Philippe predicts, they force a reaction on the other side. There's a push-pull to every relationship. After years of infighting and not much more, the Left in France is beginning to coalesce against a stronger populist Far Right. The National Front is thus helping empower the Socialists. And vice versa, one can argue.

The youth of France are also being provided with an important history lesson and are getting politicized. In addition to the antifascist movement, there are ongoing labor strikes across the country, the growth of the homeless movement, and new coalitions between the old Communists and the teenagers at ACT UP meetings. Without the threat of the National Front, how many of them would turn up to vote, never mind protest in the streets? Perhaps far fewer.

However odious, however real a threat, Le Pen is politically useful to the Left.

But one has to ask: what cost may France pay for this political lesson? And who is likely to pay the heavier price? We know the answer: all the undesirables.

~ 99

An important event has taken place, one with major implications for both France and for me, as the scribe of Sel's story. One that's thrown a serious wrench in Le Pen's ambitions for the presidency and his role in the National Front—and into my own narrative, given that Sel has been stalking the man she derisively calls La Poule. Of course, it's good news, too.

The event in question took place last June, during the campaign for the general election. Le Pen, who has a lifelong reputation for brawling, apparently attacked a Socialist deputy, Annette Peulvast-Bergeal. He jumped out of a car and began shoving her at an election rally. A lovely example of the French chivalry he often talks about. This incident has now cost him his leadership of the National Front—for a while, at least. He's been suspended from the European Parliament and can't participate in politics for a year. He's going to appeal, of course, but the verdict has caused a major feud to develop within the National Front. It immediately set the stage for his former protégé, Bruno Mégret, to vie for the party secretary and top spot in the later elections. He has been steadily gaining his own supporters in the party.

So, now, there's an internal soap opera taking place. Le Pen is bitterly upset that Mégret is trying to wrest control of the party—*the little upstart*. He's hoping to push forward his wife, Jany (née Jeanne-Marie Paschos), whom he married in 1991, into some proxy role. Or his daughters—the eldest, Marie-Caroline, the youngest, Marine, who are aspiring party members. The middle daughter, Yann, is married to Samuel Maréchal, head of the National Front's youth wing. It's all in the family, then.

So, the party faithful are split. Some worry that Le Pen has now damaged his party's hope for broader electoral appeal with his rough temper and his penchant for denying the Holocaust (*a little detail*, he's called it—and been fined as a result). Mégret, the newcomer, is a fresh, more youthful face. There are also others who don't like Le Pen trying to put his wife into power.

This is where the story gets especially rich. I've just learned from the newspapers here that Le Pen's daughter Marie-Caroline is lovers with one of Mégret's top lieutenants named Philippe Olivier. Papa Le Pen is not happy. A traitor,

right in his own family. Forget *Dallas*. This is a hometown *telenovela*! So: an unexpected advance for the antifascists. And all on account of *that damn woman*, as
Le Pen refers to the Socialist leader he assaulted.

⁓

And what does my damn woman, Sel, think of all Le Pen's fisticuffs? Ah, I see
her . . . she's sitting on a park bench this morning, near the Tuileries, her laughter
more like a hacking, tubercular cough. She found something very amusing. The
morning's newspaper, with its headlines about the court's decision.

So, Sel? Is it over, then? Is it the end of Le Pen?

She's looking up at me, shaking her head, muttering now, as if I'm slow.

What's that, Sel?

He's down but not out.

Ah, true. Le Pen has suffered a setback, but he's a survivor. He's a tough
old bird, an ex-sailor and ex-miner. A man who was repeatedly convicted of
assault for beating up communist sympathizers as a young man; a man accused
of torturing prisoners during the Algerian War; a man who lost his left eye during
an election rally brawl in 1958—the year of my birth; a man who studied law
and is well versed in manipulating it. The *fuhrer of modern France*, as the antifascists call him; the paterfamilias of a possible fascist dynasty that appears to
be imploding. Still, he's not about to let any damn woman get in his—or his
movement's—way. He'll remain on the scene, until he's out in front again, or die
trying. All of which makes my job here clear. I'll stay on the *piste*, taking my notes.

~ 100

In the news again today: Kosovo, in southern Serbia. The latest site of ethnic
cleansing, of nationalistic madness. The victims this time: Albanians. Again,
people are being mercilessly raped, tortured, shot, then loaded onto trucks and
dumped into hastily dug graves, the earth bulldozed to hide any evidence of the
crime. Fifty-one innocent people, including twenty-five women and children.
Last week, more slaughter: twenty-four ethnic Albanians from the town of
Likošane, many badly mutilated, their eyes gouged out. A town of a thousand
residents deemed a stronghold of Albanian terrorists. Raked by machine-gun
fire, mortar, and helicopter attack, houses burned. Once again, reports of
police standing silently by, or arriving only in time to bury the dead. Those
from Likošane had the luck to be buried in front of their loved ones, a mass
funeral attended by thirty thousand, many of whom had walked for hours to
reach the site.

Who's behind these killings? Slobodan Milošević, Butcher of Serbia, spiritual kin to Hitler, wanted by the international tribunal at The Hague, a free man reelected to lead his people. Who's behind these killings? The human heart and selfish ego and its craven, murderous desire for power.

Why is all this happening now? Why such a frantic grab by so many different groups at this moment in history? Why this release of stored-up resentments? Why now? That's what the television journalists ask, standing with their microphones before the scenes of slaughter.

There are many reasons, it's very complex, the pundits say: the fall of Russia; the end of the Cold War; the lack of social structure, which allows people to fall apart, to lose their bearings, to become unglued.

All of it is a testament to what I said earlier: *we are a savage species*. It's as easy for us to kill and kill again as it is to love and then hate the one we loved, and then open our hearts to love again.

I can't help but thinking of those mass graves, of typhus and cholera and other germs released from the wounded and the dead into the air, the ground, the rivers. The dead have their own ways of speaking to the living, of linking the future back to the past.

Will it rise one day, the pox of Kosovo?

~ 101

I've been wounded, a deep heart wound, and years went by without any balm to soothe the pain. The wound was Belle, a grand, ill-fated love, a leap that led to a silent crash, one that still echoes in my heart. But not as loudly, and not as often, these days. And here I am, meeting her again for a short coffee now that we've renewed our contact. She looks different, changed.

Her blonde hair is gone; her natural color is soft brown. She's heavier than before and feels self-conscious about it. I think she looks wonderful, sensual, womanly, but I think she hears my words as charity. After smoking two packs a day, she's quit. That's when the weight came on. I look at her body and love it all the more. It's hard to imagine her without a cigarette. When we were lovers, the smoke was in her hair, in the way she would rub her fingers together while smoking. Details of intimacy. But it would frighten me too, her smoker's cough. I would imagine her lungs getting yellow, then brown, spotting. I am thrilled she finally quit.

There are other changes. Her hair is longer, her makeup perfect, her clothes fancier, her style altogether more feminine. She's dating men only. She's been in love at least twice since our breakup, once with a married man, and now she's considering another affair, again to someone who's married. I sense a trend.

You're being very French, I tease her.

It's true. She's become very French, or let herself integrate into French culture more than before. Her relationship with her parents has improved, partly, I'm sure, because she stopped sleeping with women. Privately, I feel a sadness that she's conformed to external expectations, become more hetero-sexually conventional because of her social surroundings, her need to feel supported by her family. But I have to check myself against these paternalistic feelings: *who am I to say what's right for her?* She's brought herself to this point, shed earlier identities. It's only her unhappiness that makes me think the woman who sits before me is swinging on a pendulum.

When I met her, Belle was swinging hard in one direction, as a lesbian in the ACT UP–Paris nation; now she's swinging the other way. She no longer goes to ACT UP meetings and has lost touch with many of her friends in the group, though a few friendships formed in ACT UP remain strong. Gilles is still a bestie. Her true identity, I think, lies somewhere in between the girl I fell for and this more conservative Belle. When I dated her, she wore jeans and ACT UP T-shirts, with Doc Marten boots: activist gear. Her happiness was infectious, a smile that lit up a room.

Now she's adopted a professional look, tailored, put together. Still, something looks not quite right. If the suit fit well, she'd be happier wearing it, I conclude. She's happier than she was, but she's not happy-happy. But I'm happy to see her again.

~

We make plans to meet again. On the second night, after our dinner runs late, she invites me to stay over. I debate the idea. I'm afraid of the renewed intimacy, of feeling my great sadness in this same apartment where our love fell apart. But I take the chance. She makes up a little bed for me on the sofa and sleeps in the other room. In the morning, she crawls next to me and we hold each other and my eyes are full of tears. *I've missed her so much.*

Her own feelings remain veiled. If she feels sadness, I don't see it. I think she's keeping her feelings in check; all of them. Not just her feelings about me or any other lover but her overall feelings about everything. I sense that she misses me and is happy to have me back in her life. I don't need more, not now. I wanted a bridge, a reconnection, and now I have it. We can move forward from here. When we part, it's not for the last time but with the knowledge that though our lives are separate, we still love each other.

XIX

New York

~ 102

I'm back in the East Village again, back in the thicket of my life, which is how everything feels. My relationship with Bridget isn't resolved; it remains a bit of a mess. She's not happy at all, and we may break up for good after the summer, but I'm too worn out to worry about it much more than I have. I haven't finished my draft and now time's up—I have to begin producing my new HIV magazine, *HIV Plus*, a huge project. It's all on my shoulders. My idea, my baby. Still, I don't feel that stressed. I feel like making a schedule and keeping to it, cutting out time for each thing every day and making sure I take naps in the park and get in some beach time too.

The gay and lesbian film festival is coming up soon; so is another International AIDS Conference. When was the first one I went to? Twelve years ago? Something like that. And here I still am, still hammering away at that damn virus whose genetic structure I study every day for clues, for weakness. I know we will overcome it, sooner or later. When? How? And then, later, will it re-emerge? When? How? In a thousand years will this pox be a Darwinian winner or loser?

Tomorrow, I go to see my father and my sister. Bridget's coming too, which makes me very happy. Despite our problems, I think we'll have a nice time. Visit Savannah and let Bridget see a little more of my life, my family, how it's been for me to live with total heartbreak about my sister for the twenty-plus years since her nervous breakdown. My own heart flexes defensively, preparing itself for a familiar anguish.

After Savannah, Bridget is leaving for California and then to spend two months traveling alone or with a friend in Thailand and Vietnam. We'll have a separation. I might join her in Vietnam after that, if things feel better between us. For now, we both think time apart would do us good. We need a break. Not a breakup, but some space. At least that's how I feel about it. I worry Bridget will change her mind once she's away. But it's something we agree should happen.

~ 103

May Days

Almost summer. I just dyed my hair jet black, got rid of the very nice brilliant red with hints of black that I dyed it on my fortieth birthday. Three months to this day. Blood colors, very vibrant. The red matched my mood, set a tone for this decade. Bold. Anyway, I'm happy. Did I say that already? I feel good today, relaxed, enjoying my afternoon of writing, the smell of coconut pomade in my hair, my chipped, cherry-red nails, a warm cup of coffee. My body aches a little as it seems to these years. I'm older, remember, with traces of arthritis — or is it Lyme disease? — in my fingers as I type. So much not done, so much done, so much undone. *How much more time for me?*

By now, you know I think this way, with a ticking clock in my head. I don't take any of this for granted. None of it. Today is happiness, flowing. For all of these minutes.

~ 104

June 1998

Bridget and I have officially separated for the summer, but maybe forever. It's hard to write this; harder to say it. Even harder to feel it. Actually, we crumbled under pressure. The difficulties we've experienced for months have become the dance, the almost daily backdrop to our relationship. Try as we might — and we have tried — the dynamic hasn't changed enough for us to find our rhythm, our happiness.

Bridget feels more strongly than ever that she needs to be released, to release herself, to feel stronger, to get some perspective. That this isn't the relationship for her; not in its present form and not under the present circumstances. For now, we haven't canceled my trip to see her in Vietnam in August, but until then, we're apart. We're free to do or not do what we want, and with whom, on opposite sides of the planet. And we're not going to discuss any of it on the phone when we talk.

What pleases me, it seems, is work and writing. I don't want to think about relationships, except to pray (in my own way) that I'll make the right decisions in this one. I've gotten confused by the conflicts with Bridget, less certain of my own needs. The time alone will be good for me too, much as I miss her and am afraid I've lost her—or will—forever. The hope is that a radical break will preserve the future, the hope we still carry of working something out. I feel myself constantly holding my breath and have to remind myself to release it. There's the old fear of the unknown and of being alone, which makes me compare myself to other friends who are in happier, coupled relationships, who have regular passionate sex. *What's wrong with me? Nothing, you're fine. You've set up some bad dynamics with your lover. Bad timing.*

That's what friends tell me, and I know they're partly right, but I can't help blaming myself. An old, bad habit in itself, the self-blame game. Not one that's very helpful, as they remind me, but I can't shake it. I feel like a failure; like I've failed her. Rationally, I know we're in this together; that she's failed me too, in myriad big and small ways. I believe in committed love, and my love includes carrying forward exes into family. But that takes maturity and working through personal insecurity. I still believe I made the right choice, to live with Jersey, to love her in our new family way. But not at the cost of losing Bridget or making her feel anything less than adored. So I'm stuck with self-reproach, wishing my efforts had paid off. I tried. My love was and is true. It's a sad story that began with such promise. Such dizzying promise. *Is this chapter two or the end?* I don't know. I can't predict. I'm Dorothy in Oz, wishing I could click my red heels and go home again. To Bridget, that is.

⁓

I am home, of course. Home in myself. No need to be so dramatic. Grounded despite this turmoil. Trying to adopt an attitude of curiosity about the future, not anxiety. Smart advice I got from a therapist years ago. I'm doing the same with regard to Sel and my journey of research for this book. An antinovel, I sometimes think. A dubious memoir. The writing and voices that aren't separate from me. That flow when I release my brain from its wallowing. That keeps me preoccupied and increasingly excited, even though I'm not sleeping well again.

It's not only because I miss Bridget. It's because of Sel and Henri and how I've gotten closer to them and to newer characters who've sprung up when I've developed scenes for Sel's story: Lolita, a young ball-breaker; and Torn Stockings, an addict-hooker who's organized some regiment of streetwalkers; and other voices and characters with fictional biographies that spring into my mind when I take my little daily walks, my somnambulist's reveries.

Except I'm not in Paris; I'm in Manhattan, as if it mattered. It doesn't seem to. I'm obsessed, Jersey tells me, forgetting to eat and losing all track of time. Writing for hours at a stretch in a fugue of creativity. De Quincey land, without opium. It's as close to happiness as writing can make me. Time, expanding before me in the present and behind me, far into history. *Action=Life. Being=Writing.*

Two weeks later. I'm missing Bridget. A slow burn in my stomach. Hard not to call long-distance, to ask, *Hey, how are you? What are you doing today? What's new?* I'm practicing emotional discipline, a necessity and a bore. In my mind, the phone lines are humming, far under the sea. Singing, pulsing. I'm speaking to Bridget anyway, sending her my thoughts. Testing my psychic powers.

    What are you thinking, love? Are you having fun over there? Are you happy or sad? Do you feel stronger? Have you met a boy to fuck yet? I know you want to. A girl? I hope so / hope not. I do want you to be happy. I'd be jealous if you have an affair. I hope you're taking all the space you need. That you feel good alone. I'm sending you my good vibes, my protection against harm. I wish we could talk. Are you thinking about me?

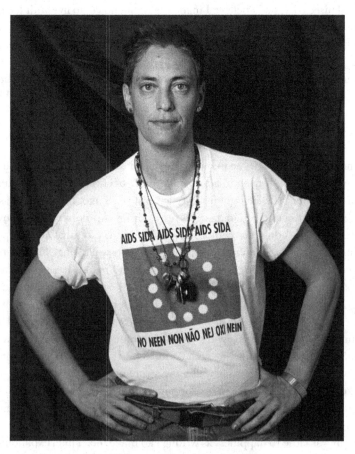

Author portrait, 1990s. (Bill Bytsura/The AIDS Activist Project)

~ 105

I talked with Sebastien today. He's become his own expert about HIV, started reading articles online. He's read some of my pieces. His hair's grown back, but now another problem has developed. After weeks on a non-nuke combo, he says his body is changing: he's got muscle definition he never had. He's lost some weight in his ass. At first, that was wonderful—he had the leaner gym body he's always dreamed of having—but now he's worried about it. The veins are popping in his arms and legs like a bodybuilder. But he hasn't lost any weight; if anything, he's gained a little in his belly. And he's freaked out.

I'm scared my coworkers will notice it, he adds. *At first I liked losing my butt, but I don't want to look like a freak. I want my old butt back. What can I do? What should I do?*

Calling Action Jackson. What can I do? What should I do? No easy answers this time either, but some clues. As luck (or fate) would have it, I've been researching this particular phenomenon called lipodystrophy. A redistribution of fat. You lose it in one place and develop it in another. It gives you a pot belly and skinny arms like someone who's been doing chemo for years. Crix belly—a side effect of Crixivan. Makes some women grow giant breasts and turns others into humpbacks with buffalo lumps of fat. You can suck it out surgically, but it may come back. It puts you at a high risk for a heart attack. Losing your ass isn't merely a cosmetic issue. This is a serious health risk. Unfortunately, no one knows exactly what causes this problem. There are theories but not much data. But, again, the drugs are clearly the culprit.

Really, Sebastien says in a small voice. *I read about the other stuff, the fat stuff, but not about the heart attack. I already have high cholesterol.*

I'll get back to you, Sebastien, I say. His body may be adjusting, but I'm concerned about one of the drugs. *But just to be safe maybe you should smoke less and cut down on the mayo.*

It's advice he's heard for years, the same advice we all get. Basic good health advice.

Yeah, I know, he says. *Not gonna happen.*

~

You have two choices, I inform Sebastien a few days later after doing more research and interviewing several leading specialists. *Same as before. Go off the meds or switch them. If the side effects go away, you'll know it's not permanent damage.* I tell him to talk to his doctor first, ask for a CAT scan. *If you've got a wad of fat around your intestines, then that's a bad sign.* There's going to be a discussion of lipodystrophy at the AIDS conference in two weeks; I'm going. If he can wait until then, and I think he can, then we'll know more.

One week later, the CAT scan results are in. Dark shapes of fat in the belly that could be mistaken for a tumor. Sebastien's voice wavers on the telephone. Major panic. Uncertainty. Fear. His new trinity.

I'm thinking of going off, he says. *I can't handle this. My doctor says going off for a short period of time isn't likely to hurt me too much. My viral load is still undetectable. If it goes back up quickly, I'll go back on. But I want my body back. I'll wait until you get back from Geneva.*

Whatever you need to do, I tell him, *I'll be there for you. I think you've made a good decision. If it feels good to you, it's right.* I add lightly, *There's no clear wrong or right here, there's only rock and roll. Keep me posted. I'll definitely call you from Geneva.*

Who made me God, even this small a god? I feel nervous after our call. I take a deep breath. There are times I want to be a real doctor like my father, not a self-taught science nerd journo. Moments like this when I want deeper knowledge and a personal experience of treating the body myself to draw on, to make me assess the state of research. The clinicians I've spoken to so far don't really understand why this lipid problem is happening as it is. There's no clear consensus for the moment, just best guesses. Protease inhibitors are still new; each body and person has a unique health history, genetic profile, evolving immune system. There's no cookie-cutter approach to HIV treatment, never has been. It more like sailing uncharted waters: catch the wind and tack, and if you hit the shoals, tack again.

~ 106

Right now there's something mysterious happening in my body, in my hands, causing my knuckles to swell and hurt a bit. Some minor inner battle and body adjustment taking place, something I've exposed myself to. It's my joints again; they're hurting a little.

I look at my hands: they're my mother's, an exact replica. But my wrists are bigger, my arms muscular from years of playing competitive tennis. I started playing at thirteen, got a scholarship to Rollins College, number two in women's tennis after Trinity. Sports kept me away from drugs and possible trouble as a teenager—my parents' initial goal. But by my sophomore year, I was bored and I had barely overcome a worsening case of anorexia from playing too many sports all day and not eating enough to compensate. Extreme exercise. It helped me cope with stress. My sister had come home, changed, suicidal, so very depressed and sick. My parents were on the verge of divorce, heartbroken, needing someone to blame. I had convinced them to have my sister live near me, at a halfway house up the street from the Rollins campus. But it was too much. She ran away, trying to get back to Harvard, to her old life. She got attacked, got returned. I was on high alert, vigilant, protective, heartbroken too. I exercised my anxiety away.

How can we know where life will take us? I was on one track, then radically on another. New York sealed my fate. M helped, thank god. She was my best friend, a rock; so was her mother, Mary. My second mother.

Then one day on a summer trip to Europe after freshman year, M surprised me, kissed me, woke me from some deep-freeze state of sexual slumber as in a fairy tale. I was that far in the closet, unaware even to myself of what I might desire, the result of Catholic repression and my father's intense disapproval of homosexuality. Or just a super-late bloomer.

New York and Barnard and M opened me up, gave me a view of what life might offer, who I might be. I didn't give up tennis immediately, but it couldn't compete as before. I wanted to head downtown with M to meet Paul, who was swishy gay and an actor and NYU student who knew the best dance clubs. I was lost, unsure what I wanted to study. But I was hungry now, for everything.

Under my thumb, where I'm pressing my wrist now, is a tattoo I got in New Orleans a long time ago: *gran vi*. As in *big life* in Kreyol, after *grande vie* in French. I designed it myself, rough-looking like a prison tattoo. There's a small cross between the words—the vodou crossroads of life. It was my Haitian grand-mother's secret religion, the one she would consider when the Catholic saints had failed to satisfy her prayers. A religion of dances, where a believer communes with the spirits, with forces at work beyond what is visible, with one's own dead in a realm between heaven and earth, between sky and sea, between life and death. She was superstitious, a closet mystic.

I didn't want the tattoo to be too neat or feminine. It's spelled *gran*, lower-case, only one *n*, not *grann*, with an extra *n* that would be the correct feminine syntax ending to the feminine word for life: *lavi (la vie)*. I deliberately misspelled it, drew it crude. I like imperfection, don't want too much polish. I don't want to be a man, but I embrace my androgyny, my masculinity. I didn't want to be a boy when I was young; I *was* a boy. I felt like one, acted like one. I refused to wear a shirt. I only had male role models. But I was a girl too, and that was okay. And when my body later changed, I loved all the girl parts. I've grown into my sexuality, my own sense of gender.

This tattoo is a personal reminder to live large, to take risks, to have faith in the power of forces beyond my control, to call forth my dead, my spirit guides. Before my mother died, I told her I would take her into my body; she would walk with me now. Before Johnny died, I told him the same. I'm carrying them inside me. I feel them without trying.

So, my mannish hands, my achy joints, the stiffness in my wrists today . . . is it Lyme or age or typing for hours? They're part of my big life. I'll just rub some arnica gel on them to relieve the stiffness now. And get back to my writing.

~ 107

I'm attending a special symposium this week on trends in HIV research with science bigwigs, some of the brains I most admire. The names that will stand out in a hundred years when the world looks back on this epidemic. David Ho, David Baltimore, Ron Desrosiers. As I meet with them, mingle, I feel Sel checking them out. *What do you think, Sel?* I want to know. *Are they as smart as they should be? Should I be impressed with them?*

Desrosiers is describing his new experiments, searching for a vaccine. Sel's distracting me. Desrosiers describes how he's deleting genes from a simian virus, SIV, the sister virus to HIV, and is injecting monkeys with the vaccine. The monkeys are fully protected. Sounds good, but I'm skeptical.

Next to him, hovering like a shadow, I spy Sel.

Oy Jesus. Sel's picking at her arm, looking at her blood under a microscope in Desrosier's lab, delighted by the swimming world she sees. She's thinking about her own experiments to come, about her slow-acting pox. Or whether Henri and his friends can steal a boat from the river police to take her to Nogent, site of a nuclear facility, to fish for giant mutant carp. Narrative questions she's mulling on my behalf, her creator, since I have to occupy myself with a life outside our imaginary shared world, support myself as a science journo. It's making me feel a bit schizo today, I have to admit, though not schizo like my sister. More like very distracted, à la De Quincey. Daydreaming, the nectar of my childhood, though I'm hardly bored. I'm fascinated by simian viruses.

During a session break, I go downstairs to discover a row of display cases with early microscopes and beautifully handblown glass flasks used to trap and grow bacteria. Here are filters used to passage rabbit viruses, to make them stronger or weaker. Sel would love to steal this equipment, test it to passage her poxes the old-fashioned way, from person to person, starting with herself.

Outside, the weather is gorgeous. Inside my mind, Sel's happy too, stretching out on the banks of the river, taking a break from me. I feel less lonely with her here, so present in my mind. Every time I think about Bridget, I hear Sel's voice saying: *Stop. Stop thinking about her and stay here with me. You have work to do.*

Yes, general. Mistress Sel. It makes me smile. I wish Bridget could share these moments. I know she would fully appreciate them.

From a distance, Sel's making a face at me. A hideous face. A face that shows me her black teeth. But her eyes aren't hard, aren't cold, aren't accusing or pitying. They're soft, a very soft gray. An expression I've never seen. Gruff but tender. That's a smile meant for me. Why? What have I done to deserve this? She's saying something, something I can't hear.

Ma folle.

My crazy? *Me . . . crazy?*

Ma folle. Pointing to me with her walking stick. With a caring look in her eyes.

I see. I'm *your* crazy. Well, all right. From one poxed creature to another, I'll take that as a compliment.

XX

Vietnam

~ 108

August 1998

I'm in flight, crossing datelines and newly created borders, heading from West to East, beyond the zone of what has been familiar territory for me, watching a string of clouds appear on the endless horizon and knit itself into shapes, into faces, valleys, and puffed-up cottony kingdoms, then dissipate into thin air again.

Time travel; my favorite. I'm en route to Vietnam, land of sorrow and survival, of endless colonization and nationalistic purges, of Buddhism and Ho Chi Minh. A land where the sweet-smelling French overthrew the Chinese warlords and, for over a hundred years, established their perfume colony, built schools, cities and railroads, and picturesque villas in the choicest valleys, while they plundered the country and the women with their language and their European white man's lust for empire.

Like all Americans, I think, I feel a certain historical connection to this faraway land, this Vietnam. A mix of curiosity and regret that comes from the recognition of America's terrible war here, the lingering trauma. But I feel interest too, in a people and culture I've learned about from a former roommate. I'm looking forward to the cities, the trains, the art, and the objects of the culture in particular—ordinary objects that I find so beautiful when I travel abroad. I'm planning days in the street markets, temples, corner noodle shops.

Most of all, I'm looking forward to seeing Bridget. The silence has gone on for too long and I'm not at all certain we're good. But she's excited to see me, she said in a recent static-filled phone call, and I'm hoping the trip has not only rejuvenated her, which she says it has, but opened her heart to us again as well. She's been in Thailand, traveling solo and with the elephants. A fantastic trip that has restored her good humor and her spirits. I'm so happy about that. I haven't had as happy a time, but I've kept myself busy too.

There's an undercurrent to our conversation having to do with the other people we may have met or spent time with during this break. I've seen a woman I met two years ago for a casual, yet intense—what should I call it?—*affairlet*. An affair that represents a past trigger of pain to Bridget. Something that took place early in our time together in New York, when we were still undefined as a couple but dating. An affair she viewed then and still views as a betrayal, a sign of my failure to be trustworthy.

I look back at that same event, the circumstances, and see that Bridget set a secret test for me; one I failed. I think it's worth going into here, because it represents, more than anything, a miscommunication—to me, anyway. A failure on my part, but on hers too; a failure to read each other right, to express ourselves clearly enough. This affair caused a fissure that became, over time, a serious rupture in our relationship and that widened as the drama with the Jersey triangle unfolded.

The initial incident occurred two months after Bridget arrived in New York. We were still undefined then, newly in lust-love and feeling our way. She had been seeing someone casually back in San Francisco; I had had Jessie. We weren't talking about monogamy yet, just about enjoying our time together. We had great passion; it wasn't easy to contain. And we're both intense people who crave connection. But at that time, we were still in a let's-get-to-know-each-other-better rhythm. By July, the tensions over my living with Jersey had already cropped up. I wanted a break, some solo time.

That's when I went to the Michigan Womyn's Music Festival, just for a day or two, as a side trip to visiting my birthplace, Marquette. I had decided to have a little vacation, to revisit the house where I was born. Jersey was going to be in Michigan too, in Ann Arbor, where she had gone to college. She was traveling to a concert with her new lover, a rising pop star and somewhat of a lesbian celebrity. I wanted to show Jersey I had moved on, and it was okay that she had moved on too. Of course, I felt some jealousy, more like envy. *Her new girlfriend is an actual rock star? Dang. She's going to meet all these fancy people in Hollywood, go to lots of parties.*

How is it that we can fail to see the obvious? I didn't and I got blindsided. Before leaving for the festival, Bridget had teased me, warned me about the wild, sexy romps that had given the Michigan Womyn's Music Festival its reputation, aside from the granola-crunchy music. *You know, everybody there sleeps with everybody else,* she had said, raising a touchy subject. *That's what happens there. So, if you meet someone, well, go ahead. Enjoy yourself. But tell me about it—that's all I'm asking.* I'm paraphrasing here, but it's her tone that I remember. My version of the rules we agreed to.

I remember protesting too, thinking that the *last thing I wanted* was to engage with someone new. I was already tense over the jealousy that was mounting between Bridget and Jersey. I remember thinking: *Why are you saying this? Is there someone you want to sleep with?* But I kept my mouth shut. *I'm not planning on that,* I told her, and I meant it. *But good to know. Glad I have your permission.*

Never say never. I think I was on the grounds of the festival for about five minutes before a woman approached me and said, with a sweet smile, *You're welcome to sleep in my tent.* It was pouring rain, and I had arrived empty-handed, without even a tent and only one night's change of clothes. Just a dainty pink umbrella. It was almost the last day of the festival, and I was planning to crash in the tent of a Seattle friend, Djayne. *Uh, no thanks,* I said, and never saw her again. But that definitely set the tone for what I discovered was, quite rightly, a lesbian bacchanal. It was indeed Woodstock for lesbians. Naked breasts everywhere. Very, *very* friendly women sticking their heads in one's tent to offer food, a massage, or an invitation to a sex or menstruation workshop.

———

Could I have avoided sleeping with someone in Michigan? Of course. But I had been given Bridget's teasing permission to have some fun. I had deliberately come on the second-to-the-last night, not certain I would like it at all. Too much estrogen; too many hairy women's legs. But I was pleasantly surprised. It was quite fun, and very easy to meet people. Especially with a little weed.

I hadn't known my friend was a major pothead, but I learned at Michfest. So was her friend. They were both stoners, single, and into having playful sex. I was trying to sleep. I felt like grandma: *Can you keep it down?* I declined the offer of a threesome, and even a twosome, with my very stoned friend, Djayne—who had suddenly gotten much friendlier. Eventually, though, I slipped over to the other side. Not with her, but with her friend from Chicago, a cute, very sweet Jewish woman with a business card that read Sex Goddess. I really should have known, shouldn't I? I know. But hey, shit happens. *As in Vegas, as at Michfest.*

And so I had my Michigan moment. It was delightful and light and everything you want those moments to be. And, afterward, I felt happy, sobered up, but just a little worried about Bridget. Before anything happened, I had given full disclosure. *I have a girlfriend,* I told the Sex Goddess. I had explained my house rules. I told her Bridget might not be thrilled, but she would probably be okay. I would just have to tell her. It was a moment of fun. That's all it was meant to be.

Wrong. Wrong. Wrong!

It wasn't okay with Bridget. *Not at all.* Unfortunately, it was a test and I had failed it. Bridget hadn't meant it, after all. She *assumed* I would understood that. When I called on the way home, finally out of the Michigan woods, I stopped at a gas station to call her. She got really, really upset. *Couldn't believe it.* Couldn't believe the woman was still with me too, because I had offered to give her and another woman a ride back to the city, to catch a plane. *She's still with you? Right now. In the car? And you're calling me to tell me this? Really?*

⌒

The incredulity in Bridget's voice will haunt me forever. Truly, I had been more than clueless in failing her test. I was an ass; an insensitive idiot!

Looking back, I can see from her perspective how it all seemed. But from my seat, it didn't feel that way. I had had a moment in a tent, with pot, with pushy naked lesbians determined to see me play too. And the Sex Goddess had asked for a ride out of the campsite at the last minute because her ride had taken off. She asked; I said yes. But no matter. Bridget was incensed. And I was so sorry—so very sorry. I had wanted to call but there was no reception in the woods; I had had to wait. I had called the minute I could. I knew it wouldn't be an easy conversation, but I didn't expect such a tsunami. Bridget, however, read this the way a new lover might: as seriously threatening; as a true betrayal. It was our first big failure—mine, anyway—in her mind.

⌒

Today, I trace the fissure that's deepened between Bridget and me to that moment, to that test and my failure to see through it. I felt terrible: guilty, and later a bit set up too. I had believed her, I had. Had she intimated how she really felt, I wouldn't have been open to a spontaneous be-free-in-the-woods Michfest moment. And maybe she was angry with herself too, privately. She hadn't wanted to appear insecure, so she had presented me with false bravado. And I had taken the bait.

She could have told me the truth. That she wanted strict monogamy. But that would have been risky: to risk appearing vulnerable, afraid; drawing a line that I might not like. Except, honestly, I would've been fine with that. I didn't need that Michigan moment. I wasn't actively seeking it. I had opened up to it in part because of our prefestival discussion. It was all a bad miscommunication, but it blew up in my face. I had really hurt Bridget. I really hurt myself too because I was in love with Bridget, and I wanted to make a life with her.

Lesson learned: I should've gotten into some other girl's tent, not a stoner pal and a cute sex goddess friend looking for naughty fun. And I need to be honest: the Sex Goddess was hot, she was. And great, and fun. And I felt for a second like, *Damn, I can't pursue this because I'm with Bridget and I want to be. But what a great girl!*

But I was also clear: I was in love with Bridget.

All of this reflects a pattern that's continued in our relationship. I can't do right; that's how it feels. And the more Bridget feels that I'm not quite right for her, not to be trusted with her sensitive heart, the more she pushes me away. So, I'll take responsibility for being a fool, as Kiki would say, for taking Bridget at her word and for getting it really wrong. For living a bit. Even for hearing what I wanted to hear, which is how she saw and still sees it. But I know we're in a dance and it takes two. Her part includes setting little traps for me to fall into, to prove I'll fail her, that I'm not a safe partner. Mine is to take the bait, to want to prove I'm worthy. Clearly, we've had plenty of fodder for a therapist.

A little while after Michigan, the Sex Goddess, who actually lives in Seattle, came to New York to visit friends. I was one, she hoped. Instead of a bundle of fun, she met an uptight, shut-down woman: me. *The timing was wrong*, I told her. I had chosen Bridget. I still wanted to sleep with her and we fooled around a little later. That was after Bridget had opened up the space for us a bit, wanting her own space to fool around with someone, a revenge space, as I thought of it. But I had cut my MichFest affair short and only resumed it, a bit, this summer. Our rules had changed, and Bridget set them this time. She wanted to be single this summer and not have to report back to me. So I was free to see the Sex Goddess.

Again, it would be dishonest to say I don't or didn't enjoy my time with the Sex Goddess; I do; I did. She's very sweet. But I miss Bridget and I'm deeply in love and heartbroken and thinking about her all the time. I miss her and I'm scared. I wanted to spend my life with her, and instead, I lost her.

What am I going to find now? Are we going to make this work? That's the question that's hung over the spring, and now the summer. That's what we agreed to think about, during our trial separation. A two-month break to be apart, think, feel, and come back together. To be free.

For me, this time without Bridget has been mixed. I've really missed her but I haven't missed the drama. I hope that if we remain lovers, we're both able to be happy. And if we can't, well, I'll try to make my peace with that too. I just wish I knew what she was thinking right now.

Postscript: It was so great to see Bridget, but also really hard. She took some major space to find herself on the trip, and she's very wary of coming closer to me again, wary of losing that center. It's so good to see her happy again, to see her laughing. For now, we're moving very slowly, taking it day by day. Our romantic relationship is in a kind of limbo. We're sort of back together but we just had a real separation and we can't just pick up where we were before. Things feel tentative. Both of us recognize that the problems we had earlier aren't gone.

The difference is that Bridget's regained her happiness, the light that she had when we first met me, the joy. And that's spilled over into her feelings for me. I can feel it—an openness that wasn't there before; that's been missing for months. It makes me so happy.

～ 109

There's another big, big reason for Bridget's happiness, something that's thrown a wrench in everything. A major event—a *huge* event—that unfurled just when I arrived to meet her. One that's changed everything for the foreseeable future—for her and for us too, in ways we aren't yet completely sure of. *What happened?* Well, here's the short version.

During her trip, Bridget decided to try for the dream she had long talked about: a baby. She had a brief affair with someone. There's a backstory to all of this—how we found out, how we felt, what it means for her, and me, and well, us. But, for now, it means that we're back together, in some fashion, as a couple, and she's definitely having a baby.

We've been talking for the last weeks about our relationship and what's going to happen. She's asked me to consider co-parenting, but only if, as she puts it, I sign on for real. Of course that's the only way I would do it, and I feel clear about my response.

A baby? A child? Yes. Of course. I would be honored and committed to helping raise this child for the long haul. Even though our romantic future is still cloudy, I tell her, I'll co-parent. But if I do, it's for the rest of my life. Because we might not work out; we could break up one day. And I take my commitments seriously.

Of course, there's another triangle involved, though not a romantic one, for once. Bridget's best friend, Sorcha, is also on the scene, and she'll be helping too. They're still living together in Brooklyn, but after the New Year, Bridget and I may get a place together. What matters most to me right now is being able to love Bridget and support her. That's what I want. The fact that she's having a baby is fantastic. That *we're* having a baby, I should say. It's a *we* now; I'm on board. I'm thrilled. I wanted to have children myself but always felt afraid to bear one, because of my family's health history, my sister's mental illness. Worried about bad genes. Plus, I don't sleep with men; that complicates baby-making a little bit. It's hard for lesbians to adopt. Still, I had always dreamed of being a parent, assumed somehow that I would have a brood.

And here now is Bridget, the woman I love, despite the rocky shoals we hit. I'm so thankful she pursued this dream and that she's invited me to share it, to build it, even if the overall shape of the future isn't completely clear.

As for me, I've started dreaming. Dreaming of the baby. *The unnamed, un-known, beautiful one that is coming.*

XXI

New York

~ 110

Spring 1999

The Crazy Girls call from France. Where have I been? Why don't I call? They've tried all the telephone numbers I've given them. *You're hiding*, says French Ann in her latest message, adding, *Où ça? Where?*

In the land of idiots. Among those who work too much, too hard, for long hours, until there is nothing left but a shell. And this they crawl into, grabbing a moment to sleep, hiding from the world they've neglected. I've been working, nonstop, for weeks.

When they finally reach me, one morning at 6:00 a.m., they apologize for the early hour. I tell them I'm just going to sleep, but for once I haven't been working—I've been talking with friends; I've been laughing; I've walked around the city noticing how much it has changed for the worse. Gentrifying. Turning Soho into a rich tourist draw, no longer a home for artists with cheap warehouse lofts. I've pulled the kind of late-night trawl that feeds my soul even though I'm tired now. I've been dreaming of a baby, and the life that is developing, with Bridget.

They give me an update on Le Pen, which I've asked for; tell me there are two new books out. One is an exposé about all the corporations that support the National Front. *Complètement dégo*, they say. The other one is a novel in which the writer has modeled his characters after Le Pen and his crowd. It sounds a bit like the idea for my book, no? they ask. *Should they just send me the books?*

Sure. Why not? I want to see what others are writing. I'm glad someone's publishing these books. They're my allies. They haven't written my book, because Sel is in my head, and her story is unique. No one else could even imagine her voice, her rants. I'm not overly concerned. Just a bit envious. I'm making progress, I'm writing, but I won't be done for some time.

French Ann confirms what I've been reading in the *Times*: that Le Pen has made a comeback, despite his political ban. The National Front has split into two camps, and wily Le Pen seems to have an edge over his ex-protégé Bruno Mégret. He went so far as to publicly denounce his eldest daughter, Marie-Caroline, on television, for abandoning him in support of Mégret and their new offshoot rival party. She was a fool in love, thinks Papa Le Pen; she was influenced by her boyfriend to jump ship. *Love makes us idiots.*

Le Pen's also made some surprise gains in the south, with the help of his youngest daughter, Marine, who's declared her plan to assume the family mantle one day. She's a lawyer and said to be tough and therefore less likely to become a fool in love, one assumes.

~ 111

The dawn at 6:00 a.m. is soft in my bedroom. I'm confronted with the passage of time. I've been too slow, haven't I? Other writers have beaten me to it—to the task of exposing the rising populist French Far Right? But that wasn't really my only goal, was it? Everyone in France knows about Le Pen. It's more his neighbor I'm concerned about. Those who would elect a wolf. The ordinary man and woman, the civil servants like old Papon whose pensions are disappearing in a troubled economy. Who live in a proud nation with hurt memories. One drummed out of colonies, with a faltering economy, rising crime, and many would-be citizens who aren't Catholic or white or speaking French as their mother tongue.

My book isn't merely about France, either. It's just as much about America and AIDS and our cultural holy wars here too. I'm talking to my inner critic, the one that keeps seeking to silence and distract my creative voice, that reminds me of pressing workaday realities, the new protests being planned to demand fast-track compassionate-use release of one of the newer drugs.

I climb into bed, fully dressed. I half-doze, listening to the Crazy Girls go on about the freezing weather in Paris, about a new apartment one of them found, about how they might stop by New York on their way to Argentina and Bolivia in March. I can feel the wine I drank earlier. Not too much, but enough to invite a minor hangover.

Someone's listening in on our gossipy conversation. A group. I can feel their silent, internal presence: Sel; then Henri; Torn Stockings; Lolita, the impudent tartelette; Madame Paule, an exile from Rwanda who's turned up in their midst recently. A seasoned ally of ethnic wars. And there is Piglet, the child with watery veins.

I feel each of them inside me, awake, ready to live. They aren't impatient or critical tonight, not frustrated that I haven't released their voices, their stories. They're simply waiting for me, the orchestra director, poised to play their song whenever I choose. *If I choose.*

The Crazy Girls and I compare notes about life as we near the new millennium: the weird weather—El Niño and La Niña—the continuing fall of the stock market in Asia; the arrest of Pinochet; the demonstrations against Rudy Giuliani in New York; the ongoing huge good news about HIV protease drugs; the celebration of Christmas in Cuba. And about our ongoing losses, in ACT UP and in my circle: the boys, the men who fought the good fight—Aldyn and Kiki and Assotto and Johnny and Oui. And the women too. We lost several beautiful souls. The multi-rooted, many-branched tree of the poxed fallen.

It's early but it's late, I tell my good friends in Paris at last, saying *adieu. Keep me posted. Keep sending pictures.*

I turn on the computer to look at new pictures they've sent over to share: snapshots of a fresh ACT UP–Paris demonstration. In the background of one of them, I see a poster for the National Front. Someone has drawn a Hitler mustache on the fearless leader, Jean-Marie Le Pen. It continues to be an effective universal haiku. *Facho!*

The pictures give me some ideas, more plotlines for Sel's campaign against the Right, more biography about the budding personalities that make up her dirty-faced clan.

It's early but it's late. Am I too late? I worry about that.

Before falling asleep, I hear the reply. Sel's voice, almost annoyed at me for raising this question. *Listen up, my friend. When it comes to truth, or justice, there's never a statute of limitations.*

~ 112

I barely remember shutting my eyes. But it's almost noon. I'm awake and being prodded to wake further. I have work to do. I should get up, get coffee. The hangover I feared hasn't hit but could still emerge. I should take an aspirin. Instead I stay put. I'm like a recovering stroke patient, alert behind closed lids, not yet ready to tempt movement. I imagine walking downstairs to the corner store to buy a to-go coffee. I think we're all out in the kitchen. A small tragedy.

But someone is up, someone's moving. I hear her talking to herself, to me, from outside the bedroom door, as clearly as ever. Her grinding voice, like the dull blade of a machete being sharpened against stone, to cut through the wine-fueled fog of my late-night reverie.

Il est beau de rêver, she says. *Mais après il faut agir.* It's great to dream. But then it's time to act.

Get up my friend. It's time.

Time for what?

Il est trop tôt, I protest. *I need to sleep some more.* But the voice is there. I can't ignore it. My inner pest.

Il est tôt, mais il est tard. It's early but it's late.

I hear a rustling on the window ledge. The pigeons aren't asleep either, apparently. It's a conspiracy, to get me up, and it's working. *Fine, I'm up,* even if my eyes are still half-closed. Outside, the world is far too awake. I want to stay dreaming.

———

Where are you taking me now?

Sel is moving faster than an old lady should move, especially one whose crooked left leg drags a little as she rounds a corner. I can glimpse where she's headed—to a party, to some street festival. I've been here before. I recognize the music. *La Marseillaise.*

I see the banners of the National Front and their youth corps, led by Jean-Marie Le Pen, dressed formally in white, wearing a French tricolor red-white-blue sash. Beside him are two of his daughters, Marie-Caroline and Marine, dressed alike in matching white business suits. Ready for God and a job as a corporate CEO. I see a choir of white schoolchildren, also wearing white: long, white skirts; long shorts; and short-sleeved shirts with neatly draped red, white, and blue French tricolor neck kerchiefs and bowties for the boys. I see rows of nuns and young seminarians, all dressed equally in white. Many have a picture of the pope pinned to their clothes.

Welcome to the new Crusades, Sel says to me. *Our friends have been busy.*

I read the flyers handed out by the children. An invitation to walk across France, from city to city, to gather the flock. A millennial Crusade. The organizers are taking their processional very seriously; they've actually brought the animal flock with them too, a Noah's Ark of sheep, horses, chickens, roosters, and doves—a dozen cages of white doves. The optics, as an advertiser would say, are fantastic.

The National Front has taken a page from ACT UP and recognized the power of drama, of theater. The True Believers will march across France, into the shopping malls of Les Halles, over to the slums they usually take pains to avoid, into the communities where many mother tongues are spoken and French is the second language of most residents, though their children and grandchildren can all swear in French as well as salty-tongued French Ann.

The Crusaders plan to march to the intersections of corner mosques across France, to confront the sons and daughters of another prophet, Mohammed, also kneeling in devotion. A war of prayers will follow. They're going to set up the Stations of the Cross, with a stop in every bidonville. They'll double as recruiting centers.

I look into the farther corners of the Place de l'Hôtel de Ville, the magnificent stage of historic events in France. It's the ultimate royalist backdrop. Perfect for the launch of the populist Right's *get-out-the-vote* campaign.

Look closely, Sel says. *Consider the future. Even our friends appear tempted to join this party.*

~

Down an alley, a contingent of the faithless, the dying, and the sick are enjoying a free meal. Some lean on a large wooden festival float on wheels—a giant icon of Saint Joan of Arc, wearing a cape with the words *Flame de la Nation* on it. Flame of the Nation. They've come for the food but they take the handout rosaries too.

Sel accepts a rosary from a young girl.

Beyond them, I see an AIDS banner. But the faces have changed. The boys of ACT UP are so much older now. The once-hot young boys who danced in after-hours clubs in short-shorts and go-go army boots, now sporting balding pates and modest potbellies. A gay couple moves past us with a pram, wiping jam off the faces of an infant. They're headed toward a baptism fountain that looms to our right. The fountain is on wheels too. It will accompany the Crusaders. A moveable Resurrection.

Several *sans papiers* homeless advocates are manning the buffet table, offering food to the elderly survivors of Vichy, the veterans of foreign wars. I spy a mound of mini-baguettes, set beside small guillotine-shaped bread slicers. The pious choir children break ranks, slip away from the nuns, squabble happily among themselves for a chance to use the tiny guillotines.

The smell of sardines overwhelms us. I see Madame Paule, a proud Tutsi survivor, born in Rukara, next to the forest park of Akagera, where the *genocidaires* are hiding, dreaming anew of Hutu Power. She's taking charge of the commerce, making sure the other members of her Rwandan family, the newer émigrés, are paying attention to the needs of fussy customers. They've grilled their salted fish, wrapped them in cellophane paper with pretty tricolored ribbons. The women take the coins and slip them into tricolored handkerchiefs, stuff these into their bosoms. They'll make a decent profit today, because, for once, the police won't harass them.

The police are here too, of course, waiting to escort the Crusaders to the edges of the city. Down a side alley, other African faces, members of local churches, sway in quiet song. They know every word of the Marseillaise, hum it through thick French accents.

⌒⌐

We'll find her here. Sel pulls me over. The crowd is thick, like the lines of tourists who flock to the Louvre and Euro Disney. Twenty feet ahead, Torn Stockings looks transformed, healthier than I could have previously imagined, no longer a bony frame with fake boobs but a modestly dressed woman well past thirty. She's wearing a lovely flowered dress and a hat. She looks like a church lady, I think, like a French mother attending the annual Easter Mass.

Torn Stockings, lifelong junkie-whore, has cleaned up her act like some of my friends in New York are doing, slowly and steadily. She's happily sipping an apple cider, chatting with her new family, a Marais chapter of Narcotics Anonymous. She's raised her hand; she wants to speak. She wants to talk about her greatest regret, her abandonment of her children, to smack.

I'm ready to atone, she tells them. *I'm ready to ask for forgiveness. I don't deserve to be forgiven, I know, but I'm asking my Higher Power anyway.* Looking past her, I see that other 12-step recovery meetings are taking place all along the side alleys of the street adjacent to the Place de l'Hôtel de Ville. A sprinkling of folding chairs with the tell-tale 12-step book placed on the seat, the contemporary sinner's Bible. Small tables with glasses and pitchers of water to help when the words dry up.

⌒⌐

We keep walking. Up ahead, standing on a small, elevated box like a town crier, Piglet is holding up brochures. He's with the hemophiliac contingent. I see he's wearing whites too. Except he's not a small, delicate boy anymore. He's become a twenty-year-old National Front youth ambassador, wearing tennis whites and sneakers with tricolored laces. He's put his name in as a mayoral candidate and is eyeing the National Assembly in a few years. He's studying the law. He's a young rising star, a neoconservative, purist poster boy.

A first wave of white doves is released. They swirl over our heads for an instant in a storm of feathers, then take their place aside their dirty cousins, the pigeons. That's where I see Henri. Squatting among the frightening gargoyles. Surveying us, holding a pair of binoculars in one hand, a walkie-talkie in the other. He's changed too, dressed like the serious shock troop security forces who are standing along a cordoned-off VIP section of the square. The president of France is expected today, and many diplomats. They may even march part of the way with the Crusaders. No one knows if the pope will show up. But they pray for it, mightily. Across the square, hundreds kneel, hundreds are giving testimony to the power of God.

Henri's older, thicker, and stronger; a contender for a gay bodybuilding contest. He looks as strong and fierce as the statues around him, his face hard, his attention focused on one thing: would-be terrorists. Henri's crossed over too, become a member of the specialist neighborhood swat team he so despises.

Even Henri. How could this happen?

Sel's wearing a familiar expression, amused at my innocence. *We're such a mutable species*, she remarks. *Hasn't the pox taught you that?*

I hear shouts, clapping. Coming across the water, having commandeered a fleet of Bateaux Mouches, are the drag queens and transwomen, escorted by drag kings and transmen. From afar, they're a fashion spectacle, beyond gorgeous, dressed up as members of successive generations of the French royal families. The queens have outdone themselves, planned a public performance beyond anything I have seen. The kings are impeccable, attired in pointed shoes, codpieces, leather hunting gloves and boots, others in light armor, armed with the weapons of a conquering, jousting nation: swords, lances, long knives.

The future is not yet written, Sel whispers. *But the past speaks so loudly, doesn't it? The question remains, who's listening?*

L'Afterword

The Circle Is Complete

~ 113

Sometimes the end is the beginning. . . .

An era has ended; a new millennium has begun. It feels so long ago that I first heard Sel's voice, felt that invasion, that inner beckoning. Now she's so fully with me I'll never lose her, I think. She's the uncensored inner voice that I can access easily now: impolitic, less concerned with the opinions of others, free to err and free to care deeply too about people and events and things others deem far in the past, perhaps not worth the effort to dig up.

For me, the more I dig, the more I learn, the more I see connections between the past and unfolding present. It helps me look ahead, consider the future.

The nineties are over; the nineties live on. *What did we do in that tumultuous decade? What did we change? What changed us? What endures? What did we learn? What do we still refuse to see? What is the legacy of this decade of activism?*

Let me turn the mirror on myself, first: On my remarkable, painful, transformative, exuberant decade. A decade of profound losses amid victories, new loves, and hard breakups; a dance of hard science, inner dreaming, and outer protest. It's one that yielded more questions than answers with every stone I turned over.

What did I learn? What am I carrying forward from the second decade of AIDS?

A lot. So much. I would need another book to capture it all. Plus, the lessons and connections continue to evolve. And some repeat themselves. Look at my love triangles in the nineties. Some lessons take longer to sink in.

Let me start with the pox, HIV—the enemy but also my teacher. The still-mysterious, utterly compelling, ever-more-complex world of AIDS and its journey in the human body. As with Sel, I've learned the rabbit holes of inquiry aren't holes; they're tunnels, an expansion; a constellation that offers a glimpse of another internal possible galaxy of connections. I'm endlessly fascinated. Even before Sel hijacked an inner track of my mind, I had come to view the whole concept of sickness differently; to reverse it by 360 degrees. I view illness

286

as natural, not foreign to my body. That doesn't mean we shouldn't strive to eradicate infections that might kill us, but it's given me a different view of our dance with the poxes, our dance with nature, with biology. We are hosts to a world more complex than we have even grasped.

⌒

My nineties journey with Sel began in a shroud of sorrow and personal loss. I was so tired that my exhaustion masked my grief, and when it broke open, it yielded older pain. Memories and people I had pushed down, pushed into a place of waiting for the emotional space to process. Now when I see Johnny or Kiki, or Jon Greenberg or Assotto, it's not through a scrim of tears or loss only but a space of light, released from their pain and suffering, inhabiting the fuller life they had. I can smile when I think of them, share this with more people. I remain haunted, but they are warmer haunts. They've joined the pantheon of my dead, a group of spirits that move with lighter energy through my heart. I like to think I'm giving them what they most sought in the end: a chance to live longer, to mean something, to not be allowed to disappear.

⌒

In the nineties, the pox shadowed everything for me and us—I say *us* meaning my personal and social circle, ACT UP, the gay and Haitian and immigrant communities of New York and Paris and Port-au-Prince that overlapped only a little. When protease inhibitors arrived in 1996, overnight, our lives changed. Although the shadow is not gone, it is lifted. It put death at bay—far less a possibility. We've witnessed a modern medical victory with protease drugs, and that's informed our response to other epidemics, most recently Ebola, now Zika. AIDS activism has offered proven strategies, connections, arguments.

The pox is a profane teacher. It reveals to us the sacredness of the body. The poxed body in all its fury to survive, to remain beautiful and functional, to be touched, and to love. The HIV-positive body, the homosexual body, the bodies of women and babies, the imprisoned body, the sex-worker body, the immigrant body, all the bodies being left outside the clinics and hospitals unable to pay for health care. The bodies across Africa and Asia and the Middle East. Each of them a person with dreams and a right to live without the threat of a pox gallows. A person and body in need of love and healing, of compassion and our collective moral action. The nineties showed us all of that.

Yet we still see repeated examples of how the first response continues to be fear, followed by denial and violence and a desire to cast out, to quarantine, to contain. That hasn't changed—not enough. The powers that be continue to think we can close our borders to contain a global epidemic like Zika. But

AIDS showed us that exclusion drives the epidemic underground, fuels its spread. It invites the state to criminalize our bodies and separate the sick from the strong, detaching us from those who most need our compassion. That is not the answer. We need to support communities to respond, empower mothers with Zika to mobilize other parents. Local solutions, supported by resources.

Today the stigma of HIV continues to be very strong; so does homophobia that prevents us from targeting the most vulnerable. It's not the taboo subject it was even in the nineties. Today, HIV treatment provides control, not a cure—though that is coming. In the past two years, we have made real advances toward a cure. Aldyn and the early long-term survivors provided critical clues about why some individuals exposed to HIV get sick and others don't. Now we know that one in a hundred people exposed to the virus has a natural immunity: they don't get sick, they don't take medicine, they remain without detectable levels of HIV in their blood, they don't pose a threat to sexual partners. They are the model for remission. We are moving toward a Cure.

Now as then, the AIDS movement changed the terms of battle. The concept of patient empowerment is ACT UP's legacy, and it has impacted all other diseases, from cancer and hepatitis and lupus and TB and malaria to neglected diseases, providing inspiration and models and tools and principles and leadership. Many hemophiliacs died in Paris due to tainted Factor VII, as did Americans and Haitians and Mexicans and others who received contaminated blood transfusions in the early years of AIDS. Now the hemophilia movement is just that: a health movement; informed, mobilized. Some joined ACT UP. Their children are adult patient advocates; leaders; teachers.

This is ACT UP's legacy: that people living with an illness are not victims but the experts in their own disease, who hold the keys to their own health, with doctors and scientists as allies to offer medicines and expertise in managing care. That's a sea change of mentality. By the time Sebastien got his diagnosis, patient empowerment was not only the playbook but the rule book. It worked to transform his fear into rapid action. It's transformed our health industry.

To me the nineties yielded a stronger voice of organized outrage, the naming of the crime, the shaming of the criminal—not the victim with HIV but the state, and the profit-driven drug industry. But it also pointed a finger at the quiet ones, the public. That continues to be important, to address silence and inaction.

The advent of protease drugs and new technologies yielded the roadmap and tools for treatment. In 1997 that revealed the next, great challenge: how to deliver these to millions living in the world's poorest regions. That's what occupied me and many ACT UP colleagues in the new millennium.

In 2000, I boarded a plane bound for Durban, South Africa, and the AIDS conference with Bridget and our gorgeous baby girl, Wave, and my colleagues from *HIV Plus*, including Jersey. Our focus was still inequity and drug access but we became students anew, as many in ACT UP did. The global AIDS movement began to tackle the complex root issues of inequality that underlie health care: gender inequity, structural violence, racism, poverty. It's not by accident that the poorest in Puerto Rico or Brazil or Mexico are most impacted by diseases like AIDS or now, Zika. It won't surprise anyone if the poor in Sierra Leone struggle to access the brand new Ebola vaccine.

Today, as then, the issues of treatment access remain highly political. ACT UP knew that in 1987, called out the greed. It's still the key human factor driving our profit-driven health system and limiting treatment access for AIDS and many diseases. It continues to lead to criminal actions and fuels our calls for justice.

In France, ACT UP helped the hemophiliacs score a partial victory. The blood scandal led to a court case and a national mea culpa from higher-up officials. The former minister of health Edmond Hervé was ruled "negligent" in the affair. But he was released without being sentenced—a virtual slap of the wrist. More recently, a special court acquitted then prime minister Laurent Fabius and two aides of manslaughter charges, though several lower-ranking officials were convicted. Is that justice? No. It's a high crime. Thousands died.

From 2000 to 2003, I traveled to a dozen countries, reporting for an amfAR HIV newsletter on the challenge of providing universal HIV treatment to people in the poorest settings. My 2004 book, *Moving Mountains*, catalogs the success of dozens of pioneering groups to do that. The research showed me just how far AIDS activism has penetrated, how profoundly it impacts health care across so many spheres and levels. I also roped two talented pals, filmmakers Ann T. Rossetti and Shanti Avirgan, into jumping on airplanes with me to capture the unfolding drama for a companion documentary, *Pills, Profits, Protest: Chronicle of the Global AIDS Movement*.

After that, I took a break from reporting to apply what I had learned from the pioneers. In 2004 I co-launched the Women's Equity in Access to Care and Treatment (WE-ACTx) project with two of the WIHS feminist HIV doctors I most admired, Kathy Anastos and Mardge Cohen. WE-ACTx in Kigali was a project born of urgency, like ACT UP: to help Rwandan women survivors of genocidal rape access free HIV drugs and care. What I learned, in a repeat of the fast-track speed of nineties lessons, was just how much a small group can do, working in coalition, armed with resources and political will.

Today, WE-ACTx is a point of pride for me—a collective pride shared by my colleagues and the seventy-plus Rwandan staffers who continue to run two clinics in Kigali. It's an all-Rwandan-run clinical project that's put thousands of women and over three hundred children on free, comprehensive therapy, and provided many more with HIV prevention, testing, and holistic services. The entire experience deserves another book.

In the decade after the nineties, I also focused on home and family. My personal life radically changed. After Durban, it was clear that Bridget and I were struggling as a couple. But we were smitten with our daughter, and committed to the difficult task of separating and reshaping our family life as co-parents.

Later, I adopted two sweetheart girls: Nibs, who I met when Wave began preschool; and in fall 2013, Flor, who I spotted on my second trip to Kigali in 2004. Like Wave, they've grown up in the blink of an eye. I have three daughters headed for college in 2017. As their lives flourish, my joy expands.

In 2010 I found myself back in Haiti, where a historic earthquake badly damaged my grandmother's gingerbread house and much of the capital and other cities, causing some three hundred thousand deaths. Here, as in Rwanda, I worked with women survivors of sexual violence and later, with V-Day. I witnessed, anew, how catastrophe and our response to humanitarian crises run along underlying currents of gender and social inequality. My 2014 book, *Beyond Shock*, captures the lessons.

What about the legacy of the lesbians, my other protest family in the nineties? That's an easy one. I see the answer every June when my teenage daughters and I head to the annual Dyke March in San Francisco. That event has become a massive march of thousands of women of all ages, and lately, a good number of straight college dudes who support gay rights too.

In 1992, when we sat around Ana Simo's table to brainstorm a fun, fierce dyke action group, the Lesbian Avengers, and began dreaming of a Washington march, we wondered who might join the party. A quarter century later, the short answer is: *everyone*. The Dyke March, which happens in many cities, remains a flash point of public visibility and pride for the *L* in the LGBT nation. This year, my teen daughters attended it and the Trans March, and other Pride events, each with their own posse of friends. Their younger generation of millennials are chill about the gays, as they put it; they easily adopt the pronoun *they* when friends or teachers—*teachers!*—who are transgender or have evolving genders make this name request. Amazeballs, as I've learned to say.

⌒⌐

Looking back, the Avengers didn't last long but triggered changes that continue to ripple out. The work on antigay ordinances stands out as exemplary. What impresses me is how many of my colleagues remain lifelong activists and leaders, true changemakers across many social movements. The buzzword today is *inter-sectional*. That's the approach many lesbians have always brought to their politi-cal organizing work. June 2017 will mark the twenty-fifth anniversary of the Avengers; a reunion is planned. I can't wait to march with the old gang.

⌒⌐

The world as we know it, then, has vastly changed from the day when I held a purple balloon, donning my *I was a lesbian child* T-shirt at our first Avenger action in 1992 at a Queens schoolyard. I'm a single parent and a co-parent. I'm part of a generational demographic. I'm not married, but many friends are. The rest are like me, single or in complex relationships, testing online dating, identifying somewhere along the spectrum from monogamish (*that's more me*) to polyamorous (*the rest of San Francisco, haha*). We continue to push the envelope of our lives, resisting easy boxes. But we have an amazing sisterhood, us Ls. And we rock as parents—and always have.

⌒⌐

What about the far right wolves, the new threat of fascism that pushed me to begin exploring my family's role in post-Vichy France, and what threat they pose now? On the family front, my search has yielded fresh nuggets and some gold. It's good news, I'm happy to report. I can now confirm that Mamie, my superstitious, slightly imperious countess grandmother, did run a boarding-house in Megève and did have a Jewish childhood friend who worked with her to house and ferret Jewish children to safety. Mamie accompanied them to the Swiss border; her friend met her on the other side, in Geneva. The details of their small underground railroad invite further research, but there's no question: my pope-loving Grand-mère Mamie did the right thing, morally, and that makes me proud of her.

Now, about Papou, my cherished grandpere. I learned he indeed profited after the war by leasing his luxury apartments to Algerian returnees, but they were rich Algerian Jews, not anti-Semite pieds noirs. He helped those still likely to face discrimination in a post-Vichy Jew-hating world. I also learned the name of the mayor of Marseille who put my grandfather behind bars: Gaston Defferre. I found him on Wikipedia.

I learned that Papou spent his year in prison working as a librarian. So that's why he learned to love books! That made me happy; it's another thing we share. Papou also had a cousin at the time, Jean Berthoin, who served as minister of the interior under de Gaulle. Apparently Jean remained unmoved by Papou's tax plight, and unmoved, too, by the Jewish clients who testified on my grandfather's behalf at his court hearing. But maybe Jean's hands were tied; he couldn't be found showing favoritism to a relative. To the Algerian Jews, though, my grandfather had been a good guy, even if he had cheated the government out of some taxes. He paid for that crime. In the big history picture—to me—he too comes out on top.

To cap off this happy update, I've learned that Jean's son, Georges, now eighty-five and living in Paris, is a retired deputy in the European Parliament who tried to block the entry of Jean-Marie Le Pen and his neo-right wolves there. Georges worked closely with David Rockefeller to help found the Trilateral Commission.

So now you see, I have solid answers, as well as more leads to pursue if I want. My parent's parents were not indifferent, after all. They stepped up. Papou might have skirted the taxman, but he helped the Jews who survived the Vichy purges in the French colonies—the extension of France's collaboration with Hitler that I had overlooked. I don't overly judge my grandfather, either; no one loves paying taxes. (Just look at Donald Trump.) Papou got caught and convicted; justice was served, more so than ordinary Vichyites who looked on as Papon cleared Marseille of Jews.

For France, the Papon trial served as a public reeducation lesson. I'm not sure what was learned by the schoolchildren, but the victims of Vichy had their day in court. They were heard; the papers covered the trial avidly, and now the truth is known. That's a form of justice already.

~⌒

There are other positive updates from the nineties to report; other victories that mark our future. The Haitians who escaped the Guantánamo camps got help; their families did too. CCR also helped in the unfinished effort to reclaim the stolen Duvalier fortune. Not long ago, Duvalier had the audacity to return to Haiti, and died there in October 2014. I ran into him at a children's choir concert in Pétion-Ville. He was older, quieter; the people in the hall stared at him but kept their distance. The stench of his regime trailed him home. Today, there's still an enormous sum of money missing. Michèle Bennett, Haiti's Eva Perón, is still residing in France. She returned to Haiti in 2010, when I did, to bury her brother Rudy, one of the many victims of the earthquake. No one had forgotten her either, she learned. She didn't stay long.

The past is not sleeping; the dead are speaking. Are you listening, Michèle?

There are other old justice cases that have been reopened. I'm happy to see that a French committee tasked by Chirac to investigate the stolen Nazi gold in Swiss banks has newly begun delving more deeply into insurance policies. Will the man from Lloyds, my grandpapa, turn up in their archives?

What else? Well, I'm also satisfied to find that my compadre Laura Flanders was right, early on, about the impact of low-dose sarin on the brains and nerve cells of Gulf War vets: these long-dismissed claims are now going forward; the wheels of justice turning anew. She's at the forefront of reporting at *Grit TV*, still breaking stories daily.

That takes me to the bigger questions of crime and justice I was asking myself in 1992. Today, Jean-Marie Le Pen is out of power, sidelined, having ceded power to his lawyer daughter, Marine. She and her niece Marion Maréchal-Le Pen lead the strongwomen of the National Front; followed by ever-fashionable Catherine Mégret. By the time my book is published, Marine may be in power. So too, may the Euroskeptic Alliance for Democracy in Germany, closely allied with PEGIDA, a newish neo-Nazi, anti-Muslim front. Despite the dark lessons of history—Hitler, the Holocaust, Vichy—a new crop of fascists advance.

They're getting help and money from Russia's Vladimir Putin, the emerging power broker of the world. And from the crisis of immigration that's followed the rise of Islamic terrorism and ISIS in the Middle East. We've witnessed horrific Jihadist attacks in Paris, in Lyon, in Nice; bombings in Brussels and Berlin. We've experienced Jihadist attacks here, too, as at the Boston Marathon. With every explosion, the far right benefits, as do jihadis. The ordinary citizens are afraid. In Boston, in Paris, in Berlin, we're witnessing a true spasm of political xenophobia. Fear is driving our global body politic.

The wolves are uniting, then, as they did before. That was Sel muttering, but it came out of my mouth. They're out in the daylight now, more emerging daily, inciting a new generation of snarling young.

Where does that lead us, the land of democracy? Will the new wolves triumph? When I began to reread my nineties diaries to shape this book months ago, Donald Trump was a billionaire populist wildcard, a real estate magnate with an orange-tinged toupee (we assume) and a bombastic ego and personality, famous for his reality television show, *The Apprentice*. Now he's our rogue Twitter president. Among my set—progressives and the LGBTQ crowd, even journalists—few saw Trump coming. It was too unthinkable, for starters, as with Jean-Marie Le Pen in 1990. It's taken the French a decade to get used to his daughter Marine, to her softer racial denunciations of African immigrants. Here, we had little preparation for "The Donald," and the shock is great. We swallowed a very bitter pill overnight.

So my muse Sel was right. The world is—was—being remade, is rooted in what the wolves were quietly seeding in the nineties. I dreamed this nightmare years ago, in my reveries with and about Sel. It was my attempt to imagine the impossible. Now it's our new reality. Our surreality, as I feel it.

Looking ahead, looking back, the past offers us a mirror to reflect on. There, I find not only lessons and weapons from the nineties but all my old comrades-in-arms, who've been quick to rally and lead the charge. We are in a new historic moment, but we've seen much of this before. The failure of our elected leaders, the criminalization of our bodies, the need to create new alliances across social movements, to rebuild safety nets for the most vulnerable . . . all of this we did in the nineties in ACT UP and won. We also lost so many lives to AIDS. So it is now, with the wolves braying their victories in many corners. Whatever thought of rest I might have had is for another day. I'm newly wearing my protest hat. On the day after Trump's election I started a Facebook group to fight the man I call Drumpf. Now, I'm meeting all the ex–ACT UP and Queer Nation and West Coast Avengers who have joined our fast-growing Bay Area Queer Anti-Fascist Network. Once again, I'm losing sleep, debating tactics, writing manifestos, and making protest art, dancing between the protests. Once again, we are taking to the streets.

ACT UP showed us—showed me—we have the answers and we have the tools to fight back and win. We had to show people the human face of those living with AIDS, and of gay people. We had to create our own resources when the state criminalized our bodies, refused us services. We had to forge new alliances. With AIDS, we had no time to wait. I feel that now. This time the virus is fascism, which threatens the core of our democracy.

Sel's given me her mantra for the new times; it's apt. *Il est tôt et il est tard. Mais j'amais trop tard. It's early and it's late. But never too late.* Not for justice, not for health, not for a cure, not for some truth-telling. Do it tomorrow if you can't do it today. Look, listen, and act. Don't sleep. Stay awake. Write it down. Do it now. Dream your Action. Put it in a manifesto. A poem. Forget your manners. Embrace your desire. Love madly. Reach out to another. I did and we did in the nineties and we'll continue to do so. The party's not over. This party of life. Mine, yours, ours. Make it count.

I repeat: It's late, but never too late. Not for this fight, not for our stories, not for our voices, or actions, not for justice. The nineties taught us that most important lesson. The arc of justice is infinite. It may not bend as quickly or exactly in the place we wish, but if we act to help it along, it will do so faster. And we'll feel much better, too. I can vouch for that. The antidote to despair is definitely action. *Informed* action, to paraphrase ACT UP.

So here I am once again. Past midnight, eluding sleep. In my mind's eye, I see my friends, alive as ever: Johnny, whirling with Boy Kelly to Bronski Beat in his living room, his pretty blue eyes perfectly clear; Aldyn, standing at the podium in Berlin, offering lessons from long-term survivors; Oui, a lithe, blond, prancing fairy with a dogged spirit, haranguing the boys of the Marais to take a condom, join a demo; Assotto, flamboyant lover of *vodou* and Toussaint L'Ouverture and James Baldwin, reciting his gay poetry in Kreyol, a rare, proud Haitian *masisi* (fag). Here now is Kiki, diva lesion liberator, carefully applying a cleansing facial at night, channeling his inner Crawford spirit to compose an editorial to Drumpf and Marine Le Pen.

Dear Fools, it begins . . .

I hear them as clearly and loudly as yesterday. I know what they'd say, eyeing the uncertain future we face, so I'll give them the last word:

> *Fuck Death and Don't Forget Us.*
> *Dance and Love Each Other.*
> *Be So Gay and Make Us Proud.*
> *Don't Let the Motherfuckers Win.*
> *ACT UP! Fight Back! Fight Hate!*

February 2017
Oakland, CA

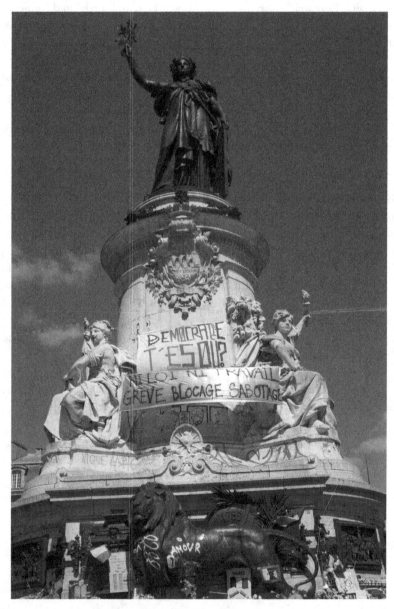

Homage to the victims of terrorist bombings and Islamophobia, Place de la République, Paris, 2016. (Kawri Juno Photography)

℘.S.

*D*id you really think she would let me have the final word?

Sel is here, whispering in my ear as always. That hot, gritty breath, that sandpaper smoker's rough voice. *Go on, finish your diary if you must. The decade is over but our journey is not, not by a long shot. You won't be rid of us that easily. Plus, there's so much more fun to be had.*

She's right. The future beckons. Sel's an inner mirror, a part of myself that arose from some place of sorrow and exhaustion to creatively revive me, to remind me, to push me, to pull me back into my life, into the love and losses I experienced in that extraordinary decade for me, the nineties. I won't lose her. I have draft pages of her own dramatic story to complete, a separate tale of fabulist historical redress, as I've come to think of it. A journey for my next decade. Or the rest of my life; we'll see where this goes. There are new battles afoot; I'm called to action, and distraction. I do know she's capable of endless mutation, so it's not a journey I can predict. But I also know it will lead to wonderland; my inner imaginarium. For now, I'm happy to host for as long as I can. She was an imperfect muse for a rough decade and now, we're entering another. I could use her no-holds-barred advice. After all, we survived the nineties together, didn't we?

I'm the scribe. The terms of engagement are clear.

Don't look away. Write it down.

Thank You

First, to the doctors who tended so well to my friends with AIDS in the nineties, who took my calls, who kept my close circle alive and with realistic hope for as long as possible, then helped them die with courage, and dignity: Paul Bellman, Joe Sonnabend, Barbara Starrett in the United States; Jean Pape and Marie Deschamps with GHESKIO in Haiti; Paul Farmer with Partners in Health.

. . . to researchers who delved deeply into the science and immunology of AIDS with me, notably: David Ho and Marty Markowitz at the Aaron Diamond AIDS Research Center; Bob Siliciano at Johns Hopkins; Tony Fauci at the National Institutes of Health; the Women's Interagency Health Study (WIHS) principal investigators Kathryn Anastos, Mardge Cohen, Ruth Greenblatt, and Michael Saag; and the late Joep Lange of the International AIDS Society.

. . . to nineties-era lawyers and Haiti human rights monitors: Anne Fuller, Johnny McCalla, Ronald Aubourg, and the late Mike Hooper at the National Coalition for Haitian Refugees; the late Michael Ratner and José Luis Morín of the Center for Constitutional Rights (CCR); the Emergency Coalition to Shut Down Guantánamo group. *Chapo*. Hats off.

. . . to AIDS activist colleagues in ACT UP chapters and the NYC Treatment and Data Committee (later Treatment Action Group, TAG), especially Garance Franke-Ruta; Richard Jefferys; AIDS Treatment Resources (ATR) with Iris Long and Jim Eigo; amfAR; the Community Research Initiative (CRI; later CRIA); People with AIDS Coalition (PWAC); PWA Health Group; Gay Men's Health Crisis (GMHC); Stand Up Harlem; Black AIDS Mobilization; the Latino Caucus of ACT UP/NY; the Latino AIDS Project; Jesus Aguais and AID for AIDS and ACT UP–Americas.

. . . to the Lesbian Avengers and my cofounders Sarah Schulman, Maxine Wolfe, Ana Maria Simo; and Marie Honan and Anne Maguire (also with ILGO) and LACROP organizers and all the glorious chapters and individual fierce fire eaters; to Women's Action Coalition (WAC); to GET SMART; to Kelly Cogswell at CITYAXE; to Marie de Cenival and La Barbe in Paris.

... to my friend, the irrepressible Chloe Dzubila of Transsexual Menace and her posse—so fierce in demanding that transwomen receive respect and care from HIV service providers.

... to the housing activists Charles King, Keith Cylar, Nina Herzog, and others at Housing Works; to the HIV-positive pioneers Iris de la Cruz at Iris House, Rebecca Denison with WORLD in San Francisco, and Esther Boucicault in Haiti; and to ally Marie St. Cyr.

... to the art-activist collectives: Dyke Action Machine; to Gran Fury, with Vincent Gagliostro and Avram Finkelstein (and Marisa Cardinale—our posse at *x-x-x fruit* mag); Visual AIDS; to curators Linda Chapman, Split Britches, and all the theater gals at WOW Cafe; Mark Russell at PS122; Ellie Covan at Dixon Place.

... to the spaces for queer artists: Danspace; the Kitchen; Circus Amok; to Lady Bunny and the *fabulous* crew at Wigstock; to the Wessel O'Connor gallery for groundbreaking work by and about HIV and queer bodies.

... to the owners and promoters of Wonder Bar; Boy Bar; the Boiler Room; the Pyramid Club; Life Café; Meow Mix; Clit Club; Art Bar; and the incomparable Florent Morellet at Florent.

⁓

... to my late close friend, adventure pal, and editor at *OutWeek* and *Out*, Sarah Pettit, who shared the nineties with me on a daily basis; and to Michael Goff, *Out* cofounder, for their strong support of my AIDS reporting.

... to fellow editors and staff writers at *OutWeek* and *Out* (Bruce Steele, James Conrad, Mary Connelly, Elise Harris, Ellen Marin, Michael Kaminer, George Slowik Jr., Debi Farmer, Amy Steiner, the late Harry Taylor, Sally Chew, Henry Scott); *POZ* (Sean Strub, Walter Armstrong); *HIV Plus* (Emily Bass, Cindra Feuer, Stanya Kahn); *Gai Pied* (Christophe Martet); Mark Schoofs; David France; the zine *Diseased Pariah News*; and Liz Highleyman.

... to community documentarians: DIVA TV and James Wentzy at AIDS Community Television, Paper Tiger TV, Alex Juhasz and the Women's AIDS Video Enterprise (WAVE); photo/videographers: Dona Ann McAdams, Donna Binder, Bill Bytsura, Harriet Hirshorn, Carolina Kroon, Jack Louth, Amy Steiner, Ellen Neipris, Mary Patierno, James Wentzy, Charles Rosenberg.

... to the nineties filmmakers Lisa Cholodenko, Cheryl Dunye, Su Friedrich, Robert Hilferty, Jim Hubbard, Kim Peirce, Rose Troche, Guin Turner; and to my journo and writer pals Michael Cunningham, Hilton Als, Heather Lewis, Alex Chee, Ann Rower; book editors Amy Scholder and Ira Silverberg at High Risk books . . . and more.

If I forgot you, forgive me. You know who you are. We know what you did, what you do.

⁓

You rock. You changed the world, baby: mine, all of ours.

⁓

Let me add a personal thanks to my blood family, for their support and love. My siblings: Kathy, Serge, and Philippe; my cousin Claude Berthoin; my nephew Eric d'Adesky; my nieces Viviane d'Adesky, Lara and Claudia Berthoin. Let me honor two relatives I've lost without being able to say a proper good-bye: Carole d'Adesky and her son Fulton (Ti Zwing). Let me recognize my far-flung relatives — the ever-expanding d'Adesky-*plus* clan: our sense of family roots us; even when we disagree politically, we remain family.

Let me thank my own children. Being your maman gives me ground to walk on, a ship to sail, a shared future to invest our best dreams. And let me welcome V., sister to Wave, in our tent of bigger, blended family. We are blessed.

A special *merci* to my other *proches*; friendships and love are the glue of my life (*in alphabetical order*): Kathy Brady, Cindra Feuer, Susie Frankel, Angela Garcia, Karina Hodoyan, Ann Maniglier, Kelly McKaig, Megan McLemore, Peter Mcquaid, Max Miller, Paul Outlaw, Soeurette Policar, Judy Sisneros, Kate Sorensen, Sophie Russell, Anthony Viti, Nicole Whear, Pascale Willi. Let me remember my lovely friends Martine Aumaître and Heather Lewis, lost too early, and the late Philippe Madelin, my Paris journo comrade in arms.

Let me thank my nineties romantic partners and *affaires de coeur*: passion is the flight of the soul into that higher place. I will keep only the best memories.

And a special thanks to friends who helped read, review, and prepare this book: Marsh Agobert, Sally Engelfried, Laura Flanders, Katia Noyes, Shelley Marlow, Michele Rudenko, Ann Rower, David Ryan, David Walter; to editor Rebecca Peters-Golden; and to University of Wisconsin Press staff Raphael Kadushin, Amber Rose, Carla Marolt, and their team for their support. I'm incredibly grateful to Julie Sutherland and Juno (Amy) Rosenhaus for their un-flagging help and support of this project.

And finally, to Rabbit, who brought a bit of last magic to journey into and out of my inner wonderland.

In Memory and Action

*f*or colleagues and friends who died of AIDS and fought homophobia:

Terry Beirn | Michael Botkin | Michael Callen | Bob Carr | Iris de la Cruz | Spencer Cox | Peter Cucich | Keith Cylar | Keri Duran | David Feinberg | Stephen Gendin | Robert Massa | Jim Matthews | Lungi Mazibuko | Jeffrey Schmalz | Bob Rafsky | Sylvia Rivera | Randy Shilts | Darrell Yates Rist | Phil Zwickler

And others lost who inspire me with their lives, words, creativity, and courage:

Kathy Acker | Reinaldo Arenas | Melvin Dixon | Gugu Dlamini | Nkosi Johnson | Fela Anikulapo Kuti | Cookie Mueller | Haoui Montaug | Robert Mapplethorpe | Flores (Flo) McGarrell | Simon Nkoli | Michael Ratner | Marlon Riggs | David Wojnarowicz | Pedro Zamora

And those who we lost to homophobic violence and mourned in the nineties:

Hattie Mae Cohens | Brian Mock | Marsha Johnson

Suggested Readings

French Far Right and Fascism

Froment, Pascale. *René Bousquet*. Paris: Stock, 1994.

Klarsfeld, Serge. *Vichy-Auschwitz: Le rôle de Vichy dans la solution finale de la question juive en France*. Vol. 2, *1943–44*. Paris: Fayard, 1985.

Konopnicki, Guy. *Les filières noires*. Paris: Éditions Denoël, 1996.

Milza, Pierre. *Fascisme français: Passé et présent*. Paris: Flammarion, 1987.

Monzat, René. *Enquêtes sur la droite extrême*. Paris: Le Monde-Editions, 1992.

Rigoulot, Pierre. *Les enfants de l'épuration*. Paris: Plon, 1993.

Shields, James. *The Extreme Right in France: From Pétain to Le Pen*. New York: Routledge, 2007.

Haiti, the Duvaliers in France

Abbott, Elizabeth. *Haiti: A Shattered Nation*. New York: Overlook, 2011.

d'Adesky, Anne-christine. *Under the Bone*. New York: Farrar, Straus and Giroux, 1994.

Diederich, Bernard. *Papa Doc and the Tontons Macoutes*. New York: Penguin, 1969.

Dubois, Laurent. *Haiti: The Aftershocks of History*. New York: MacMillan, 2012.

Katz, Jonathan. *The Big Truck that Went By*. New York: St. Martin's, 2013.

Madelin, Philippe. *L'or des dictatures*. Paris: Fayard, 1993.

Smartt Bell, Madison. *The Haitian Revolution Trilogy*. *All Soul's Rising* (1995); *Master of the Crossroads* (2000); *The Stone that the Builder Refused* (2004). New York: Pantheon.

Wilentz, Amy. *The Rainy Season*. New York: Simon & Schuster, 1989.

AIDS and Activism

ACT UP/New York Women and AIDS Book Group, eds. *Women, AIDS, and Activism*. Boston: South End Press, 1990.

Burkett, Elinor. *The Gravest Show on Earth: America in the Age of AIDS*. New York: Houghton Mifflin, 1995.

Casteret, Anne-Marie. *L'affaire du sang*. Paris: Éditions La Découverte, 1992.

———. "Le rapport qui accuse le Centre National de la Transfusion Sanguine." *L'Événement du Jeudi*, April 25, 1991, 52–54.

Cogswell, Kelly. *Eating Fire: My Life as a Lesbian Avenger*. Minneapolis: University of Minnesota Press, 2014.
d'Adesky, Anne-christine. *Moving Mountains: The Race to Treat Global AIDS*. New York: Verso, 2004.
Duberman, Martin. *Hold Tight Gently: Michael Callen, Essex Hemphill, and the Battlefield of AIDS*. New York: New Press, 2016.
Farmer, Paul. *AIDS and Accusation: Haiti and the Geography of Blame*. Berkeley: University of California Press, 2006.
——. *Infections and Inequality: The Modern Plagues*. Berkeley: University of California Press, 2001.
Kushner, Tony. *Angels in America: A Gay Fantasia on National Themes*. New York: Theatre Communications Group, 1993–94.
Levenson, Jacob. *The Secret Epidemic: The Story of AIDS and Black America*. New York: Pantheon Books, 2004.
Mason, Kiki. "Manifesto Destiny." *POZ*, June/July 1996.
Monette, Paul. *Borrowed Time: An AIDS Memoir*. San Diego: Harcourt Brace Jovanovich, 1988.
Saint, Assotto. *Spells of a Voodoo Doll: The Poems, Fiction, Essays and Plays of Assotto Saint*. New York: Masquerade Books, 1996.
Schulman, Sarah. *After Delores*. New York: Dutton, 1988.
——. *The Cosmopolitans*. New York: Feminist Press, 2016.
——. *My American History: Lesbian and Gay Life during the Reagan/Bush Years*. New York: Routledge, 1994.
Shilts, Randy. *And the Band Played On: Politics, People and the AIDS Epidemic*. New York: St. Martin's, 1987.
Strub, Sean. *Body Counts*. New York: Simon & Schuster, 2014.
White, Edmund. *The Flâneur: A Stroll through the Paradoxes of Paris*. New York: Bloomsbury, 2008.
Wojnarowicz, David. *Close to the Knives: A Memoir of Disintegration*. New York: Vintage Books, 1991.
——. *Seven Miles A Second*. New York: DC Comics, 1996.
——. *The Waterfront Journals*. New York: Grove Press, 1996.

Historical France

Allan, Tony. *Paris: The Glamour Years, 1919–40*. New York: Gallery Books, 1977.
Ehrlich, Blake. *Paris on the Seine*. New York: Atheneum, 1962.
Laffont, Robert. *The Illustrated History of Paris and the Parisians*. New York: Doubleday, 1958.
Lecat, Jacques. *Ici sont les Halles et le Marais et l'Île Saint-Louis*. Paris: Le Cadratin, 1986.
Le Moël, Michel, and Jean Dérens. *La Place de Grève*. Edited by La Délégation à l'Action Artistique de la Ville de Paris. Paris: Hachette, 1991.
Levy, Barbara. *Legacy of Death: The Remarkable Saga of the Sanson Family, Who Served as Executioners of France for Seven Generations*. Englewood Cliffs, NJ: Prentice-Hall, 1973.
Péan, Pierre. *Une jeunesse française: François Mitterrand, 1934–1947*. Paris: Fayard, 1994.
Quétel, Claude. *History of Syphilis*. Baltimore: Johns Hopkins University Press, 1990.

Victorian Drugs, the Pox, and Miscellany

De Quincey, Thomas. *Confessions of an Opium Eater*. Edited by Alethea Hayter. New York: Penguin Classics, 1971. First published in the *London Magazine*, 1821.

Gerould, Daniel. *Guillotine: Its Legend and Lore*. New York: Blast Books, 1992.

Lewis, W. H. *The Splendid Century: Life in the France of Louis XIV*. New York: Doubleday Anchor, 1953.

Strausbaugh, John, and Donald Blaise. *The Drug User: Documents, 1840–1960*. New York: Blast Books, 1991.

Printed in the United States
By Bookmasters